Clinical Cases in
INTERNAL MEDICINE

Clinical Cases in
INTERNAL MEDICINE

SAMY AZER

MB, BCh, MSc Medicine, PhD (Syd), MEd (NSW), FACG, MPH (NSW)
Professor of Medical Education
College of Medicine, King Saud University, Saudi Arabia
Formerly Professor of Medical Education, Universiti Teknologi MARA, Malaysia
Visiting Professor of Medical Education, University of Toyama, Japan
Formerly Senior Lecturer of Medical Education, Faculty of Medicine, Dentistry and Health Sciences, the University of Melbourne and School of Medicine, the University of Sydney, Australia

ELSEVIER

Elsevier Australia. ACN 001 002 357
(a division of Reed International Books Australia Pty Ltd)
Tower 1, 475 Victoria Avenue, Chatswood, NSW 2067

ISBN: 978-0-7020-8049-4

National Library of Australia Cataloguing-in-Publication Data

 A catalogue record for this book is available from the National Library of Australia

Content Strategist: Larissa Norrie
Content Project Manager: Subodh Kumar
Proofread by Annabel Adair
Cover by Georgette Hall
Index by Innodata Indexing
Typeset by GW Tech India
Printed in India by Multivista Global Pvt. Ltd

Last digit is the print number: 9 8 7 6 5 4 3 2 1

To
The memory of my parents

To
My family for their love and support, and

To
My grandchildren – Jemimah, Elizabeth, Christopher, Asher

FOREWORD

To face the challenges of modern health care, future physicians must master not only an extensive knowledge base but also the analytical and integrative thinking skills needed to provide safe, comprehensive patient care in the context of clinical complexity.

While many textbooks present the content of this comprehensive knowledge base, *Clinical Cases in Internal Medicine* additionally guides learners on the *process* to apply knowledge and scientifically understand the various concerns (expressed in lay terms) that patients entrust their physicians to address. In this textbook, the concise and memorable case discussions highlight the differential diagnoses that must be systematically considered and review the mechanisms that explain the patient's signs and symptoms and the basis for why certain treatments work. The tables and figures are truly high-yield and helpful in practice. The questions, throughout the chapter, are framed very thoughtfully around queries that arise in clinical decision-making, in education of patients and families and in preparation for standardised examinations.

This textbook is ideal for students – in both problem-based learning (PBL) and traditional curricula – hoping to deepen their learning through case-based and interactive learning approaches.

Professor Samy Azer is an internationally renowned medical educator, who currently serves as Professor of Medical Education at the College of Medicine, King Saud University in Saudi Arabia. He has formerly served as Professor of Medical Education at the Universiti Teknologi MARA in Malaysia; Visiting Professor of Medical Education at the University of Toyama in Japan; and Senior Lecturer of Medical Education at the Faculty of Medicine, Dentistry and Health Sciences at the University of Melbourne and at the School of Medicine at the University of Sydney in Australia.

Through his commitment to innovations that optimise clinical learning and teaching and through publications and other connections that make these innovations graspable and accessible, Professor Azer has been an inspiration to the global community of medical educators and students alike. I join Professor Azer in his hope that educator colleagues, students and future patients will all benefit from the journey of learning through the cases presented in this text.

Anthony P. S. Guerrero, M.D.
Professor and Chair, Department of Psychiatry
The Char, McDermott, and Andrade Endowed
University of Hawai'i John A. Burns School of Medicine
United States

FOREWORD

Medical curricula have changed worldwide to reflect the changing roles of health systems and the challenges faced by graduating doctors. The advances in technology and the overwhelming increase in scientific and medical publications add to these challenges and the need to prepare our doctors at the best international standards and reassuring their continuing professional development.

This book addresses these needs as a learning resource to be used by students and other recommended and prescribed resources and enables them to study 50 clinical cases and apply knowledge to clinically relevant topics in their undergraduate curriculum.

Practising clinicians tend to use 'schema' in their reasoning to arrive at a diagnosis based on pattern recognition and previous experience. However, undergraduate students did not have sufficient experience and seeing patients in the wards may not be available for their clinical training. Furthermore, most hospitals are moving to minimally invasive techniques and one-day care and minimising the length of hospital stay with the new developments in diagnosis and patient management. These days there are changes in hospital admission because of the COVID-19 pandemic. These changes have affected bedside teaching worldwide and the need for alternative teaching/learning methods to address the students' learning needs and enhance their clinical skills.

Professor Azer, the chair of the curriculum development and research unit at King Saud University, has written this book with these challenges in mind. The book reflects his international expertise in the field and addresses this area of need. International experts have reviewed the book and provide the core clinical cases taught in internal medicine. Students may use this book together with their clinical sessions and seeing patients in the wards presenting with illnesses described. Students may critically compare between clinical findings they identified in the patient and what was discussed in the clinical cases in the book. They may also answer questions and revise the MCQs at the end of each case.

Together with reading recommended resources and reviewing their lectures, such preparation will help in their clinical learning.

I am proud that Professor Azer is an academic at King Saud University for his achievement and contribution to the medical profession at the global, local and international levels. I want to congratulate the author on this achievement, and it is my pleasure to commend this book as an additional resource to medical students and clinical teachers. This book will be a valuable resource to medical libraries, students and clinicians, medical educators and curriculum designers.

Professor Badran AlOmar
President, King Saud University

PREFACE

Clinical Cases in Internal Medicine is not a textbook covering the whole undergraduate curriculum in internal medicine. Although reading texts and daily engagement with simulated patients and actual patients is vital to enhance your competency in medicine, students also need to complement their learning through case-based learning.

This book is written for students as a learning resource to use with other standard textbooks and resources recommended in this discipline. It comprises 50 cases in internal medicine covering different body systems and focuses on common diseases that all medical students should know.

Learning through cases helps students to master several skills and deepen their understanding by applying theoretical knowledge. It brings factual knowledge to what they face in practice. Case scenarios also stimulate students' thinking to interpret the history findings and clinical findings, generate hypotheses, construct a differential diagnosis, relates basic knowledge from physiology and pathology to the clinical picture, interprets laboratory findings and design a management plan.

Clinical Cases in Internal Medicine can be used on an individual basis or in small-group tutorials with or without a tutor. After reading the case scenarios, students could start answering each question that follows the scenario—one student in the group summarise critical points raised in the group discussion- act as the group scribe, and guiding the group discussion. During this process, students may identify gaps in their knowledge or issues they do not know. Also, questions raised could stimulate further thinking, search for answers/evidence and turning the discussion into a meaningful session. Through active learning, and self-regulated learning and examining other resources, students could deepen their understanding of the case, explore relationships, and turn their learning into engaging and stimulating behaviour.

After completing the case discussion, a section titled 'back to basics' has been included in each case. This section aims at linking knowledge from physiology, pathology, pathogenesis, microbiology and pharmacology with the case clinical discussion. Students may try answering the short-answer questions in this section, then compare their responses with the answers provided. Each case discussion ends with 5-6 multiple-choice questions that students could try on their own, then check at the end their performance against model answers and justification given. At last, the case discussion ends with 'a take-home message'. and 'further readings' from the literature. These resources are recommended for students to dig deeper and read more about current knowledge related to the case.

I wish success to all my current students and graduates at different universities where I was honoured to teach and other universities worldwide enforcing active learning practices.

Samy Azer
Melbourne
2021

ACKNOWLEDGEMENTS

I am particularly indebted to my undergraduate and postgraduate medical students at the University of Sydney and the University of Melbourne in Australia, the University of Toyama in Japan, the Universiti Teknologi MARA in Malaysia and my current students at King Saud University in Saudi Arabia. Their engagement, questions and areas that they found difficult to understand have been an excellent source for me as I prepared the manuscript of this book.

I am indebted to the work of many individuals, particularly the publication team of Elsevier, for providing a professional standard during the book production. I thank Laurence Hunter, the content strategist, Elsevier Oxford, the United Kingdom. He was the first content strategist who handled the book before retiring. I thank Nimisha Goswami, the head of the content strategy, Elsevier India, who also dealt with the book content. I also thank Larissa Norrie, head of content strategy, Australia, who made significant help and support in the book production. Also, I thank Annabel Adair for the proofreading of the book as a freelance proofreader. I deeply appreciate and thank Subodh Kumar, who carried out the content development and project management responsibility. His hard work in preparing the proofs at professional standards is appreciated.

ABBREVIATIONS

5-HT	5-hydroxytryptamine
ACE	Angiotensin-converting enzyme
AChR	Anti-acetylcholine receptor
ACTH	Adrenocorticotrophic hormone
ADH	Antidiuretic hormone
AFB	Acid-fast bacillus
AHR	Airway hyper-reactivity
AIDS	Acquired immunodeficiency syndrome
ALT	Alanine aminotransferase
ANA	Antinuclear antibody
Anti-La (or SS-B) autoantibodies	These occur in 10%–20% of patients with systemic lupus erythematosus and 50% of patients with primary or secondary Sjögren syndrome; maternal anti-La (SS-B) autoantibodies are associated with neonatal lupus syndromes, particularly congenital heart block
Anti-Ro (anti-SS-A) autoantibodies	These are anti–Sjögren-syndrome-related antigen A autoantibodies; also called anti-Ro
Anti-U1-RNP	It is a serological marker for MCTD; It can be also detected in patients with systemic sclerosis or SLE
APACHE-II	Acute Physiology and Chronic Health Evaluation II
APC	Adenomatous polyposis coli
AST	Aspartate aminotransferase
ATP	Adenosine triphosphate
AV node	Atrioventricular node
B. burgdorferi	*Borrelia burgdorferi*
BCG	*Bacillus Calmette–Guérin* vaccine
BCR-ABL	It is a mutation formed by the combination of two genes, known as BCR and ABL; the mutated chromosome 22 is called the Philadelphia chromosome (referring to the city where researchers first discovered Ph chromosome)
BG	Blood glucose
BMD	Bone mass density
BMI	Body mass index
BNP	Brain natriuretic peptide
BPPV	Benign paroxysmal positional vertigo
C, T, L, S nerve roots	C, cervical; T, thoracic; L, lumbar; S, sacral nerve roots
C. jejuni	*Campylobacter jejuni*

C. trachomatis	*Chlamydia trachomatis*
C3, C4	Complement fragments C3 and C4
C3NeF	C3 nephritic factor
cAMP	Cyclic 3′,5′-adenosine monophosphate
CAP	Community-acquired pneumonia
CD4$^+$	A T-helper white blood cell
CD8$^+$	It is a cytotoxic T-cell; also known as T-killer cell or cytotoxic T-lymphocyte
CEA	Carcinoembryonic antigen
CFU	Colony-forming unit
CK–MB	Creatine kinase myocardial band
CML	Chronic myeloid leukaemia
CMV	Cytomegalovirus
CNS	Central nervous system
COPD	Chronic obstructive pulmonary disease
COX	Cyclooxygenase
CRF-1	Corticotrophin-releasing factor-1
CRP	C-reactive protein
CSF	Cerebrospinal fluid
CT scan	Computed tomography scan
cTn	Cardiac troponin
cTnI	Cardiac troponin I
cTnT	Cardiac troponin T
CTPA	Computed tomography pulmonary angiography
CURB-65 score	C, confusion; U, urea; R, respiratory; B, blood pressure; 65, age > 65
CXCL	Chemokines playing a role in chemoattractant for several immune cells, and angiogenesis/arteriogenesis and cancer progression
CYP2E1	It is a member of the cytochrome P450, which is involved in metabolism of xenobiotics
D receptor	Dopamine receptor
Delta wave	In ECG, the delta wave is a slurred upstroke in the QRS complex, commonly associated with pre-excitation syndrome such as WPW
DHEAS	Dehydroepiandrosterone sulphate
DIP	Distal interphalangeal joints
DKA	Diabetic ketoacidosis
DMARDs	Disease-modifying antirheumatic drugs
DNA	Deoxyribonucleic acid

DR4	It is a serotype of HLA, which is associated with extra-articular rheumatoid arthritis, obstructive hypertrophic cardiomyopathy, IgA nephropathy, certain types of systemic lupus erythematosus and polymyalgia rheumatica
dsDNA	Double-stranded DNA
DVT	Deep venous thrombosis
DXA (or DEXA)	Dual-energy x-ray absorptiometry
E. coli	*Escherichia coli*
EBV	Epstein-Barr virus
ECG	Electrocardiogram
ECL	Enterochromaffin-like cells
EHEC	Enterohaemorrhagic *Escherichia coli*
EIEC	Enteroinvasive *Escherichia coli*
ELISA	Enzyme-linked immunosorbent assay
ELISpot	Enzyme-linked immunospot
EMG	Electromyogram
EML4-ALK	EML4 is echinoderm microtubule-associated protein-like 4 gene that has been fused to the anaplastic lymphoma kinase (ALK) gene; this fusion leads to the production of a protein, EML4-ALK; first isolated from small cell lung cancer
eNOS	Endothelial nitric oxide synthase
EPEC	Enteropathogenic *Escherichia coli*
ERCP	Endoscopic retrograde cholangiopancreatography
ESR	Erythrocyte sedimentation rate
ESRD	End-stage renal disease
ETEC	Enterotoxigenic Escherichia coli
FAP	Familial adenomatous polyposis
FEV_1	Forced expiratory volume of 1 second
FGF23	Fibroblast growth factor 23
FRAX	Fracture Risk Assessment Tool
FVC	Forced vital capacity
G6PD deficiency	Glucose-6-phosphate dehydrogenase deficiency
GABA	Gamma-aminobutyric acid
GADA	Glutamate decarboxylase alpha
GDP	Guanosine diphosphate or guanosine 5'-diphosphate
GGT	Gamma-glutamyl transferase
GH	Growth hormone
GINA	Global Institute for Asthma
GN	Glomerulonephritis
GnRH	Gonadotrophin-releasing hormone
GP	Globus pallidus
GTP	Guanosine-5'-triphosphate

H. influenzae	*Haemophilus influenzae*
H. pylori	*Helicobacter pylori*
H1-receptor	Histamine antagonist receptor-1
HAP	Hospital-acquired pneumonia
HAV	Hepatitis A virus
Hb	Haemoglobin
HbA_{1c}	Haemoglobin A_{1c}
HBsAg	Hepatitis B surface antigen
HBV	Hepatitis B virus
HCO_3^-	Bicarbonate
HCV	Hepatitis C virus
HDL	High-density lipoprotein
HDV	Hepatitis D virus
HEV	Hepatitis E virus
HGPRT	Hypoxanthine-guanine phosphoribosyltransferase
Hib	*Haemophilus Influenzae* type b
HIV	Human immunodeficiency virus
HLA	Human leukocyte antigen
hs-cTnT	High-sensitivity cardiac troponin T
IA2A	Insulinoma-associated protein 2 autoantibody
IAA	Islet cell autoantigen
IBD	Inflammatory bowel disease
IBS	Irritable bowel syndrome
IBS-C	Constipation-predominant IBS
IBS-D	Diarrhoea-predominant IBS
IBS-M	Mixed bowel pattern IBS
IBS-U	Unclassified IBS
ICA	Islet cell antibodies
Ig	Immunoglobulin
IGF-1	Insulin-like growth factor type 1
IL	Interleukin
IM	Intramuscular
INR	International normalised ratio
ITP	Immune thrombocytopenic purpura
IU	International unit
IV	Intravenous
JVP	*Jugular venous pressure*
K. pneumoniae	*Klebsiella pneumoniae*
Kv1−4 antibodies	These are the antibodies directed to the potassium voltage-gated channel; subfamily members 1−4
LA	Left atrium
LDDST	Low-dose dexamethasone suppression test

LDH	Lactate dehydrogenase
LDL	Low-density lipoprotein
LMWH	Low-molecular-weight heparin
LRP$_4$	Lipoprotein receptor-related peptide 4
LTB$_4$	Leukotriene B$_4$
LTD$_4$	Leukotriene D$_4$
LV	Left ventricle
M. catarrhalis	*Moraxella catarrhalis*
MALT	Mucosa-associated lymphoid tissue
MCHC	Mean corpuscular haemoglobin concentration
MCTD	Mixed connective tissue disease
MCV	Mean corpuscular volume
MEN type 1	Multiple endocrine neoplasia type 1
MERS-CoV	Middle East respiratory syndrome coronavirus
MGDF	Megakaryocyte growth and development factor
MGUS	Monoclonal gammopathy of undetermined significance
MHC	Major histocompatibility complex
MRI	Magnetic resonance imaging
MuSK	Muscle specific tyrosine kinase
N. meningitides	*Neisseria meningitidis*
NADP$^+$	Nicotinamide adenine dinucleotide phosphate
NADPH	Reduced nicotinamide adenine dinucleotide phosphate; it used in anabolic cellular reactions
NAPQI	*N*-acetyl-*p*-benzoquinone imine
NICE	National Institute for Health and Care Excellence
NLRP3	NLRP3 inflammasome complex is implicated as a regulator of the innate inflammatory phenotype of several diseases, including gout and type 2 diabetes
NPA	Neutral protamine aspart
NPH	Neutral protamine Hagedorn
NPL	Neutral protamine lispro
NSAIDs	Nonsteroidal anti-inflammatory drugs
OP receptor	Opioid receptors
OPG	Osteoprotegerin
OS	Opening snap
P wave	In ECG, the P wave represents atrial depolarisation, atrial contraction or atrial systole
P. aeruginosa	*Pseudomonas aeruginosa*
P. falciparum	*Plasmodium falciparum*
P. jirovecii	*Pneumocystis jirovecii*
P. malariae	*Plasmodium malariae*
P. mirabilis	*Proteus mirabilis*

P. ovale	*Plasmodium ovale*
P. vivax	*Plasmodium vivax*
p53	Tumour suppressor gene p53 (a 53-kilodalton [kDa] protein)
PAS stain	Periodic acid–Schiff stain
pCO_2	The partial pressure of carbon dioxide
PCR	Polymerase chain reaction
PCV	Packed cell volume
PDGFR	Platelet-derived growth factor receptor
PE	Pulmonary embolism
PEF	Peak expiratory flow
PET scan	Positron emission tomography scan
PfEMP1	*P. falciparum* erythrocyte membrane protein 1
PG	Prostaglandin
PGE_2	Prostaglandin E_2
pH	Potential of hydrogen or power of hydrogen; it is a scale to specify the acidity or basicity of an aqueous solution
Ph chromosome	Philadelphia chromosome
PIP	Proximal interphalangeal joints
PKCiota (PKCI)	Protein kinase Ciota
PLA2R	Phospholipase A2 receptor
PO	Per oral
POEMS syndrome	It is a syndrome characterised by polyneuropathy, organomegaly, endocrinopathy, monoclonal gammopathy and skin changes
PTH	Parathyroid hormone
Q wave	In ECG, the Q wave represents left-to-right depolarisation of the interventricular septum
R wave	In ECG, the R wave is the first upward deflection after the P wave; it represents early ventricular depolarisation
RA	Right atrium
RANKL	Receptor activator of nuclear factor $\kappa\beta$ ligand
RBCs	Red blood cells
RF	Rheumatoid factor
RNA	Ribonucleic acid
RV	Right ventricle
S. aureus	*Staphylococcus aureus*
S. flexneri	*Shigella flexneri*
S. pneumoniae	*Streptococcus pneumoniae*
S. saprophyticus	*Staphylococcus saprophyticus*
S. typhimurium	*Salmonella typhimurium*
S1 + S2 heart sounds	First and second heart sounds

S3 heart sound	The third heart sound, is an extra heart sound, also known as the ventricular gallop; it occurs just after S2
S4 heart sound	The fourth heart sound, is an extra heart sound, also known as the atrial gallop; it occurs just before S1 when the atria contract to force blood into the left ventricle; it can be heard in acute myocardial infarction, cardiomyopathy, aortic stenosis and left bundle branch block
SA node	Sinoatrial node
SAH	Subarachnoid haemorrhage
SaO_2	Oxygen saturation
SARS-CoV	Severe acute respiratory syndrome
SARS-CoV-2	Severe acute respiratory syndrome coronavirus 2
SC	Subcutaneous
SIADH	Syndrome of inappropriate antidiuretic hormone secretion
SLE	Systemic lupus erythematosus
SPEP	Serum protein electrophoresis
SSTR2	Somatostatin receptor type 2
ST segment	In ECG, the ST segment represents the interval between ventricular depolarisation and repolarisation
T wave	In ECG, the T wave represents the repolarisation of the ventricles
T3	Tri-iodothyronine
T4	Thyroxine
TB	Tuberculosis
TGF-ß	Transforming growth factor-beta
Th-1 or T_{h1} cell	T-helper cell-type 1
TH1	T-helper type 1 cells are a lineage of $CD4^+$
TH2	T-helper type 2 cells are a distinct lineage of $CD4^+$
TIA	Transient ischemic attack
TIBC	Total iron-binding capacity
TNF-α	Tumour necrosis factor-alpha
TNM staging	Staging of cancer: T, tumour size; N, spread to lymph nodes; M, metastasis
TP53 gene	It is located on the short arm of chromosome 17 (17p13.1) and its mutation plays a role in cancer development
TPMT	Thiopurine methyltransferase
TRAb	TSH receptor IgG antibody, also known as thyrotrophin receptor antibody
TRAs	Thrombopoietin receptor agonists
TSH	Thyroid-stimulating hormone
tTG	Tissue transglutaminase

TTP	Thrombotic thrombocytopenic purpura
UGI	Upper gastrointestinal
UPEP	Urine protein electrophoresis
UTI	Urinary tract infection
V/Q scan	Ventilation/perfusion scan
VAP	Ventilation-associated pneumonia
WBC	White blood cell
WPW syndrome	Wolff–Parkinson–White syndrome
Y. enterocolitica	*Yersinia enterocolitica*
ZN stain	Ziehl–Neelsen stain

CONTENTS

Gastroenterology and Hepatobiliary Systems

CASE 1.1

'I Have Tummy Pain …'

Lilian Murad, a 70-year-old retired teacher, is brought by an ambulance to the emergency department of a local hospital because she is suffering from mild upper abdominal pain for the last 2 days and feeling unsteady during walking. Mrs Murad has severe osteoarthritis and she takes 600 mg of ibuprofen three times a day for the arthritis pains. On examination, her resting pulse rate is 110/min, and her blood pressure is 140/75 mm Hg, lying flat (100/50 mm Hg, sitting). She looks pale but not jaundiced. On abdominal palpation, mild tenderness in the epigastrium is found. The liver and spleen are not palpable. Per rectum examination reveals soft black tarry stool on the gloved examining finger. The cardiovascular and respiratory examination reports are normal.

CASE DISCUSSION

Q1. On the basis of Mrs Murad's presentation, what is your diagnosis?

Q2. What is your differential diagnosis?

Q3. What are the key clinical features of this disease? What are the scientific bases for these features?

Q4. What is the pathophysiology underlying these changes?

Q5. What are your management goals and management options?

ANSWERS

1. The findings of using ibuprofen, a nonsteroidal anti-inflammatory drug (NSAID), tachycardia, postural drop of blood pressure, tenderness in the epigastrium, pallor and the presence of soft black tarry stool (melaena stool) are suggestive of bleeding from a gastric ulcer. Upper gastrointestinal (UGI) bleeding is a common clinical problem and has been associated with increasing NSAID use and the high prevalence of *Helicobacter pylori* infection in patients with bleeding peptic ulcer. Rapid assessment and resuscitation should precede the diagnostic evaluation, particularly in patients with haemodynamic changes (such as elevated heart rate and postural changes in blood pressure) due to severe bleeding.

2. The differential diagnosis:
   - Peptic ulcer bleeding (60%–65% of cases)
   - Gastritis and duodenitis (8% of cases)
   - Oesophageal varices (6% of cases)

- Mallory–Weiss tear (4% of cases)
- Gastric malignancy (1%–2% of cases)
- Arteriovenous malformation (angiodysplasias) (10% of cases)
- Oesophagitis or oesophageal ulcer
- Duodenal ulcer
- Pancreatic cancer (rare cause)
- No identified cause

The following are essential for the diagnosis of peptic ulcer bleeding:
- Haematemesis, melaena stool, history of aspirin or NSAID use, abdominal pain, nocturnal symptoms, history of peptic ulcer bleeding or confirmed *H. pylori* infection.
- Early upper endoscopy (within 24 hours) confirms the diagnosis and allows for targeted treatment (e.g. injection of a sclerosant or epinephrine, thermocoagulation, allocation of metallic clips and rubber banding).

3. Symptoms and signs:
- Abdominal pain, coffee ground–like emesis, haematemesis, dyspepsia, soft black tarry stools, bright red blood per rectum (occurs when there is a loss of more than 1000 mL of blood), warfarin, aspirin, NSAIDs, selective serotonin reuptake inhibitors (SSRIs) or corticosteroid use, or history of peptic ulcer disease.
- Previous abdominal surgery, previous episodes of UGI bleeding, alcohol use and smoking.
- Ask about and assess for chronic renal or liver diseases, or chronic obstructive pulmonary disease.
- Heavy alcohol ingestion may be suggestive of Mallory–Weiss tear.
- Signs of chronic liver disease may indicate that the bleeding is due to portal hypertension.

4. Pathophysiological and laboratory features:
- The common causes of peptic ulcer disease are (i) use of NSAIDs: about 5%–20% of patients who use NSAIDs over long periods develop peptic ulcer disease, particularly in elderly patients; (ii) *H. pylori* infection (Gram-negative mobile spiral rod) is found in 48% of patients with peptic ulcer disease; (iii) acid hypersecretory states (e.g. Zollinger–Ellison syndrome); and (iv) stress-induced ulcers, e.g. after acute illness, multiorgan failure, ventilator support, extreme burns (Curling ulcer), head injury (Cushing ulcers). Fig. 1.1.1 shows pathology and pathogenesis of peptic ulcer disease – injurious and defence mechanisms.
- *H. pylori* infection causes peptic ulcer disease through several mechanisms including (i) the presence of an outer inflammatory protein in the bacterium, (ii) the presence of a functional cytotoxin-associated gene island in the bacterial chromosome causing virulence and ulcerative changes, (iii) decreased gastric mucosal production and decreased duodenal mucosal bicarbonate secretion and (iv) increased resting and meal-stimulated gastrin levels. Fig. 1.1.2 shows *H. pylori* adherent to gastric mucosa.
- NSAIDs cause inhibition of the cyclooxygenase (COX) and inhibition of prostaglandins and their protective COX-2–mediated effects. This results in decreased

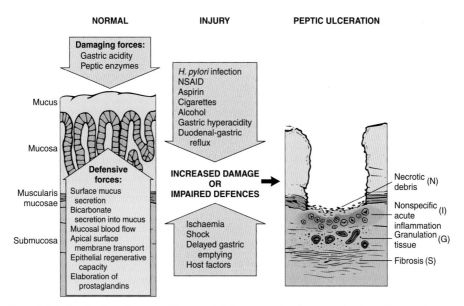

Figure 1.1.1 Peptic ulcer disease pathogenesis. Injurious and defence mechanisms. The peptic ulcer is characterised by necrotic tissues (N), acute inflammatory changes (I), granulation tissues (G) and fibrosis (S). *(Source: Kumar V, Abbas AK, Fausto N, Mitchell R. Robbins Basic Pathology, 8th Edition. London, UK: Elsevier; 2007.)*

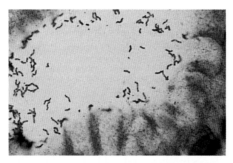

Figure 1.1.2 *H. pylori* silver stain showing spiral-shaped organisms adherent to the gastric mucosa. *(Source: Goering R, Dockrell N, Zuckerman M, Wakelin D, Roitt I, Mims C, Chiodini P. Mims' Medical Microbiology. 4th ed. London, UK: Elsevier; 2007.)*

mucus secretion and bicarbonate secretion, decreased mucosal blood flow and disturbed epithelial cell proliferation, and hence peptic ulcer disease.
• There is evidence that coexisting *H. pylori* infection increases the likelihood of intensity of NSAID-induced damage.
• Laboratory tests needed to assess the condition of Mrs Murad include complete blood count, platelet count, prothrombin time, international normalised ratio (INR), serum creatinine, liver function tests and blood typing and screening. Remember that haematocrit is not a reliable indicator of severity of acute bleeding.

5. Management goals:
- Correct any haemodynamic changes.
- Assess risks.
- Stop bleeding.
- Manage the cause of bleeding.

A. Correct any haemodynamic changes. (i) Patients with haemodynamic compromise should be given 0.9% saline or lactated Ringer injections and crossmatched for 2–4 units of packed red blood cells. (ii) Blood transfusion should be administered to those with a haemoglobin level of 70 g/L or less. The haemoglobin should be maintained at 90 g/L. (iii) Patients with active bleeding and coagulopathy (and INR > 1.8) should be considered for fresh frozen plasma. If there is thrombocytopenia, platelet transfusion should be considered.

B. Assess risk. Clinical assessment should be for whether the bleeding is from upper or lower GI tract. Assess the patient's age, presence of shock, systolic blood pressure, heart rate and comorbid conditions. Assess risk for rebleeding. Review the Rockall risk scoring system (for further reading, check Rockall et al., 1996).

C. Stop bleeding. Nasogastric tube is placed for aspiration. Intravenous proton-pump inhibitor is used in patients admitted for active bleeding. Early upper endoscopy (within the first 24 hours of presentation) should be considered. Gastric lavage to clear the stomach of blood increases the success of localisation of the source of bleeding. Early endoscopy confirms the diagnosis and allows for targeted treatment (e.g. injection of a sclerosant or epinephrine, thermocoagulation, allocation of metallic clips and rubber banding).

BACK TO BASIC SCIENCES

Q1. What are the functions of the main cells in the stomach?
- Mucous neck cells → produce soluble mucus that lubricates the chime.
- Stem cells → proliferate to replace all the specialised cells lining the fundic glands.
- Parietal (oxyntic) cells → produce hydrochloric acid (HCl) and the gastric intrinsic factor (IF), which is essential for the absorption of vitamin B12, mainly in terminal ileum.
- Peptic (chief) cells → secrete pepsinogen.
- Enterochromaffin cells → store serotonin (5-HT).
- Enterochromaffin-like (ECL) cells → synthesise and secrete histamine.
- Pyloric glands contain mucus and endocrine cells including gastrin cells (G-cells), which release gastrin, usually in response to gastric distension and the presence of nutrients (amino acids and amines).
- D-cells (endocrine cells) → release somatostatin in response to HCl. Somatostatin inhibits the release of HCl from the parietal cells.

Q2. What are the noxious factors that may expose the gastric mucosa to damage?
- HCl, pepsinogen, pepsin, bile salts.
- Medications, alcohol, bacteria.

Q3. Briefly discuss the gastric mucosal defence system.
It comprises three level barriers:
- Pre-epithelial: Represented by a physicochemical barrier comprising a mucus–bicarbonate–phospholipid layer. This barrier forms a pH gradient ranging from 1 to 2 at the gastric luminal surface and reaching 6–7 along the epithelial cells.
- Epithelial: Represented by (i) mucus production, epithelial cell ionic transporters and intracellular tight junctions; (ii) epithelial cells, which generate heat shock proteins that prevent protein denaturation; (iii) production of growth factors and prostaglandins. These growth factors include epidermal growth factor (EGF), transforming growth factor (TGF) and fibroblast growth factor (FGF) that promote epithelial protection. Prostaglandins and growth factors play a role in epithelial cell renewal and formation of new vessels (angiogenesis).
- Subepithelial: The production of HCO_3^-, which neutralises the acid generated by the parietal cells. The formation of effective microcirculatory bed, the removal of toxic by-products and the continuing supply of oxygen and micronutrients.

Prostaglandins provide central role in the protection. A key enzyme that regulates the rate-limiting step in prostaglandin synthesis is cyclooxygenase (COX), which is present in two isoforms (COX-1 and COX-2).

Q4. What are the main differences between COX-1 and COX-2?
- Cyclooxygennase-1 (COX-1) is expressed in a host of tissues including stomach, platelets, kidneys and endothelial cells. This enzyme is important for maintaining the integrity of the renal function, platelet aggregation and the GI mucosal integrity.
- Cyclooxygenase-2 (COX-2) is inducible by inflammation stimuli. Therefore, it is expressed in inflammatory cells including macrophages, leukocytes, fibroblasts and synovial cells.

The applications of these differences are as follows:
  (i) Aspirin and NSAIDs demonstrate their anti-inflammatory effects by inhibiting COX-1. Therefore, toxicity such as mucosal ulceration and renal dysfunction can occur in relation to COX-1 inhibition.
  (ii) Aspirin even in small doses can inhibit platelet aggregation via inhibiting COX-1 isoenzyme.
  (iii) The highly selective COX-2 NSAIDs have the potential effects of decreasing inflammation without causing toxicity to the stomach mucosa or the kidney. However, selective COX-2 drugs have adverse effects on the cardiovascular system such as myocardial infarction.

Q5. What are the most common causes of peptic ulcer disease?
H. pylori infection and the use of NSAIDs are the most common causes of peptic ulcer disease.

Q6. What are the other diagnoses that should be considered in the differential diagnosis of peptic ulcer disease?
The other diagnoses are oesophagitis, functional dyspepsia, gastritis, gastro-oesophageal reflux, cholangitis, cholecystitis, cholelithiasis, oesophageal perforation, inflammatory bowel disease, coeliac disease, irritable bowel syndrome, gastric cancer, viral hepatitis and Zollinger–Ellison syndrome.

Q7. What do you know about *Helicobacter pylori*?
H. pylori is a Gram-negative helical rod-shaped bacterium that colonises in the gastric mucosa. It is estimated to be present in one-half of the world population. It is present in >90% of patients with duodenal ulcers and in 30%–60% of patients with gastric ulcers. Infection occurs via the faecal–oral route and during early childhood and persists for decades. Infection with *H. pylori* is one of the common causes of peptic ulcer disease and is a risk factor for mucosa-associated lymphoid tissue (MALT) lymphoma and gastric adenocarcinoma.

Q8. What are the two most accurate tests for identifying *H. pylori* infection?
The urea breath test and the stool antigen test.

Q9. What are the advantages and disadvantages of the serologic tests?
The serologic tests aim at detecting immunoglobulin G specific to *H. pylori* in the serum. Therefore, the test cannot distinguish between an active infection and a past infection. The serologic tests can be used in mass population surveys and in patients who cannot stop taking proton-pump inhibitors (e.g. those with GI bleeding).

Q10. What are the main complications of peptic ulcer disease?
The main complications are bleeding, perforation, gastric outlet obstruction and gastric cancer.

REVIEW QUESTIONS

Q1. Which *one* of the following gastric cells is responsible for HCl secretion?
A. Enterochromaffin cells
B. Enterochromaffin-like (ECL) cells
C. D-cells
D. Peptic (chief) cells
E. Parietal cells

Q2. Regarding COX-1, which *one* of the following statements is correct?
A. Inducible by inflammation
B. Expressed in macrophages
C. Expressed in the stomach
D. Its inhibition causes platelet aggregation

Q3. Which *one* of the following is correct about *H. pylori*?
A. Is Gram-positive
B. Causes peptic ulcer disease in >90% of infected patients
C. Produces uric acid
D. Causes gastric cancer
E. Causes Zollinger–Ellison syndrome

Q4. Patients with bleeding gastric ulcers due to low-dose aspirin taken for secondary cardiovascular prevention should: (*select one response*)
A. Stop taking aspirin.
B. Take an antiplatelet drug instead.
C. Take low-dose aspirin twice weekly after bleeding stops.
D. Resume the use of aspirin together with a proton-pump inhibitor.

Q5. There is evidence from randomised trials that administration of a proton-pump inhibitor to patients with UGI bleeding soon after presentation is associated with: (*select one response*)
A. Significant reduction of the risk of further bleeding.
B. Significant reduction of the need of surgery to manage bleeding.
C. No significant reduction in death.
D. No reduction of the need for endoscopic therapy.

Q6. In patients with UGI bleeding, which *one* of the following is *not* associated with increased risk of further bleeding?
A. Tachycardia > 100 beats/min
B. Hypotension – systolic < 100 mm Hg
C. Age > 60 years
D. Major coexisting condition
E. White blood cell count > 13×10^9/L

ANSWERS

A1. **E.** Parietal cells in the stomach are responsible for HCl secretion.

A2. **C.** COX-1 is expressed in the stomach. Other items are correct for COX-2.

A3. **D.** *H. pylori* cause gastric cancer.

A4. **D**. If aspirin was used for primary prevention, aspirin has been shown to result in a small reduction in the absolute risk of cardiovascular events. However, the absolute reduction in cardiovascular events is much greater when aspirin is used for secondary prevention. Therefore, aspirin should be resumed within 1–7 days after bleeding stops. Co-therapy with a proton-pump inhibitor should be considered (for further reading, check Bhatt et al., 2008).

A5. **C**. A meta-analysis of six randomised trials showed that the use of a proton-pump inhibitor soon after presentation was associated with no significant reduction of the risks of further bleeding, surgery or death. However, the administration of a proton-pump inhibitor was associated with a decrease in the frequency of high-risk endoscopic findings (e.g. active bleeding) and the need for endoscopic therapy (for further reading, check Sreedharan et al., 2010).

A6. **E**. Higher risk of further bleeding or death in relation to UGI bleeding is calculated from Glasgow-Blatchford score (range from 0 to 23). The score comprises blood urea, haemoglobin level, systolic blood pressure, heart rate and other variables including melaena, syncope and evidence of hepatic disease and cardiac failure. White blood cell count is not a parameter in such assessments (for further reading, check Gralnek et al., 2015).

TAKE-HOME MESSAGE

- Peptic ulcers due to *H. pylori* infection or the use of NSAIDs are the most common causes of UGI bleeding.
- The differential diagnosis includes peptic ulcer disease (60%–65%), gastritis/duodenitis (8%), oesophageal varices (65%), Mallory–Weiss tear (4%), gastric malignancy (1%–2%) and arteriovenous malformation (10%).
- The clinical picture is characterised by abdominal pain, dizziness, haematemesis and melaena stool (soft black tarry stool).
- Management goals are to correct haemodynamic changes, assess risks, stop bleeding and manage the cause of bleeding.

FURTHER READINGS

Bhatt DL et al. ACCF/ACG/AHA 2008 expert consensus document on reducing the gastrointestinal risks of antiplatelet therapy and NSAID use: a report of the American College of Cardiology Foundation Task Force on Clinical Expert Consensus Documents. American College of Cardiology Foundation Task Force on Clinical Expert Consensus Documents. *J Am Coll Cardiol*. 2008;52(18):1502-1517.

Gralnek IM, Barkun AN, Bardou M. Management of acute bleeding from a peptic ulcer. *N Engl J Med*. 2008;359(9):928-937. Review.

Gralnek IM, Dumonceau JM, Kuipers EJ, et al. Diagnosis and management of nonvariceal upper gastrointestinal hemorrhage: European Society of Gastrointestinal Endoscopy (ESGE) Guideline. *Endoscopy*. 2015;47(10):a1-a46.

Laine L. Clinical Practice: Upper gastrointestinal bleeding due to a peptic ulcer. *N Engl J Med*. 2016; 374(24):2367-2376. Review.

Lanas A, Chan FKL. Peptic ulcer disease. *Lancet*. 2017;390(10094):613-624.

Rockall TA, Logan RF, Devlin HB, Northfield TC. Risk assessment after acute upper gastrointestinal haemorrhage. *Gut*. 1996;38(3):316-321.

Sreedharan A, Martin J, Leontiadis GI, et al. Proton pump inhibitor treatment initiated prior to endoscopic diagnosis in upper gastrointestinal bleeding. *Cochrane Database Syst Rev*. 2010;(7):CD005415.

CASE 1.2

'I Am Losing Weight ...'

Asma Ali, a 7-year-old primary school student, comes in with her mother to see a general practitioner because she is suffering from chronic diarrhoea and abdominal discomfort. She has been feeling tired over the last few months and has lost 3 kg in body weight over the last 8–9 months. On examination, nothing significant is found. Laboratory tests show that she has a haemoglobin level of 90 g/L (normal = 115–160 g/L) with an iron-deficiency picture on the blood film. Serum ferritin is low, confirming iron-deficiency anaemia. Her stool analysis shows undigested food and fat globules.

CASE DISCUSSION

Q1. On the basis of Asma's presentation, what is your diagnosis?

Q2. What is your differential diagnosis?

Q3. What are the key clinical features of this disease? What are the scientific bases for these features?

Q4. What is the pathophysiology underlying these changes?

Q5. What are your management goals and management options?

ANSWERS

1. The findings of chronic diarrhoea, abdominal discomfort, tiredness, loss of body weight and iron-deficiency anaemia are suggestive of malabsorption. The presence of undigested food and fat globules in the stool analysis is also consistent with the diagnosis of malabsorption, such as coeliac disease. However, further assessment is needed to confirm the diagnosis.
2. The differential diagnosis:
   - Autoimmune enteropathy
   - Bacterial overgrowth
   - Crohn disease
   - Giardiasis
   - Occult gastrointestinal bleeding
   - Intestinal lymphoma
   - Lactose intolerance
   - Soy protein intolerance

- Tropical sprue
- Tuberculosis

The following are essential for the diagnosis of coeliac disease:
- Typical presentations: Weight loss, chronic diarrhoea, tiredness, abdominal distension, abdominal discomfort and flatulence.
- Atypical presentation: Iron-deficiency anaemia, osteoporosis, low serum albumin and dermatitis herpetiformis.
- The diagnosis is confirmed by serologic tests (IgA endomysial antibody and IgA tTG antibody tests), both of which have a >90% sensitivity and >95% specificity for the diagnosis of coeliac disease. Endoscopic mucosal biopsy of the proximal jejunum is the standard method for confirming the diagnosis.
- Clinical improvement on gluten-free diet.

3. Symptoms and signs:
   - The classic symptoms of malabsorption such as coeliac disease include chronic diarrhoea, steatorrhoea, weight loss, abdominal distension, weakness, muscle wasting or growth retardation. These symptoms are usually present in young children (younger than 2 years).
   - Adults are less likely to present with gastrointestinal symptoms. They may have dyspepsia, chronic diarrhoea or flatulence. Usually adults present with extraintestinal 'atypical' manifestations including fatigue, depression, tiredness, iron-deficiency anaemia, osteoporosis, delayed puberty or reduced fertility.
   - Clinical examination may be normal or shows signs of malabsorption such as loss of body weight, loss of muscle mass or subcutaneous fat, pallor due to anaemia, easy bruising (due to vitamin K deficiency), ankle oedema (due to low serum albumin), hyperkeratosis (due to vitamin A deficiency), bone pain (due to osteomalacia), osteoporosis (due to vitamin D deficiency) or peripheral neuropathy. Abdominal examination may reveal abdominal distension and hyperactive bowel sounds.

4. Pathophysiological and laboratory features:
   - The common causes of steatorrhoea (malabsorption of fats) are (i) conditions affecting the pancreas such as chronic pancreatitis and pancreatic cancer; (ii) conditions affecting bile salt availability such as primary biliary cirrhosis and intrahepatic cholestasis; and (iii) conditions affecting the small intestine and interfering with absorption such as coeliac disease, tropical sprue, giardiasis and bacterial overgrowth syndrome.
   - Regardless of the cause, a 72-hour quantitative stool collection, preferably on a defined diet, must be obtained to determine stool fat content to establish the diagnosis of steatorrhoea.
   - Coeliac disease is an autoimmune disease triggered by exposure to dietary gluten in genetically susceptible individuals. Gliadin, the alcohol-soluble protein of gluten, cannot be fully broken down in the intestine and generally this protein remains in the intestinal lumen of all individuals. In genetically sus-

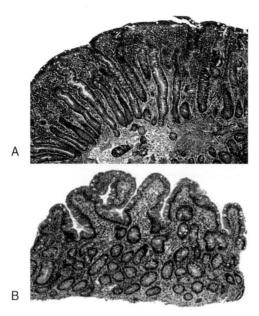

Figure 1.2.1 (A) Intestinal biopsy showing changes consistent with coeliac disease (flattened villi, hyperplasia of crypts and increased intestinal lymphocytes). (B) Regeneration of intestinal villi after starting the patient on a gluten-free diet. *(Source: Goldman L, Schafer AI. Goldman-Cecil Medicine. 25th ed. Elsevier; 2016.)*

ceptible patients, the gliadin particle passes through the epithelial layer of the small intestine and stimulates immune response. The gliadin proteins then bind to the human leukocyte antigen class II DQ2 or DQ8 molecules, which activates CD4 T-cells in the intestinal mucosa. This autoimmune activation produces chronic inflammation of the proximal small bowel mucosa leading to villus atrophy and malabsorption, mainly of fats, iron and fat-soluble vitamins (Fig. 1.2.1A and B).

- The severity of the clinical picture depends on the severity and extent of intestinal damage.
- Persons at an increased risk of coeliac disease are (i) first-degree relatives of a person with coeliac disease, (ii) second-degree relatives of a person with coeliac disease, (iii) those with Down syndrome, (iv) those with Turner syndrome, (v) those with autoimmune thyroid disorders, (vi) those with immune globulin A deficiency and (vii) those with type 1 diabetes mellitus.
- Serologic testing and small bowel biopsy are highly sensitive and specific in diagnosing coeliac disease. Those at an increased risk should be investigated including (i) patients with a family history of coeliac disease; (ii) those with associated autoimmune disorders; (iii) patients presenting with gastrointestinal symptoms such as abdominal pain, chronic diarrhoea, malabsorption, weight loss and bloating; and (iv) patients with premature osteoporosis, iron-deficiency anaemia, low serum albumin and unexplained abnormal liver function tests.

- Other laboratory tests needed to assess the condition of Asma include complete blood count, blood film, iron studies, B12 and blood folate levels, prothrombin time, international normalised ratio (INR), liver function tests, serum albumin, blood calcium and electrolytes, and blood urea and creatinine.

5. Management goals:
   - Adherence to a gluten-free diet (serologic monitoring for coeliac disease could help in assessing adherence)
   - Patient education
   - Monitoring for associated conditions (osteoporosis, autoimmune thyroiditis)
   - Monitoring for complications

BACK TO BASIC SCIENCES

Q1. Briefly discuss the epidemiology of coeliac disease.

- Coeliac disease affects 0.6%–1.0% of the population worldwide. It shows a high prevalence in North Africa and the Middle East population. It is rare in black Africans.
- It is more common in females (female to male ratio is 2–3:1).
- The frequency of coeliac disease is rising in developing countries because of changes in wheat production and possibly increased consumption of Western foods and awareness of the disease.
- The disease is increased in persons who have a first-degree relative affected, type 1 diabetes mellitus, Hashimoto thyroiditis or other autoimmune disorders.
- Coeliac disease can present at any age. It is commonly diagnosed in early childhood. However, the diagnosis may be delayed up to 10 years from the time of first presentation.
- Genetic background plays a role in the disease and HLA-DQ2 haplotype is expressed in the majority of patients. HLA-DQ8 is expressed in 5%–10% of patients.

Q2. Briefly discuss the pathogenesis of coeliac disease.

- The disease occurs as a result of an inappropriate immune body response to an external trigger (dietary gluten protein) found in wheat, rye and barley in individuals who are genetically predisposed to the disease.
- The disease in the majority of patients is associated with HLA-DQ2 or HLA-DQ8 haplotype but other genes have been identified and involved in the disease susceptibility.
- The disease is immune mediated and is dependent on the presentation of gluten peptides to T-cells. This process necessitates prior deamidation of glutamine residue by tissue transglutaminase.
- Although the HLA expression is important in the pathogenesis, there is evidence of non-HLA genetic component with over 40 regions harbouring susceptibility genes for coeliac disease.

- The immunological changes result in chronic inflammatory changes of the mucosa of the small intestine, infiltration of the lamina propria, increased intraepithelial lymphocytes, crypt hyperplasia and intestinal mucosal atrophy (loss of villi). These changes impair the absorptive functions of the small intestine, resulting in malabsorption of fat- and lipid-soluble vitamins (A, D, E and K) as well as iron, folate and calcium.

Q3. Briefly discuss the clinical picture of coeliac disease.
- The disease is frequently asymptomatic.
- Although it is commonly diagnosed in early childhood (usually because of profuse diarrhoea and failure to thrive after weaning), the disease may be diagnosed at any age and the diagnosis may be delayed up to 10 years after the first presentation.
- Common presenting signs and symptoms:
  1. Loose bowel motions and steatorrhoea (excessive loss of fats in stools because of failure of fat absorption)
  2. Bloating, recurrent abdominal pain and symptoms similar to those of irritable bowel syndrome (therefore, all patients with irritable bowel syndrome should be serologically investigated for coeliac disease)
  3. Weight loss
  4. Tiredness and chronic fatigue
  5. Iron-deficiency anaemia (in those with duodenal and early jejunum involvement)
  6. Anaemia due to deficiency of vitamin B12 (terminal ileum involvement) and folate (early jejunum involvement)
  7. Vitamin D deficiency, reduced bone mineral density and osteomalacia in adults and rickets in children
  8. Peripheral neuropathy, proximal muscle pains, gluten ataxia and epilepsy
  9. Dermatitis herpetiformis (rare)

Q4. Briefly discuss the complications associated with untreated coeliac disease.
1. Osteoporosis
2. Impaired splenic functions
3. Infertility and recurrent abortions in females
4. Cancer and T-cell lymphoma
5. Adenocarcinoma of the jejunum (rare)
6. Peripheral neuropathy and gluten ataxia
7. Ulcerations and inflammation of the jejunum and ileum
8. Refractory coeliac disease despite strict gluten-free diet over 12 months

Q5. Would you expect to find elevated serum coeliac antibodies and intestinal mucosal atrophy in all patients with coeliac disease?
No. Patients may show positive coeliac autoantibodies in their sera, whereas intestinal mucosa on biopsies may be normal.

Overt intestinal mucosal atrophy may develop later over time. The serum antibodies usually appear earlier.

Mucosal atrophy may not be seen early in the disease development.

Q6. What are the investigations recommended for the diagnosis of coeliac disease?

1. Serological tests: Serum IgA anti-tissue transglutaminase (tTG) antibodies. In patients with concomitant IgA deficiency, IgG anti-tissue transglutaminase antibodies can be measured instead.
2. Biopsy of the small intestine and histological examination may be done.
3. Testing for HLA-DQ2 and DQ8 may be used to investigate people at risk (family members of a person with coeliac disease). The disease is unlikely in persons who are negative for both HLA-DQ2 and HLA-DQ8.
4. Other investigations may be performed for assessing complicated cases such as magnetic resonance imaging.

Q7. What are the intestinal histological changes characteristics of coeliac disease?

1. Increased number of intraepithelial lymphocytes
2. Elongation and changes in crypts
3. Total villous atrophy

REVIEW QUESTIONS

Q1. Which *one* of the following statements about coeliac disease is correct?
A. Negative serologic results exclude the diagnosis
B. A biopsy of small intestine is required in all patients
C. HLA-DQ2 haplotype is expressed in majority of patients
D. The disease is particularly common in black Africans

Q2. Which *one* of the following is *not* involved in the pathogenesis of coeliac disease?
A. The HLA-DQ2 haplotype
B. Non-HLA genes
C. Enzymatically modified gluten protein
D. Coeliac serum autoantibodies
E. IgA deficiency

Q3. Which *one* of the following is *not* among the clinical presentation of coeliac disease?
A. Iron-deficiency anaemia
B. Anaemia due to vitamin B12 and folate deficiency
C. Peripheral neuropathy
D. Osteomalacia
E. Acute renal failure

Q4. Which *one* of the following laboratory test results will help in the diagnosis of coeliac disease in patients with IgA deficiency?
A. Raised serum AST and ALT levels
B. Low serum vitamin D level
C. Raised serum alkaline phosphatase
D. Positive IgG antibodies against tissue transglutaminase
E. Raised fat content in the stools

Q5. Which *one* of the following skin lesions may be found with coeliac disease?
A. Allergic dermatitis
B. Dermatitis herpetiformis
C. Erythema multiforme
D. Hyperpigmentation
E. Livedo reticularis

ANSWERS

A1. **C.** HLA-DQ2 haplotype is expressed in 90% of patients. The HLA-DQ8 haplotype is expressed in 5% of patients. Negative serologic results do not exclude the diagnosis particularly if the clinical picture is consistent with coeliac disease. Intestinal biopsy is needed in these patients.

Patients, particularly children, with positive serological tests (anti-tTG antibody titre more than 10 times the upper limit of normal) and a clinical picture suggestive of coeliac disease do not need intestinal biopsy for confirmation of the diagnosis.

Coeliac disease is commonly seen in North Africans and in the Middle East population. It is rare in black Africans.

A2. **E.** Although IgA deficiency may occur concomitantly with coeliac disease, there is no evidence that IgA deficiency is involved in the pathogenesis of the disease.

A3. **E.** Acute renal failure is not among the clinical picture of coeliac disease.

Patients with coeliac disease commonly present with steatorrhoea, weight loss, chronic fatigue, depression, iron deficiency, vitamin B12 and folate deficiency, peripheral neuropathy, gluten ataxia, osteomalacia, fractures and proximal muscle weakness and pains.

A4. **D.** In patients with IgA deficiency and clinical presentation suggestive of coeliac disease, IgG rather than IgA anti-tissue transglutaminase antibodies are recommended for the diagnosis.

A5. **B.** Dermatitis herpetiformis is closely related to coeliac disease. It occurs in 2%–5% of patients with coeliac disease and consists of itchy vesicular skin rash on elbows, knees, buttocks and scalp.

TAKE-HOME MESSAGE

- The typical presentation of malabsorption includes weight loss, chronic diarrhoea, tiredness, abdominal distension, abdominal discomfort and flatulence.
- Atypical presentation may include iron-deficiency anaemia, osteoporosis, low serum albumin and/or dermatitis herpetiformis.
- The diagnosis is confirmed by serologic tests (IgA endomysial antibody and IgA tTG antibody tests).
- Both tests have a >90% sensitivity and >95% specificity for the diagnosis of coeliac disease. Endoscopic mucosal biopsy of the proximal jejunum is the standard method for confirming the diagnosis.
- Clinical improvement on gluten-free diet also supports the diagnosis.
- In patients with IgA deficiency and clinical presentation suggestive of coeliac disease, IgG rather than IgA anti-tissue transglutaminase antibodies are recommended for the diagnosis.
- Complications associated with untreated coeliac disease may include osteoporosis, impaired splenic functions, infertility and recurrent abortions in females, cancer and T-cell lymphoma, adenocarcinoma of the jejunum (rare), peripheral neuropathy and gluten ataxia.

FURTHER READINGS

Armstrong C. ACG releases guideline on diagnosis and management of coeliac disease. *Am Fam Physician.* 2014;89(6):485-487.

Fasano A, Catassi C. Clinical practice. Coeliac disease. *N Engl J Med.* 2012;367(25):2419-2426.

Green PH, Cellier C. Coeliac disease. *N Engl J Med.* 2007;357(17):1731-1743. Review.

Lebwohl B, Sanders DS, Green PHR. Coeliac disease. *Lancet.* 2018;391(10115):70-81.

Lionetti E, Castellaneta S, Francavilla R, et al. Introduction of gluten, HLA status, and the risk of coeliac disease in children. *N Engl J Med.* 2014;371(14):1295-1303.

Pelkowski TD, Viera AJ. Coeliac disease: diagnosis and management. *Am Fam Physician.* 2014;89(2):99-105.

Rubio-Tapia A, Hill ID, Kelly CP, Calderwood AH, Murray JA; American College of Gastroenterology. ACG clinical guidelines: diagnosis and management of coeliac disease. *Am J Gastroenterol.* 2013;108(5): 656-676.

Seehusen DA. Comparative accuracy of diagnostic tests for coeliac disease. *Am Fam Physician.* 2017;95(11): 726-728.

CASE 1.3

'Not Regular . . . '

Michael West, a 58-year-old salesman, comes in to see his general practitioner because his recent complete blood count showed a haemoglobin level of 80 g/L and a picture suggestive of iron-deficiency anaemia. Michael used to be healthy and his annual blood test results are usually within the normal range. During the consultation, Michael says, 'I noticed changes in my bowel habits over the last 3–4 months; at times I have constipation for 4–5 days followed by loose bowel motions for another 2–3 days. I used to open my bowels once a day.' He also lost 3 kg in body weight over the last 8 months. Recently he started to feel tired and thought it to be related to his work demands. Over the last few days, he noticed blood in his stools, which triggered his worries. Clinical examination reveals nothing significant except pallor of his conjunctivae. His doctor arranges a referral for a colonoscopy, which reveals a 4 × 6 cm ulcerated mass located in the sigmoid region.

CASE DISCUSSION

Q1. On the basis of Mr West's presentation, what is your diagnosis?

Q2. What is your differential diagnosis?

Q3. What are the key clinical features of this disease? What are the scientific bases for these features?

Q4. What is the pathophysiology underlying these changes?

Q5. What are your management goals and management options?

ANSWERS

1. The findings of iron-deficiency anaemia after the age of 50, together with changes in the bowel habits, abdominal discomfort, tiredness, loss of body weight (may indicate metastasis) and the presence of blood in stools or passing blood per rectum are suggestive of colorectal cancer. The colonoscopy confirms the presence of an ulcerated tumour mass in the sigmoid region.
2. The differential diagnosis:
   * Diverticular disease
   * Diverticulitis
   * Haemorrhoids
   * Iron-deficiency anaemia due to other causes

- Infectious colitis
- Inflammatory bowel disease
- Adenomatous polyps

The following are essential for the diagnosis of colorectal cancer:

- Typical presentation: This depends on the location of the tumour. (i) Tumours arising in the caecum and right colon usually do not cause obstructive symptoms or noticeable changes in the bowel habits. Patients usually present with iron-deficiency anaemia, palpitations and tiredness. The anaemia is usually related to the chronic intermittent blood loss from the tumour mass. Therefore, the stools of these patients usually do not show blood and random faecal occult blood tests may be negative. (ii) Tumours arising from the transverse colon and descending colon may present with abdominal cramping pains and sometimes obstruction. (iii) Tumours arising from the rectosigmoid may present with bleeding per rectum (haematochezia), tenesmus, changes in bowel habits (alternate constipation followed by diarrhoea), narrowing of the calibre of stool and anaemia.
- Therefore, adults, other than premenopausal women, presenting with anaemia should be investigated by thorough endoscopy and visualisation of the whole large intestine.
- The presence of a family history of adenomatous polyps or colorectal cancer is an important risk factor.
- Colonoscopy is essential for the diagnosis.

3. Symptoms and signs:
   - The classic symptoms of colorectal cancer depend on the location of the tumour.
   - Right-sided colon cancers cause iron-deficiency anaemia and tiredness. Left-sided colon cancers cause obstructive symptoms, abdominal pain, changes in bowel habits and stool streaked with blood. Rectal cancers cause rectal tenesmus, urgency and recurrent haematochezia.
   - Weight loss is not common. It may indicate metastasis.
   - Clinical examination usually does not show abnormalities apart from pallor in the presence of anaemia. An abdominal mass may be felt in thin people. Hepatomegaly may indicate the presence of liver metastasis.

4. Pathophysiological and laboratory features:
   - The risk factors for developing colon cancer are (i) a diet rich in red meat and animal fat; (ii) obesity and the presence of insulin resistance: the insulin resistance results in higher concentrations of insulin-like growth factor type 1 (IGF-1) in these patients and hence stimulation of intestinal mucosa proliferation; (ii) family history of colon cancer; (iv) the presence of any of the following two conditions: familial adenomatous polyposis (FAP) or hereditary nonpolyposis colorectal cancer; (v) inflammatory bowel disease; (vi) patients with ureterosigmoidostomy; and (vii) tobacco use.
   - Pathophysiology: Most colorectal cancers arise from adenomatous polyps.
   - A polyp may be non-neoplastic (juvenile polyp), hyperplastic or adenomatous polyp.

- Adenomatous polyps are premalignant. Only <1% of all polyps become malignant.
- Polyps are usually asymptomatic.
- Dysplastic lesions may develop in a polyp and microscopic foci of malignant tumour cells develop (the development of carcinoma in situ). The mechanisms responsible for these changes are as follows:
  - **(i)** Mutation of the p53 tumour suppressor gene
  - **(ii)** Activation of an oncogene
  - **(iii)** Loss of genes that normally suppress tumourigenesis
  - **(iv)** Potent mutation in the κ-*ras* proto-oncogene
  - **(v)** Changes in DNA methylation resulting in gene activation
  - **(vi)** Loss of DNA at the site of tumour suppressor gene
- Cancer frequently develops in sessile polyps.
- Villous adenomas (usually sessile) are three times as often to turn to malignant changes as tubular adenomas.
- The size of the polyp is an important determinant of malignant changes (10% in polyps greater than about 2.5 cm).
- Colonoscopy and follow-up is needed (every 2–3 years). Fig. 1.3.1 shows pathological and molecular colonic adenoma–carcinoma sequence of changes.
- Laboratory investigations and diagnostic procedures:
  - Laboratory tests: These include (i) complete blood cell count, blood film and iron studies (a picture of iron-deficiency anaemia); (ii) liver function tests (raised alkaline phosphatase levels may indicate metastasis); and (iii) carcinoembryonic antigen (CEA): the levels return to normal range after surgical resection of the tumour. They are useful in follow-up after surgery. Persistent and high levels necessitate further assessment of the patient.

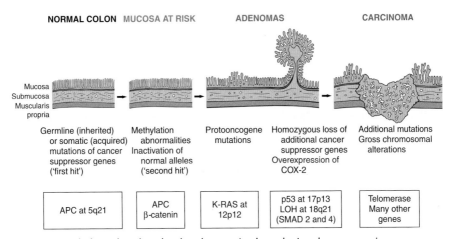

Figure 1.3.1 Pathological and molecular changes in the colonic adenoma–carcinoma sequence. *(Source: Kumar V, Abbas AK, Fausto N, Mitchell R. Robbins Basic Pathology, 8th Edition. London, UK: Elsevier; 2007.)*

  – Radiological studies: These include (i) barium enema or CT colonography; (ii) chest, abdomen and pelvic CT scan (for staging); and (iii) pelvic magnetic resonance imaging (MRI) and endorectal ultrasonography.
  – Procedure: This includes colonoscopy (visualises the whole colon and enables the examiner to take tissues for histological examination).

5. Management goals:
  • Staging
  • Deciding on management treatment to reduce tumour mass (medical, surgical, adjuvant chemotherapy or adjuvant radiotherapy; this depends on the stage)
  • Follow-up to detect recurrence early (CEA is commonly used)

BACK TO BASIC SCIENCES

Q1. What are the risk factors for the development of colorectal cancer?
• Intake of red and processed meat
• Obesity
• Alcohol and smoking
• History of adenomatous polyps
• Past history of colorectal cancer
• Inflammatory bowel disease
• FAP
• Hereditary nonpolyposis colorectal cancer (Lynch syndrome)
  The inherited forms (FAP and Lynch syndrome) are responsible for 5% of cases of colorectal cancer. Usually they develop cancer before the age of 40.

Q2. Are there any means to protect against colorectal cancer?
• Reduction of red meat and processed meat in diet
• Increasing dietary fibre
• Ceasing smoking
• Exercise and increased physical activities
• Aspirin

Q3. Briefly discuss the role of genetics in the development of colorectal cancer.
Several mechanisms may be responsible:
• Chromosomal instability: This includes changes in the chromosomal copy number and structure, e.g. loss of the tumour suppressor genes APC and p53.
• DNA repair defects: This defect usually occurs due to inactivation of genes responsible for repairs of DNA (mismatch repair genes). This may occur in Lynch syndrome and is responsible for the development of colorectal cancer in these patients.
• Aberrant DNA methylation: Methylation of aberrant DNA is a way to cause gene inactivation. This aberrant DNA-associated methylation can induce epigenetic silencing of gene expression.

- Activation of the Wnt signalling pathway is considered an initiating event in the development of colorectal cancer.
- Inactivation of the p53 pathway by mutation of the p53 gene is the second step in colorectal cancer development.
- Inactivation of the TGF-beta signalling is the third step in the progression to colorectal cancer.
- Other mechanisms include activation of the oncogene pathways (pathways promoting cancer, e.g. oncogenic mutation of *RAS* and *BRAF*).

Q4. Briefly discuss the clinical presentation of colorectal cancer.

1. Carcinoma of the left side of the colon
   - Progressive intestinal obstruction
   - Increased lower abdominal pain
   - Abdominal distension
   - Changes in bowel habits (alternate diarrhoea and constipation)
   - Rectal bleeding
2. Carcinoma of the sigmoid region
   - Progressive intestinal obstruction
   - Tenesmus and passage of mucus and blood
   - Bladder symptoms (colovesical fistula)
3. Carcinoma of the transverse colon
   - A mass in the upper abdomen
   - May be mistaken as cancer stomach
   - Anaemia
4. Carcinoma of the caecum and ascending colon
   - Anaemia
   - Tiredness and fatigue
   - A mass in the right iliac fossa
   - Intermittent obstruction
5. Carcinoma of the rectum
   - Rectal bleeding
   - Tenesmus
6. Metastatic disease
   - Jaundice
   - Ascites
   - Hepatomegaly
   - Tiredness and pain
   - Metastasis to the lungs, skin, bones and brain, which may produce symptoms

Q5. Discuss the distribution of colorectal cancer by site.

- Descending colon including splenic flexure: 28%–30%
- Sigmoid colon: 20%

- Rectum: 38%–40%
- Transverse colon: 5%
- Caecum and ascending colon and hepatic flexure: 15%–17%

However, in Lynch syndrome, the proportion of distribution of cancer is reversed with caecal cancer being the most common.

Q6. Discuss the differential diagnosis of colorectal cancer.

- Alteration of bowel habits: Irritable bowel syndrome, coeliac disease, inflammatory bowel disease and infections
- Iron-deficiency anaemia: Coeliac disease, gastric ulcers, poor diet and other sources of bleeding
- Rectal bleeding: Haemorrhoids, anal fissure, inflammatory bowel disease, infection and diverticulitis
- Abdominal distension: Irritable bowel syndrome, coeliac disease and malabsorption

Q7. How do we screen for early detection of colorectal cancer?

i. Faecal occult blood test

ii. Colonoscopy

Early detection of colorectal cancer and polyp cancers are managed by polypectomy alone.

Q8. What are the investigations used in the diagnosis of colorectal cancer?

The following investigations are indicated:

i. Full blood count, blood film and iron studies – anaemia.

ii. Liver function tests.

iii. Sigmoidoscopy: Helps in examination of the rectum and distal sigmoid.

iv. Colonoscopy: This is the gold-standard investigation, which helps in detecting cancers and polyps, and enables therapeutic removal of polyps and taking biopsies.

v. CT scan: A noninvasive means of investigation, which is useful in elderly people and helps in staging the disease.

vi. CT colonography: A multislice volume acquisition CT, which is useful in detecting colorectal cancers and polyps with sensitivity similar to that of colonoscopy.

vii. Biopsy and histological examination of masses and polyps removed.

Q9. What are the principles of the management of colorectal cancer?

i. Determine the local and distal tumour spread.

ii. Assess whether synchronous tumours are present before surgical intervention.

iii. The aim of surgery is to remove the primary tumour with a margin of healthy tissue as well as lymph nodes.

iv. Perform histological examination of removed tumour mass and use the information obtained in deciding the need for adjuvant chemotherapy.

v. Follow up the patient after surgery and perform chemotherapy by regular measurement of CEA.

REVIEW QUESTIONS

Q1. Which *one* of the following areas of the colon has the highest percentage of developing cancer?
A. Caecum
B. Ascending colon
C. Transverse colon
D. Rectum
E. Sigmoid colon

Q2. Which *one* of the following is the commonest metastatic site of colorectal cancer?
A. Brain
B. Liver
C. Skin
D. Bones
E. Peritoneum

Q3. An obese man with a colon cancer involving the caecum is expected to present with
A. Abdominal pain.
B. Abdominal distension.
C. Alteration of bowel habits.
D. Anaemia.
E. Bleeding per rectum.

Q4. Which *one* of the following is the gold standard for investigating a patient with colorectal cancer?
A. Faecal occult blood test
B. CEA
C. Sigmoidoscopy
D. Barium studies
E. Colonoscopy

Q5. Which *one* of the following is *not* a risk factor for the development of colorectal cancer?
A. Cholecystectomy
B. Dietary animal fat
C. Inflammatory bowel disease
D. Wilson disease
E. Lynch disease

ANSWERS

A1. **D.** The rectum is the commonest site of developing colorectal cancer (38%–40%).

A2. **B.** The liver is the most common metastatic site in these patients. The metastasis reaches the liver via the portal venous circulation.

A3. **D.** The caecum allows the tumour mass to grow without causing obstruction and in obese patients it is difficult to detect the tumour mass by palpation. The ulceration and bleeding of tumour mass results in blood loss and the development of iron-deficiency anaemia. Because the caecum is far from the anus, the lost blood changes as it travels in the colon and the altered blood may be detected only by faecal occult blood test. No changes of bowel habits occur in these patients.

A4. **E.** Colonoscopy is the gold standard for investigating colorectal cancer.

A5. **D.** Wilson disease is a risk factor for the development of liver cancer, and not colorectal cancer.

TAKE-HOME MESSAGE

- The clinical presentation depends on the location of the tumour.
- Right-sided colon cancers cause iron-deficiency anaemia and tiredness. Left-sided colon cancers cause obstructive symptoms, abdominal pain, changes in bowel habits and stool streaked with blood. Rectal cancers cause rectal tenesmus, urgency and recurrent haematochezia.
- Weight loss is not common. It may indicate metastasis.
- Clinical examination usually does not show abnormalities apart from pallor in the presence of anaemia. An abdominal mass may be felt in thin people. Hepatomegaly may indicate the presence of liver metastasis.
- The differential diagnosis may include diverticular disease, diverticulitis, iron-deficiency anaemia due to other causes, infectious colitis, inflammatory bowel disease, other causes of bleeding per rectum and adenomatous polyps.
- Colonoscopy is important for the diagnosis.
- Risk factors include intake of red and processed meat, obesity, alcohol and smoking, history of adenomatous polyps, past history of colorectal cancer, inflammatory bowel disease, FAP and hereditary nonpolyposis colorectal cancer (Lynch syndrome).
- The genetic mechanisms contributing to the development of colorectal cancer may include chromosomal instability, DNA repair defects, aberrant DNA methylation, activation of the Wnt signalling pathway, inactivation of the p53 pathway and other mechanisms.
- The goals of management are (i) staging; (ii) deciding on management treatment to reduce tumour mass (medical, surgical, adjuvant chemotherapy or adjuvant radiotherapy; this depends on the stage); and (iii) follow-up to detect recurrence early (CEA is commonly used).

FURTHER READINGS

Brenner H, Kloor M, Pox CP. Colorectal cancer. *Lancet*. 2014;383(9927):1490-1502. Review.

Gaskie S. Colorectal cancer screening. *Am Fam Physician*. 2005;71(5):959-960. Review.

Inadomi JM. Screening for colorectal neoplasia. *N Engl J Med*. 2017;376(2):149-156.

Lynch HT, de la Chapelle A. Hereditary colorectal cancer. *N Engl J Med*. 2003;348(10):919-32. Review.

Markowitz SD, Bertagnolli MM. Molecular origins of cancer: molecular basis of colorectal cancer. *N Engl J Med*. 2009;361(25):2449-2460.

CASE 1.4

'As Dark as Coffee Grounds . . . '

Aaron William, a 58-year-old unemployed man, is brought by an ambulance to a local hospital because of vomiting about half a litre of blood. This is the first time for him to vomit blood and he describes its colour as dark as coffee grounds. Mr William has a long history of alcoholism and he gives an 8-month history of progressive increases of his abdominal girth. On examination, he looks cachectic, his resting pulse is 110/min, his blood pressure is 110/70 mm Hg and his sclera is icteric. There are several spider naevi over his face, shoulders and arms and he has palmar erythema of both hands. He has gynaecomastia and prominent abdominal veins. Abdominal examination reveals a significant protuberant abdomen, shifting dullness and enlarged spleen (about 6 cm below the left costal margin). The lower liver margin is difficult to detect, and he has testicular atrophy. He has pitting oedema of the ankles. Laboratory investigations show low haemoglobin, leukopenia and thrombocytopenia. He also has low serum albumen, a serum bilirubin of 100 μmol/L, elevated alkaline phosphatase and γ-glutamyl transferase, and elevated prothrombin time. Ultrasound of the abdomen shows a shrunken liver, splenomegaly and significant free fluid in the peritoneal cavity (ascites).

CASE DISCUSSION

Q1. On the basis of Mr William's presentation, what is your diagnosis?

Q2. What is your differential diagnosis?

Q3. What are the key clinical features of this disease? What are the scientific bases for these features?

Q4. What is the pathophysiology underlying these changes?

Q5. What are your management goals and management options?

ANSWERS

1. The findings of chronic alcoholism, vomiting blood, jaundice, spider naevi, palmar erythema, gynaecomastia, prominent abdominal veins, testicular atrophy, increased abdominal girth (due to ascites), splenomegaly, shrunken liver and peripheral oedema are consistent with the diagnosis of liver cirrhosis, portal hypertension and impairment of the liver functions. The laboratory investigation results of anaemia, leukopenia and thrombocytopenia are consistent with hypersplenism; the increased

serum alkaline phosphatase and serum bilirubin are consistent with cholestatic changes in the liver due to cirrhosis. The raised γ-glutamyl transferase is induced by alcohol and reflects cholestasis. The coagulopathy is due to impaired liver functions.

2. The differential diagnosis:
   * Chronic viral hepatitis
   * Chronic alcoholism
   * Haemochromatosis
   * Wilson disease
   * α_1-Antitrypsin deficiency
   * Primary biliary cirrhosis
   * Secondary biliary cirrhosis
   * Nonalcoholic fatty liver disease
   * Heart failure
   * Constrictive pericarditis

3. Clinical features
   Symptoms:
   * Asymptomatic
   * Fatigue
   * Anorexia
   * Weight loss
   * Muscle wasting
   * Jaundice
   * Abdominal distension (increased abdominal girth)
   * Increased pruritus and itching marks
   * Bulging in flanks
   * Abdominal pain
   * Vomiting blood
   * History suggestive of the cause (e.g. tattooing, blood transfusion, intravenous drug use, alcohol consumption and travelling to countries where viral hepatitis is endemic)
   * Severe symptoms and end-stage liver disease

   Signs:
   * Hands: Palmar erythema, pallor, white nails and finger clubbing; jaundice all over the skin in severe cases
   * Eyes: Jaundice (yellowish discolouration of the sclerae) and pallor of the conjunctivae
   * Spider naevi (on arms, shoulders, above the nipple lines, neck and face)
   * Gynaecomastia in males
   * Loss of axillary and pubic hair in males and females
   * Abdominal distension and caput medusae
   * Splenomegaly
   * Decreased liver span and increased nodularity of the liver
   * Shifting dullness and evidence of the presence of ascites

- Oedema of lower limbs
- Testicular atrophy in males
- Hepatorenal syndrome – oliguria/anuria
- Pleural effusions
- Hepatopulmonary syndrome
- Signs of hepatic cell failure
- Signs suggestive of encephalopathy

4. Laboratory investigations:
   - Full blood count – low haemoglobin and thrombocytopenia (hypersplenism)
   - Liver function tests – low serum albumin and raised international normalised ratio (INR)
   - Liver transaminases and serum alkaline phosphatase – usually mildly elevated
   - Blood electrolytes – decreased serum sodium
   - Blood urea – may be within normal limits (because of liver failure and loss of urea cycle)
   - Serum creatinine – elevated (when serum creatinine >130 mmol/L, it indicates poor prognosis)
   - Serum iron studies including serum iron, total iron-binding capacity, ferritin and serum transferrin
   - Serum folate and B12 level (folate deficiency may be present; B12 is usually within normal limits)
   - Viral markers to exclude viral hepatitis as the cause
   - Serum immunoglobulins
   - Serum autoantibodies
   - Serum α_1-antitrypsin
   - Serum copper and ceruloplasmin to exclude Wilson disease
   - Genetic markers
   - α-Fetoprotein, to early detect hepatocellular carcinoma

   Radiological investigations:
   - Ultrasound examination – size and shape of the liver, fatty infiltration, fibrosis, echogenicity and nodularity
   - FibroScan and transient elastography – to assess liver fibrosis
   - CT scan of the upper abdomen – hepatosplenomegaly, dilated collaterals and enhanced scans, which can show defects of hepatocellular carcinoma
   - Endoscopy – upper gastro-oesophageal endoscopy to detect oesophageal varices, and treatment (colonoscopy may be indicated)
   - MRI to differentiate benign from malignant masses
   - MRI angiography for vascular anatomy/changes

   Liver biopsy:
   - This is the 'gold standard' that helps in the diagnosis of severity and the staging of chronic liver hepatitis

- Histological assessment, and chemical assessment of iron (to exclude or confirm haemochromatosis) and copper (Wilson disease)
- Digital analysis of picrosirius red staining for collagen content in the specimens

5. Pathological features:

The causes of cirrhosis:

- Alcohol
- Chronic viral hepatitis (B or C)
- Nonalcoholic fatty liver disease
- Primary biliary cirrhosis
- Primary sclerosing cholangitis
- Autoimmune liver disease
- Haemochromatosis
- Wilson disease
- α_1-Antitrypsin deficiency

It is important to note here that the most common three causes are (i) chronic viral hepatitis B or C, (ii) nonalcoholic fatty liver disease and (iii) chronic alcohol consumption.

The major complications of cirrhosis:

- Ascites
- Hepatic cell failure
- Hepatic encephalopathy
- Hepatocellular carcinoma
- Hepatorenal syndrome
- Hepatopulmonary syndrome
- Hepatic hydrothorax
- Portal vein thrombosis (may be associated with hepatocellular carcinoma)
- Spontaneous bacterial peritonitis (fever, abdominal pain, abdominal tenderness, altered mental status, sepsis)
- Variceal haemorrhage (haematemesis, melaena)
- Portal hypertension
- Portal hypertensive gastropathy (substantial bleeding, diffuse mucosal oozing, no other lesions can be found to explain anaemia)

The mechanisms involved in the pathogenesis of ascites in cirrhosis are as follows:

- Portal hypertension $\rightarrow$ portosystemic shunt $\rightarrow$ $\uparrow$ nitric oxide $\rightarrow$ splanchnic vasodilation
- Portosystemic shunt $\rightarrow$ decrease in systemic arterial pressure $\rightarrow$ activation of the renin–angiotensin system $\rightarrow$ elevation of aldosterone $\rightarrow$ salt and water retention by the kidneys
- Shift of blood to splanchnic circulation $\rightarrow$ underfilling of systemic circulation $\rightarrow$ sympathetic activation

- Underfilling of circulation → elevated atrial natriuretic hormone secretion → increased glomerular filtration → ↑ loss of water and sodium → inhibition of renin–angiotensin system
- Cirrhosis → decreased albumin synthesis → decreased oncotic pressure → transduction of fluid → ascites
- Increased blood in splanchnic circulation → vasodilation of splanchnic circulation + increased capillary permeability of the intestinal capillaries → ascites

The pathophysiological changes involved in the development of varices in patients with liver cirrhosis are as follows:

- Portal hypertension
- Increased resistance to portal blood flow and increased portal venous blood flow
- Increased portal-pressure gradient (the differences between portal vein pressure and hepatic vein pressure)
- Distortion of vascular architecture by fibrosis
- Endothelial dysfunction and decreased nitric oxide bioavailability
- Formation of portosystemic collaterals (gastro-oesophageal varices form the important collateral development as a result of the changes)

6. Management goals and options:
   - Prevention: Hepatitis A and B vaccination
   - Treatment of the cause of cirrhosis
   - Management of complications
   - Regular measurement of α-fetoprotein and ordering ultrasound of the liver (every 6 months) for early detection of hepatocellular carcinoma
   - Salt restriction
   - Stopping alcohol
   - Avoiding taking aspirin or nonsteroidal anti-inflammatory drugs (NSAIDs) because of the risks of bleeding
   - Patient education

   Fig. 1.4.1 summarises the management of cirrhosis.

BACK TO BASIC SCIENCES

Q1. What are the risk factors for alcoholic liver disease?

- Gender: Women are at a higher susceptibility to alcoholic liver disease.
- Quantity and duration: 40–80 g/day of ethanol produces fatty liver and 160 g/day for 10–20 years produces cirrhosis.
- Hepatitis C: Together with higher intake of ethanol, it increases the severity of liver pathology at a younger age and decreases survival. Alcohol also decreases the efficacy of interferon-based antiviral therapy.
- Genetics: Gene polymorphism of alcohol dehydrogenase may lead to alcoholic liver disease.

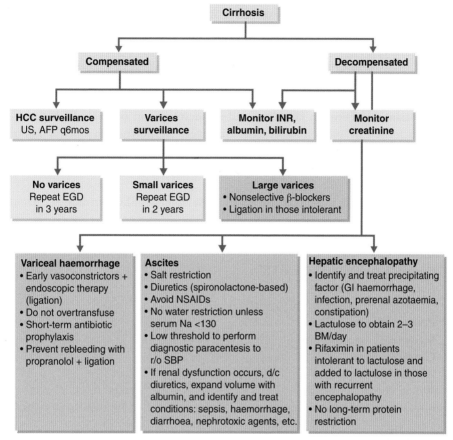

Figure 1.4.1 Management of cirrhosis. AFP, α-fetoprotein; BM, bowel movement; d/c, discontinue; EGD, oesophagogastroduodenoscopy; GI, gastrointestinal; HCC, hepatocellular carcinoma; INR, international normalised ratio; Na, sodium; NSAIDs, nonsteroidal anti-inflammatory drugs; r/o, rule out; SBP, spontaneous bacterial peritonitis; US, ultrasound. *(Source: Goldman L, Schafer Al. Goldman-Cecil Medicine. 25th ed. Elsevier; 2016.)*

- Obesity/fatty liver: It may play a role by affecting fatty acid synthesis and transport.
- Beverage type: It is not clear whether beverage type is a risk factor.

Q2. What is the threshold for developing alcoholic liver disease?
- Men: Intake of >60–80 g/day of alcohol for 10 years (about 5–7 beers/day)
- Women: Intake of 20–40 g/day of alcohol for 10 years (about 1.5–3 beers/day)

Q3. Describe the pathogenesis of alcoholic liver disease.
a. Three pathological processes are involved: (i) autoimmune response (as a result of adduct formation), (ii) fibrotic response as a result of stellate cell activation and collagen production and (iii) inflammatory response (involving Kupffer cells and the release of TNF-α, IL-1, IL-6, TGF-β).

b. Alcohol has a direct hepatotoxic effect and also causes the production of toxic protein–aldehyde adducts.

c. Alcohol increases lipogenesis and inhibits fatty acid oxidation. These changes trigger fatty liver changes and stellate cell activation.

d. Endotoxins, oxidative stress, immunological activity and proinflammatory cytokines contribute to liver injury.

e. The transition between fatty liver and the development of alcoholic hepatitis is characterised by ballooning degeneration, necrosis, polymorphonuclear infiltration and fibrosis in the periventricular and perisinusoidal space of Disse. Mallory bodies may be present but their presence is neither specific nor necessary for the diagnosis.

f. Alcoholic hepatitis is the precursor of the development of liver cirrhosis.

Q4. What are the causes of cirrhosis?

- Alcoholism
- Chronic viral hepatitis (B and C)
- Autoimmune hepatitis
- Nonalcoholic steatohepatitis
- Primary biliary cirrhosis
- Secondary biliary cirrhosis
- Cardiac cirrhosis
- Haemochromatosis
- Wilson disease
- α_1-Antitrypsin deficiency

Q5. What is the definition of cirrhosis?

- Cirrhosis is defined as histopathological changes associated with a variety of clinical manifestations and complications. The histopathological changes comprise fibrosis and architectural distortion, with the formation of regeneration nodules, resulting in a decrease in hepatocellular mass and altered blood supply and liver functions. The pathological changes may start with fatty liver infiltration, transition to hepatitis and activation of hepatic stellate cells to produce collagen and liver fibrosis.
- The histopathological changes in the liver can be staged (stage 3, characterised by nodularity and bridging fibrosis; and stage 4, cirrhosis).
- These changes will interfere with liver functions. Patients with decompensated liver will need liver transplantation.
- Cirrhosis may be (i) micronodular cirrhosis: regenerating nodules <1 cm (this is typical of alcoholic liver disease); and (ii) macronodular cirrhosis: larger regenerating nodules up to several centimetres in diameter (this is typical of cirrhosis caused by viral hepatitis and postnecrotic [posthepatic] cirrhosis).

Q6. What is portal hypertension?

- Portal hypertension is a complication of decompensated liver and comprises (i) development of ascites; (ii) bleeding from oesophageal varices; (iii) splenomegaly; (iv) loss of hepatic function (decompensation) causing jaundice, coagulopathy, hypo-albuminaemia and interference with oestrogen metabolism; and (v) contribution to the development of portosystemic encephalopathy.

Q7. What is Zieve syndrome?

It is a type of haemolytic anaemia with spur cells and acanthocytosis commonly observed in patients with severe alcoholic hepatitis.

Q8. What are the causes of hyperbilirubinaemia?

  (i) Prehepatic causes: Haemolytic anaemia (autoimmune, enzyme deficiency, haemo-globinopathy), blood transfusions and haematoma
 (ii) Hepatic causes: Hereditary disorders such as Gilbert syndrome and Crigler–Najjar syndrome types I and II, drug-induced liver injury, hepatocellular diseases, viral hepatitis, chronic hepatitis, cirrhosis, alcohol-induced liver injury, alcoholic hepa-titis, cholestasis and recurrent jaundice of pregnancy
(iii) Posthepatic causes: Drugs interfering with bilirubin efflux, extrahepatic cholestasis, cholecystitis, cancer of the head of the pancreas, bile duct cancer and biliary stones

Q9. Discuss the mechanisms underlying the development of ascites in patients with cirrhosis.

- The main underlying mechanisms are related to portal hypertension and renal salt and water retention.
- Portal hypertension and increased resistance to blood flow is caused by the following mechanisms: (i) development of hepatic fibrosis and disruption of the normal hepatic architecture causing resistance to normal blood flow in the liver; (ii) activation of hepat-ic stellate cells resulting in fibrogenesis causing smooth muscle contraction and fibrosis; and (iii) decreased endothelial nitric oxide synthetase (eNOS) production, resulting in decreased nitric oxide production and increased intrahepatic vasoconstriction.
- On the other hand, the circulating levels of nitric oxide are increased (contrary to the low intrahepatic levels), together with increased levels of vascular endothelial growth factor and tumour necrosis factor. These three factors cause splanchnic arte-rial vasodilation and pooling of blood and decreased renal perfusion.
- The kidneys respond by (i) stimulation of the renin–angiotensin system; (ii) increased antidiuretic hormone release; and (iii) decreased natriuretic hormone release.
- Hypoalbuminaemia: The decreased synthesis of albumin due to liver cell failure results in decreased intravascular oncotic pressure and the leakage of albumin through the lymph into the peritoneal cavity. The increased levels of albumen in the peritoneal cavity favour ascites formation.

- Plasma vasopressin and epinephrine levels are elevated as a result of volume depletion, causing reinforcement of the kidneys and vascular mechanisms.

Q10. Discuss portosystemic encephalopathy in patients with cirrhosis and needed management.

Generally this includes neuropsychiatric changes associated with portosystemic shunting with hepatocellular failure. There are three types of hepatic encephalopathy:

Type A: Hepatic encephalopathy associated with acute liver failure.

Type B: Hepatic encephalopathy associated with portosystemic bypass with no hepatic failure.

Type C: Hepatic encephalopathy associated with cirrhosis and portosystemic shunting.

So type C is the type related to our question.

The pathogenesis of hepatic encephalopathy in cirrhosis and portosystemic shunting is as follows:

- Hyperammonaemia (the failing liver cannot metabolise ammonia)
- Portal hypertension → inflow of toxins produced in the gut (phenols, thiols = mercaptans, short-chain fatty acids, fatty acids) to systemic circulation and end in the brain
- Cytokines and bacterial endotoxins
- Enterally produced γ-aminobutyric acid (GABA) and endogenous benzodiazepines resulting in GABAergic signalling
- Production of false transmitters (octopamine and diazepam)
- Cerebral ischaemia and loss of cerebral autoregulatory blood flow
- Changes in cerebral vascular resistance

Management:

- Eliminate ammoniagenic luminal bacteria – give nonabsorbable antibiotics such as neomycin.
- Restrict protein intake.
- Regulate luminal acidification – give lactulose.
- Treat constipation.
- There is no need for treatment with mannitol or hyperventilation unless there is evidence of cerebral oedema.
- Perform trials of branched-chain amino acids such as isoleucine, leucine and valine to reduce the production of false transmitters.

Q11. What is hepatorenal syndrome?

- This refers to acute renal failure with advanced chronic liver disease (cirrhosis and ascites).
- There is evidence of renal failure and decreased urine output but no proteinuria.
- No histopathological changes in the kidneys occur. The whole change is physiological affecting the renal function. The condition is reversible and renal functions are resumed after liver transplantation.

- Renal function impairment is related to intense systemic arteriolar vasodilation, reduced systemic vascular resistance and renal circulatory vasoconstriction and reduced renal blood flow.
- Other factors involved in the pathogenesis are renin–angiotensin–aldosterone system, sympathetic nervous system and renal prostaglandins.
- The renal failure in these patients is irreversible unless liver transplantation is performed.

REVIEW QUESTIONS

Q1. Which *one* of the following is *not* part of the mechanisms underlying the formation of ascites in cirrhosis?
A. Portal hypertension
B. Hypoalbuminaemia
C. Stimulation of renin–angiotensin
D. Elevated antidiuretic hormone release
E. Elevated intrahepatic nitric oxide

Q2. Which *one* of the following is associated with direct (conjugated) hyperbilirubinaemia?
A. Haemolytic anaemia
B. Drugs interfering with hepatic bilirubin uptake
C. Intrahepatic cholestasis
D. Gilbert syndrome

Q3. Which *one* of the following is *not* a mechanism underlying liver injury caused by chronic ethanol intake?
A. Formation of adducts
B. Decreased TNF-α and IL-1
C. Stimulation of stellate cells
D. Lipid peroxidation
E. Autoimmune response

Q4. Which *one* of the following is *not* a cause of liver cirrhosis?
A. Viral hepatitis C
B. Alcoholism
C. Primary biliary cirrhosis
D. α_1-Antitrypsin deficiency
E. Epstein–Barr virus

Q5. Which *one* of the following is the function of the hepatic stellate cells?
A. Metabolism of vitamin A
B. Production of collagen
C. Synthesis of albumin

D. Immunological response
E. Conjugation of bilirubin

ANSWERS

A1. **E.** The intrahepatic nitric oxide is reduced in liver cirrhosis and this contributes to intrahepatic vascular vasoconstriction. This is because of decreased eNOS production. On the other hand, the extrahepatic nitric oxide is elevated causing splanchnic arterial vasodilation and pooling of blood.

A2. **C.** Intrahepatic cholestasis causes direct (conjugated) hyperbilirubinaemia.

A3. **B.** Chronic ethanol intake causes Kupffer cell stimulation and the release of TNF-α, IL-1, IL-6 and TGF-β.

A4. **E.** Epstein–Barr virus infection may cause hepatitis. However, usually patients recover without long-term complications such as cirrhosis. There are some reports that Epstein–Barr virus infection may cause liver cancer.

A5. **B.** Stimulation of hepatic stellate cells results in collagen production and liver fibrosis. This is part of the mechanisms involved in liver cirrhosis.

TAKE-HOME MESSAGE

- Patients with cirrhosis may be asymptomatic. However, the following symptoms may be present: fatigue, anorexia, weight loss, muscle wasting, jaundice, abdominal distension, increased pruritus, itching marks, bulging in flanks, abdominal pain, vomiting blood, a history suggestive of the cause (e.g. tattooing, blood transfusion, intravenous drug use, alcohol consumption) or severe symptoms and end-stage liver disease.
- The clinical signs in cirrhosis are (i) hands: palmar erythema, pallor, white nails and finger clubbing (in severe cases, jaundice is all over the skin); (ii) eyes: jaundice (yellowish discolouration of the sclerae) and pallor of the conjunctivae; (iii) spider naevi (on the arms, shoulders, above the nipple lines, neck and face); (iv) gynaecomastia in males; (v) loss of axillary and pubic hair in males and females; (vi) abdominal distension and caput medusa; (vii) splenomegaly; (viii) decreased liver span and increased nodularity of the liver; (ix) shifting dullness and evidence of the presence of ascites; (x) oedema of the lower limbs; (xi) testicular atrophy in males; (xii) hepatorenal syndrome – oliguria/anuria; (xiii) pleural effusions; (xiv) hepatopulmonary syndrome; and (xv) signs of hepatic cell failure and signs suggestive of encephalopathy
- The causes of cirrhosis are alcohol, chronic viral hepatitis (B or C), nonalcoholic fatty liver disease, primary biliary cirrhosis, primary sclerosing cholangitis, autoimmune liver disease, haemochromatosis, Wilson disease, α_1-antitrypsin deficiency and cryptogenic cirrhosis.

- The most common three causes of cirrhosis are (i) chronic viral hepatitis B or C; (ii) nonalcoholic fatty liver disease; and (iii) chronic alcohol consumption.
- Portal hypertension is a complication of decompensated liver and comprises (i) development of ascites; (ii) bleeding from oesophageal varices; (iii) splenomegaly; (iv) loss of hepatic function (decompensation) causing jaundice, coagulopathy, hypoalbuminaemia and interference with oestrogen metabolism; and (v) contribution to the development of portosystemic encephalopathy.
- The pathophysiology underlying the development of portal hypertension in patients with cirrhosis includes (i) increased resistance to portal blood flow and increased portal venous blood flow; (ii) increased portal-pressure gradient (the differences between portal vein pressure and hepatic vein pressure); (iii) distortion of vascular architecture by fibrosis; (iv) endothelial dysfunction and decreased nitric oxide bioavailability; and (v) formation of portosystemic collaterals.
- The goals and options of management are (i) prevention: hepatitis A and B vaccination; (ii) treatment of the cause of cirrhosis; (iii) management of complications; (iv) regular measurement of α-fetoprotein and ultrasound of the liver (every 6 months) for early detection of hepatocellular carcinoma; (v) salt restriction; (vi) stopping alcohol; (vii) avoiding taking aspirin or NSAIDs because of the risks of bleeding; and (viii) patient education.

FURTHER READINGS

Carey EJ, Ali AH, Lindor KD. Primary biliary cirrhosis. *Lancet*. 2015;386(10003):1565-1575. Review.

Garcia-Tsao G, Bosch J. Management of varices and variceal hemorrhage in cirrhosis. *N Engl J Med*. 2010;362(9):823-832. Review.

Ge PS, Runyon BA. Treatment of patients with cirrhosis. *N Engl J Med*. 2016;375(8):767-777. Review.

Granito A, Bolondi L. Non-transplant therapies for patients with hepatocellular carcinoma and Child-Pugh-Turcotte class B cirrhosis. *Lancet Oncol*. 2017;18(2):e101-e112. Review.

Kohli A, Shaffer A, Sherman A, Kottilil S. Treatment of hepatitis C: a systematic review. *JAMA*. 2014; 312(6):631-640. Review.

Powell LW, Seckington RC, Deugnier Y. Haemochromatosis. *Lancet*. 2016;388(10045):706-716. Review.

Richter J, Bode JG, Blondin D, et al. Severe liver fibrosis caused by Schistosoma mansoni: management and treatment with a transjugular intrahepatic portosystemic shunt. *Lancet Infect Dis*. 2015;15(6):731-737. Review.

Rinella ME. Nonalcoholic fatty liver disease: a systematic review. *JAMA*. 2015;313(22):2263-2273. Review.

Rosen HR. Clinical practice. Chronic hepatitis C infection. *N Engl J Med*. 2011;364(25):2429-2438. Review.

Tripodi A, Mannucci PM. The coagulopathy of chronic liver disease. *N Engl J Med*. 2011;365(2):147-156. Review.

CASE 1.5

'There Is Blood in My Stool . . . '

Sue Erving, a 38-year-old manager, presents to her local general practitioner because she is suffering from abdominal pains all over her tummy and urgency to go to the toilet. She has had six to seven loose bowel motions a day for the last 5–7 days and has noticed that her stools contain blood. She feels incomplete emptying her bowels. She also has mild joint pains. She had similar episodes in the past. On examination, her pulse rate is 90/min, her blood pressure is 110/80 mm Hg and her body temperature is 37.8°C. Abdominal examination shows tenderness all over her abdomen but no rigidity. Per rectum examination shows blood on the examining gloved finger. The complete blood count reveals a haemoglobin level of 90 g/L (normal = 115–160 g/L) and an erythrocyte sedimentation rate (ESR) of 45 (normally <20). Further assessment, after hospital admission, including colonoscopy and biopsy, reveals that her colonic mucosa, particularly the rectum and the descending colon, is inflamed.

CASE DISCUSSION

Q1. On the basis of Sue's presentation, what is your diagnosis?

Q2. What is your differential diagnosis?

Q3. What are the key clinical features of this disease? What are the scientific bases for these features?

Q4. What is the pathophysiology underlying these changes?

Q5. What are your management goals and management options?

ANSWERS

1. The findings of bloody diarrhoea, abdominal pain all over, urgency, tenesmus, fever, arthralgia, abdominal tenderness, past history of similar episodes together with anaemia, raised ESR and colonoscopic findings of inflammation limited to the colonic mucosa are suggestive of ulcerative colitis. Further assessment is needed to confirm the diagnosis.
2. The differential diagnosis:
   - Infectious colitis (*Salmonella, Shigella, Campylobacter*, enteroinvasive *Escherichia coli*)
   - Crohn disease
   - Colon cancer
   - Amebiasis

- Antibiotic-associated diarrhoea (*Clostridium difficile* infection)
- Ischaemic colitis
- Radiation colitis
- Cytomegalovirus colitis (in immunocompromised patients)
- Infectious proctitis (gonorrhoea, chlamydia, herpes, syphilis)
- Microscopic colitis
- Viral or parasitic colitis (in immunocompromised patients)

The following are essential for the diagnosis of ulcerative colitis:

- Bloody diarrhoea, lower abdominal pain, tenesmus, urgency, anaemia, negative stool analysis (for *C. difficile* toxins, bacteria, ova and parasites) and negative stool cultures
- Sigmoidoscopy showing inflammation limited to colonic mucosa

3. Symptoms and signs:

- Diarrhoea, rectal bleeding, crampy abdominal pain, faecal urgency (due to colonic inflammation and changes in colonic motility), tenesmus, passage of mucus and evidence of malnutrition.
- When the disease extends beyond the rectum, the blood is usually mixed with stool.
- Diarrhoea is usually nocturnal and postprandial.
- Other symptoms in moderate or severe disease include fever, anorexia, nausea, vomiting and weight loss.
- The clinical course of ulcerative colitis is marked by exacerbations and remissions.
- The main signs are tenderness of the abdomen, tender anal canal and blood on rectal examination. Signs of peritonitis may be found if there are complications such as colonic perforation.
- Extracolonic signs may be present during disease activity (present in 40%–50% of patients) such as arthralgia, oral ulcers, erythema nodosum, pyoderma gangrenosum, episcleritis, uveitis, ankylosing spondylitis and sclerosing cholangitis. Fig. 1.5.1 summarises the complications of inflammatory bowel disease.
- Laboratory findings: During disease activity, acute-phase reactants are elevated: Elevated ESR, elevated platelet count, elevated C-reactive proteins (CRPs) and low haemoglobin are also noted.
- Faecal calprotectin and lactoferrin levels are sensitive and correlate with histological inflammation and predict relapse.
- Serum albumin levels drop rapidly in severe inflammation and severely ill patients.
- Leukocytosis may be present but it is not specific.
- Sigmoidoscopy is used to assess the severity and extent of the disease: (i) mild disease: erythema, decreased vascular pattern and mild friability; (ii) moderate disease: marked erythema, absent vascular patterns and moderate friability; and (iii) severe disease: bleeding and ulcerations. Colonoscopy should not be

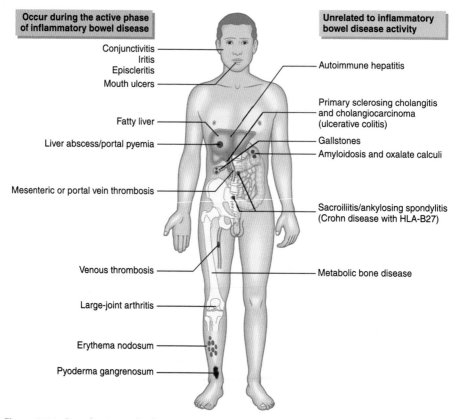

Figure 1.5.1 Complications of inflammatory bowel disease. *(Source: Ralston S, Penman I, Strachan M, Hobson R. Davidson's Principles & Practice of Medicine. 23rd ed. UK: Elsevier; 2018.)*

performed in patients with fulminant disease (risk of perforation) but be indicated after improvement.

- Abdominal radiology: Limited use. Barium enema may precipitate toxic megacolon (colonic dilatation >6 cm on radiographs together with toxic signs and risk of perforation).
- CT scan is not as useful as endoscopy.

4. Pathological features:
- The disease starts in the rectum and extends proximally to involve the colon.
- About 40%–50% of patients have the rectum and rectosigmoid involved, 30%–40% have the inflammation beyond the rectosigmoid and only 20% have the whole colon affected.
- The terminal ileum (2–3 cm) may be inflamed in 10%–20% of patients (backwash ileitis).
- In mild disease, the mucosa is erythematous and has a granular surface.
- In more severe disease, the mucosa is haemorrhagic, ulcerated and oedematous.

- In long-standing cases, the colon becomes featureless, shortened and narrowed.

5. The goals of management are as follows:
   - Induction of remission
   - Maintenance of remission (maintain symptom-free status)
   - Surgical management in patients with complications or patients who failed to respond to medical treatment

   A. Induction of remission: Managed according to the level of clinical activity and extent of the disease
   - 5-Aminosalicylates (orally, rectally)
   - Glucocorticoids (topical, orally)
   - Immunosuppressive agents (cyclosporine, azathioprine, 6-mercaptopurine)
   - Infliximab (a monoclonal antibody against tumour necrosis factor-alpha [TNF-α])

   B. Maintenance of remission
   - There is no place for glucocorticoids in the maintenance of remission because of the marked side effects associated with long-term use.
   - Maintenance of remission is usually achieved with the use of 5-aminosalicylates orally and/or rectally.
   - Azathioprine and 6-mercaptopurine can be used in the maintenance of remission if 5-aminosalicylates are ineffective.

   C. Indications for surgery in ulcerative colitis
   - Failure of medical therapy
   - Toxic megacolon
   - Perforation of colon
   - Uncontrolled bleeding
   - Side effects of medications
   - Development of strictures that cannot be resolved via endoscopy
   - Development of dysplasia or mass of cancer (colorectal cancer)

Surgical options:
- Traditional proctocolectomy with ileostomy
- Total proctocolectomy with ileal pouch–anal anastomosis
- Proctocolectomy with ileorectal anastomosis
- Proctocolectomy with the formation of a continent ileostomy or Koch's pouch

BACK TO BASIC SCIENCES

Q1. Summarise the main differences between ulcerative colitis and Crohn disease.

There are several differences between ulcerative colitis and Crohn's disease. Table 1.5.1 summarises these differences regarding pathology, clinical picture, endoscopic findings, and management.

Table 1.5.1 Differences between ulcerative colitis and Crohn's disease

Parameter	Ulcerative colitis	Crohn disease
1. Pathology	• Inflammation is restricted to mucosal layer • Continuous inflammation (no 'skip' areas) • Mucosa is infiltrated with lymphocytes and plasma cells • Goblet cells are characteristically absent • Distorted crypts, crypt abscess	• All layers are affected (transmural) • Inflammation is not continuous (skip areas) • Epithelioid granulomas are present
2. Clinical picture	• Rectal bleeding • Bloody diarrhoea • Fatigue • During active disease: Systemic symptoms such as fever, arthritis, erythema nodosum, conjunctivitis, episcleritis, scleritis, mouth ulcers (in 25%–30% of patients)	• Abdominal pain • Fatigue • Nausea, vomiting • Symptoms similar to those of acute appendicitis • Any part of the gastrointestinal tract can be affected (mouth to anus)
3. Endoscopic	• Rectum and descending colon are commonly affected (left > right colon) • Early signs: Loss of vascular patterns with hyperaemia, and mucosal oedema • Mild cases: Mucosa is granular and there is mucopus and contact bleeding • Advanced (severe) cases: Deep ulceration and bleeding	• Ileum is commonly affected (right > left colon) • Rectum is typically spared • Segmental: Skip areas • Aphthoid or confluent deep serpiginous pleomorphic ulcers • Cobblestone pattern • Deep fissures, fistulas, strictures • Increased wall thickness

4. Management	Medical treatment
	  1. Induction of remission (5-aminosalicylates, corticosteroids, cyclosporine, infliximab)
	  2. Maintenance of remission (5-aminosalicylates, azathioprine, 6-mercaptopurine, methotrexate)
	Surgical treatment
	  1. Indications: Failure of medical therapy, toxic megacolon, perforation, uncontrolled bleeding, cancer
	  2. Options: Traditional proctocolectomy with ileostomy, total proctectomy with ileal pouch–anal anastomosis, proctocolectomy with ileorectal anastomosis, proctocolectomy with the formation of a continent ileostomy or Koch's pouch
		Aims
		  • Induction and maintenance of remission
		  • Heal the mucosa
		  • Optimise the quality of life for the patient
		  • Patient education
		Management depends on the site, extent, activity of the disease and presence of complications
		Drugs commonly used in management: Prednisolone, budesonide, azathioprine, 6-mercaptopurine, methotrexate, infliximab, adalimumab, certolizumab
		Surgical management and options

Q2. What are the roles of ESR and CRP in the diagnosis of ulcerative colitis?
The diagnosis of ulcerative colitis is based on the clinical picture, stool analysis and stool culture, and sigmoidoscopy findings. Abnormally raised ESR and CRP are relatively insensitive and should not be relied on to exclude the diagnosis.

Q3. What is the role of faecal levels of calprotectin and lactoferrin in detecting inflammatory bowel disease?
Elevated faecal calprotectin and lactoferrin levels are sensitive for detecting inflammatory bowel disease. Faecal calprotectin and lactoferrin levels are sensitive and correlate with histological inflammation and predict relapse. However, these tests do not replace the role of endoscopy.

Q4. Discuss the differential diagnosis of ulcerative colitis. What are the clinical features of each disease/condition you mention? How would you exclude each disease?
The differential diagnosis of ulcerative colitis includes infectious colitis, Crohn disease, ischaemic colitis, microscopic colitis and radiation colitis (Table 1.5.2).

Table 1.5.2 Differential diagnosis and clinical features Crohn disease, with evaluating actions of each disease/condition

Disease/condition	Clinical features	Evaluation/exclusion
1. Bacterial colitis	Loose bowel motions Abdominal pain, tenderness	Stool culture Stool testing for *E. coli* O157:H7
2. Amoebic colitis	Exposure or travel to endemic area Tenesmus, loose motions, mucus and blood in stool, nausea, abdominal tenderness	Stool microscopy Respond to antiamoebic medications
3. *Clostridium difficile* infection	History of antibiotic treatment	Stool examination for *C. difficile* toxins
4. Crohn disease	Shares similar presentation and should be always considered in the differential diagnosis	Endoscopy and histological examination of biopsies
5. Ischaemic colitis	Patients have risk factors for vascular disorders	Endoscopy and histological examination of biopsies
6. Microscopic colitis	Usually no blood in stools	Endoscopy and histological examination of biopsies
7. Viral or parasitic colitis	Patients are immunocompromised	Endoscopy and histological examination of biopsies
8. Radiation colitis	Patients are exposed to radiation therapy of the abdomen or pelvis	Endoscopy and histological examination of biopsies for grading the severity of the disease

Q5. What are the main complications of ulcerative colitis?

- Massive severe bleeding (occurs in less than 1% of patients)
- Toxic megacolon: Diameter >6 cm, affecting the transverse or right colon, may be triggered by electrolyte imbalance and use of narcotics (about 50% of patients recover, and it is managed by urgent colectomy)
- Perforation (as a result of toxic megacolon)
- Strictures
- Colon cancer (the risk increases after 8–10 years of diagnosis)

Q6. How would you rank the severity of active ulcerative colitis?

The severity of active ulcerative colitis could be mild, moderate or severe (Table 1.5.3).

Table 1.5.3 Differential diagnosis of ulcerative colitis

Severity	Number of bowel motions (per day)	Blood in stool	Fever	ESR (mm)	Systemic toxicity
Mild	<4	Small	None	<30	None
Moderate	4–6	Moderate	About 37.5°C		Absent
Severe	7–10	Severe	>37.5°C	>30	Present

ESR, erythrocyte sedimentation rate.

Q7. What is the scientific basis of using infliximab in the treatment of moderate to severe cases?

Infliximab is an anti-TNF-α antibody. The treatment is based on the pathogenesis of ulcerative colitis and the fact that one of the major proinflammatory cytokines involved in the pathogenesis is TNF-α. Experimental and human studies showed that blocking TNF-α moderates the course of the disease.

Q8. Summarise the medical treatment of ulcerative colitis.

The medical treatment of ulcerative colitis, including mechanism of action, dosage and adverse effects, is summarised in Table 1.5.4.

Table 1.5.4 Medical treatment of ulcerative colitis

Medication (route)	Mechanism of action	Dosage in active disease	Maintenance dosage	Adverse effects
5-aminosalicylic acid (oral)	• Unknown • Modulation of inflammatory mediators • Inhibition of tumour necrosis factor (TNF)	2–4.8 g/day in three divided doses	1.2–2.4 g/day	Interstitial nephritis

Table 1.5.4 Medical treatment of ulcerative colitis—cont'd

Medication (route)	Mechanism of action	Dosage in active disease	Maintenance dosage	Adverse effects
5-aminosalicylic acid (enema)		1–4 g/day	2–4 g daily, every third day	Rectal irritation Difficult to retain
Prednisone (oral)	• Anti-inflammatory and immunosuppressive effects • Suppression of cell-mediated immunity • Suppression of humoral immunity causing B-cells to express lower amounts of IL-2 and IL-2 receptors • Inhibit the gene coding for several cytokines and TNF-α	40–60 mg/day until clinical improvement, and then gradual taper by 5–10 mg/week	Not recommended	Adrenal suppression Osteoporosis Cushingoid changes Infection Peptic ulcer Depression Impaired wound healing
Hydrocortisone (enema)		100 mg	Not recommended	Rectal irritation Difficult to retain
Hydrocortisone (10% foam)		90 mg once or twice per day	Not recommended	Rectal irritation
Cyclosporine (IV)	• Immunosuppression • Inhibition of T-lymphocytes (mainly inhibition of T1-helper and T1-suppressor) • Inhibition of lympho-kine production	2–4 mg/kg/day	Not recommended	Infection Cardiovascular changes Nephrotoxicity
Azathioprine (oral)	• It has cytotoxic and immunosuppressive activities • Azathioprine is a prodrug, converted in the body to active 6-mercaptopurine • It inhibits purine synthesis → inhibits cell proliferation, particularly lymphocytes and leukocytes	Not recommended	1.5–2.5 mg/kg/day	Infection Bone marrow suppression Allergic reaction

Continued

Table 1.5.4 Medical treatment of ulcerative colitis—cont'd

Medication (route)	Mechanism of action	Dosage in active disease	Maintenance dosage	Adverse effects
Infliximab (IV)	• Not clearly understood • Blocking TNF-α via apoptosis of TNF-α-expressing inflammatory cells • Apoptosis of inflammatory cells including T-cells and monocytes	5–10 mg/kg on 0, 2 and 6 weeks	5–10 mg/kg every 4–8 weeks	Expensive Infection Lymphoma

REVIEW QUESTIONS

Q1. Which *one* of the following is the first line of treatment of ulcerative colitis?
A. 6-Mercaptopurine
B. Infliximab
C. Cyclosporine
D. 5-Aminosalicylates
E. Glucocorticoids

Q2. Which *one* of the following decreases the incidence of ulcerative colitis?
A. High fat in the diet
B. Appendectomy in early life
C. Smoking cessation
D. Being of North European descent

Q3. Which *one* of the following is *not* involved in the pathogenesis of ulcerative colitis?
A. A breakdown in gut immune system tolerance
B. Alteration in the composition of the gut microbiota
C. Abnormalities in humoral and cellular adaptive immunity
D. Autoimmunity
E. Atypical Th1 response as evident by increased production of interferon-gamma

Q4. Which *one* of the following is *not* a complication of ulcerative colitis?
A. Small intestinal fistulas
B. Autoimmune liver disease
C. Toxic megacolon
D. Colorectal cancer
E. Clotting abnormalities

Q5. Which *one* of the following medications is recommended as maintenance treatment of ulcerative colitis?
A. Prednisone orally
B. Hydrocortisone enema
C. Cyclosporine intravenously
D. Hydrocortisone foam
E. 5-Aminosalicylic acid orally

Q6. Which *one* of the following histological features is *not* found in ulcerative colitis?
A. Infiltration of colonic mucosa with lymphocytes
B. Infiltration of colonic mucosa with plasma cells
C. Epithelioid granulomas
D. Mucosal ulcerations
E. Crypt abscess

ANSWERS

A1. **D.** The first line of treatment of ulcerative colitis is 5-aminosalicylates. The treatment is designed with consideration for the level of clinical activity and extent of disease.

A2. **B.** Appendectomy (surgical removal of an inflamed appendix) in early life is reported to be associated with a decreased incidence of ulcerative colitis. Smoking cigarettes is associated with milder disease, fewer hospitalisations and reduced need for medications. The incidence of ulcerative colitis is lowest in Asia, although there is recent progressive rise in the incidence.

A3. **E.** In Crohn disease, there is atypical Th1 response as evident by increased secretion of interferon-gamma. However, in ulcerative colitis, there is atypical Th2 response as shown by the presence of nonclassical natural killer T-cells in the colon and increased IL-13 production.

A4. **A.** Small intestinal fistulas occur in Crohn disease. They are less likely to be seen in ulcerative colitis.

A5. **E.** Corticosteroids should not be used in maintenance treatment because of their side effects. Usually 5-aminosalicylic acid is preferred.

A6. **C.** Epithelioid granulomas are characteristically seen in Crohn disease and not in ulcerative colitis.

TAKE-HOME MESSAGE

- Inflammatory bowel disease comprises ulcerative colitis and Crohn disease. The incidence and prevalence of ulcerative colitis are higher compared to those of Crohn disease.

- Smoking is associated with milder ulcerative colitis, fewer hospitalisations and a reduced need for hospitalisation. Also appendectomy in early years reduces the incidence of ulcerative colitis.
- Several mechanisms are involved in the pathogenesis of ulcerative colitis including genetics (genetics are less important, environmental factors are more important in ulcerative colitis), breakdown in gut immune system tolerance, alteration in the composition of gut microbiota, abnormalities in humeral and cellular adaptive immunity, autoimmunity and atypical Th2 response (increased production of IL-13 and nonclassical natural killer T-cells).
- Ulcerative colitis starts in the rectum and extends proximally to involve the colon.
- On the other hand, Crohn disease may involve any part of the gastrointestinal tract from the mouth to the anus (commonly involves the ileocaecal region).
- Clinically patients with ulcerative colitis commonly present with bloody diarrhoea, lower abdominal pain, tenesmus, urgency and anaemia.
- Sigmoidoscopy shows that inflammation limited to colonic mucosa is essential for confirming the diagnosis. Abdominal radiographs and CT scans of the abdomen may be needed but not informative when compared with endoscopy and histological examinations.
- Ulcerative colitis is associated with several complications including toxic megacolon, perforation, uncontrolled rectal bleeding, development of strictures, development of dysplasia and colorectal cancer.
- Ulcerative colitis is associated with systemic, extracolonic complications including arthritis, erythema nodosum, pyoderma gangrenosum, mouth ulcers, autoimmune liver disease, fatty liver, sclerosing cholangitis, eye changes (anterior chamber – conjunctivitis, scleritis, episcleritis, uveitis, iritis), thrombosis, clotting abnormalities and thromboembolic events.
- 5-Aminosalicylic acids (orally and locally) are the first line of treatment. However, in severe cases, other medications are used including corticosteroids (orally and locally), cyclosporine and infliximab.
- Surgical management is limited to cases that failed to respond to medical treatment, or developed complications including colorectal cancer.

FURTHER READINGS

Abraham C, Cho JH. Inflammatory bowel disease. *N Engl J Med.* 2009;361(21):2066–2078. Review.

Danese S, Fiocchi C. Ulcerative colitis. *N Engl J Med.* 2011;365(18):1713–1725. Review.

Ma C, Panaccione R, Fedorak RN, et al. A systematic review for the development of a core outcome set for ulcerative colitis clinical trials. *Clin Gastroenterol Hepatol.* 2017 Aug 23. pii: S1542-3565(17)30991-6. Review.

Podolsky DK. Inflammatory bowel disease. *N Engl J Med.* 2002;347(6):417–429. Review.

van der Sloot KWJ, Amini M, Peters V, Dijkstra G, Alizadeh BZ. Inflammatory bowel diseases: review of known environmental protective and risk factors involved. *Inflamm Bowel Dis.* 2017;23(9):1499–1509.

CASE 1.6

'It Is Itching All Over . . . '

Lilly Arnold, a 23-year-old university student, presents to a local practitioner 1 week after arrival from a visit to India. She has a fever, nausea, vomiting and loose bowel motion, and has lost her appetite. She has abdominal pain and noticed that her urine is as dark as tea. She is itching all over her body. On examination, her pulse rate is 98/min, her blood pressure is 110/70 mm Hg and her body temperature is 37.8°C. She is jaundiced and her skin shows itching marks. On abdominal examination, tenderness of the upper right region of the abdomen and palpable and tender liver and spleen are found. Her serum alanine aminotransferase (ALT) is 5000 units/L (normal: 3–36 units/L) and her serum aspartate aminotransferase (AST) is 4100 units/L (normal: 0–35 units/L).

CASE DISCUSSION

Q1. On the basis of Lilly's presentation, what is your diagnosis?

Q2. What is your differential diagnosis?

Q3. What are the key clinical features of this disease? What are the scientific bases for these features?

Q4. What is the pathophysiology underlying these changes?

Q5. What are your management goals and management options?

ANSWERS

1. The findings of fever, nausea, vomiting, diarrhoea, abdominal pain, dark urine, itching, and palpable and tender liver and spleen after a visit to India are suggestive of acute viral hepatitis. The raised serum ALT and serum AST in the range of 4000–5000 units/L are consistent with hepatitis A. Blood tests to determine immunoglobulin M (IgM) anti-HAV antibodies are needed to confirm the diagnosis. This test becomes positive after 5–10 days.
2. The differential diagnosis of acute hepatitis:
   - Cytomegalovirus infection
   - Epstein–Barr virus infection
   - Hepatitis A, B, C, D and E (all RNA viruses, except hepatitis B, which is a DNA virus)
   - Herpes simplex
   - Varicella

- Drugs (e.g. acetaminophen, rifampin, isoniazid)
- Alcohol
- Leptospirosis
- Q fever
- Typhoid fever
- Autoimmune hepatitis

Table 1.6.1 summarises viruses responsible for acute viral hepatitis and those accountable for evolution to chronic liver disease.

The following are essential for the diagnosis of hepatitis A:

- Symptoms of infection: Fever, nausea, vomiting, loss of appetite, abdominal pain and dark urine, together with palpable and tender liver and spleen
- Loss of desire for cigarette smoking or alcohol
- Raised serum ALT and serum AST in the range of 400–5000 units/L or more
- Detection of serum IgM anti-HAV antibodies

3. Symptoms and signs:
   - The onset is abrupt after an incubation period of approximately 28 days (range 15–50 days).
   - The disease may be asymptomatic and unapparent in young children. Symptoms vary but are usually present in adults. The disease may be fulminant and fatal.
   - Main symptoms: These include fever, nausea, vomiting, loss of appetite, abdominal pain, diarrhoea, dark urine, itching (due to cholestasis) and loss of weight.
   - There is loss of desire for cigarette smoking and alcohol.
   - Jaundice (variable on the sclera or the skin) and itching marks may be observed. Abdominal examination reveals tenderness but no rigidity. The liver and spleen may be palpable and tender.
   - Laboratory findings: When jaundice is present, the serum bilirubin rises to 90–340 μmol/L. Serum ALT and serum AST usually start rising earlier before

Table 1.6.1 Viruses responsible for acute viral hepatitis and likelihood of chronic evolution

Virus	Evolution to chronic viral hepatitis
Hepatitis A virus	Never
Hepatitis B virus	>90% (perinatal acquisition) to <1% (adult infection)
Hepatitis C virus	50%–80%
Hepatitis D or delta virus	2% (coinfection) to 90% (superinfection)
Hepatitis E virus	Occasionally in immunosuppressed patients

Other viruses
    Human cytomegalovirus
    Epstein–Barr virus
    Herpes simplex virus
    Human herpesvirus 6
    Parvovirus B$_{19}$
	May establish chronic infection, not associated with chronic hepatitis

Source: Goldman L, Schafer AI. Goldman-Cecil Medicine. 25th ed. Elsevier; 2016.

the elevation of serum bilirubin. The level of the serum aminotransferase is in the range of 400–5000 units/L or higher.

- ALT levels are usually higher than AST levels.
- Neutropenia and lymphopenia are usually present early, and may be followed with lymphocytosis with atypical lymphocytes (2%–20%).
- A prolonged prothrombin time (PT) may indicate severe necrosis of liver cells and worse prognosis.
- Hypoglycaemia may be present (vomiting, inadequate carbohydrate intake and inadequate stored glycogen).
- Serum alkaline phosphatase level may be normal or mildly raised.
- Hypoalbuminaemia is uncommon.
- Mild rise in γ-globulin usually occurs during the acute phase. Serum IgM is usually raised during the acute phase of hepatitis. Serum IgG is raised later.
- The diagnosis is based on the detection of serum IgM anti-HAV antibody during the acute phase.

4. Pathological features:

The virus genome (a single open reading frame) acts as a messenger RNA → attachment to a specific receptor at hepatocytes → invasion of the hepatocytes → uncoated → translation of the single frame into a mature viral protein → generation of viral genomes → viral protein production → secretion of the virus into the bile and serum.

5. Management goals:
- Provide supportive treatment, including bed rest.
- Ameliorate the patient's symptoms.
- Minimise the transmission of infection (the patient should not return to work or school until fever and jaundice subside).
- Educate the patient.

BACK TO BASIC SCIENCES

Q1. What are the complications of hepatitis A?
- Patients usually recover with no chronic liver disease or development of cirrhosis.
- Complications are more common in adults >50 years old and who have other comorbidities or liver disorders.
- Fulminant hepatitis is rare.
- Some patients (10%–15%) may have a relapse (up to 6 months after their recovery).
- Rare complications such as vasculitis, thrombocytopenia, autoimmune haemolytic anaemia, acute renal failure and Guillain–Barré syndrome may occur.

Q2. Discuss active and passive immunisation in hepatitis A.

1. Active immunisation:
- The vaccines used are single antigen vaccines or the combined vaccine TWINRIX containing HAV and HBV antigens.

- The vaccine should be administered intramuscularly in the deltoid muscle.
- The immunity is lifelong.
- The vaccine is recommended to all infants and adults who are at high risk of being infected.

2. Passive immunisation:
   - Immunoglobulin is most commonly used for pre-exposure or postexposure.
   - It is 80%–90% protective for up to 5 months depending on the dose.

Q3. Discuss how serological tests can be of help in diagnosing patients presenting with acute hepatitis.

Table 1.6.2 summarises the changes in serological tests and their use in diagnosis of acute hepatitis.

Table 1.6.2 Changes in serological tests and their use in diagnosis of acute hepatitis

Serological tests				
IgM anti-HAV	IgM anti-HBV	HBsAg	Anti-HCV	Most likely diagnosis
+	−	−	−	Acute hepatitis A
−	+	+	−	Acute hepatitis B
+	+	+	−	Acute hepatitis A and B
−	−	+	−	Chronic hepatitis B
+	−	+	−	Acute hepatitis A in a patient with chronic hepatitis B
−	−	−	+	Acute hepatitis C

Q4. Discuss the epidemiological and clinical differences between hepatitis A virus (HAV), hepatitis B virus (HBV), hepatitis C virus (HCV), hepatitis D virus (HDV) and hepatitis E virus (HEV).

Table 1.6.3 summarises the epidemiology and clinical differences between different types of viral hepatitis.

Table 1.6.3 Epidemiology and clinical differences between different types of viral hepatitis

Item	HAV	HBV	HCV	HDV	HEV
Incubation period	15–50 days (on average 28 days)	1–3 months	1–2 months	Usually coinfection with HBV (1–3 months)	1–2 months
Serum markers	Anti-HAV	HBsAg, HBcAg, HBeAg, anti-HBs, anti-HBc	Anti-HCV (IgG, IgM), RYBA, PCR assay for HCV RNA	Anti-HDV, RNA	Anti-HEV

Table 1.6.3 Epidemiology and clinical differences between different types of viral hepatitis—cont'd

Item	HAV	HBV	HCV	HDV	HEV
Transmission	Faecal–oral, rarely parenteral	Transfusion, sexual	Transfusion, parenteral	Similar to that of HBV	Faecal–oral (endemic and/or epidemic)
Fulminant liver failure	Rare	<1% unless coinfection with HDV	Uncommon	2%–20%	20%
Persistent infection	No	5%–10%	85%	2%–70%	No
Risk of hepatocellular carcinoma	No	Yes	Yes	No	No

REVIEW QUESTIONS

Q1. A 35-year-old patient is presenting with fever and jaundice. His ALT is 3000 units/L and AST is 2800 units/L. Which *one* of the following is the likely diagnosis?
A. Cirrhosis
B. Chronic hepatitis
C. Alcoholic hepatitis
D. Acute viral hepatitis

Q2. In a patient with hepatitis A, which *one* of the following statements is correct?
A. ALT levels peak before the appearance of clinical illness.
B. Prolonged PT reflects the degree of liver necrosis.
C. IgM anti-HAV appears after the return of ALT to normal levels.
D. Faecal HAV peaks around weeks 11–12.

Q3. Which *one* of the following is the incubation period of hepatitis A?
A. 15–50 days
B. 60–80 days
C. More than 80 days
D. 1 week

Q4. Which *one* of the following is correct about HAV?
A. It is a 3.2-kb DNA virus
B. It is a 1.7-kb RNA virus
C. It is a 7.5-kb RNA virus
D. It is an RNA, circular virus

ANSWERS

A1. **D.** In cirrhosis, aminotransferases are in the range of 15–30 units/L, in chronic hepatitis they are in the range of 30–120 units/L, in alcoholic hepatitis they are in the range of 100–350 units/L and in acute viral hepatitis they are in the range of 400–3000 units/L.

A2. **B.** Prolonged PT is a good indicator of hepatic necrosis. ALT levels peak during the clinical illness. IgM anti-HAV appears early in the disease and is used in diagnosis. Faecal HAV peaks early about week 3; that is why patients are usually infectious before the appearance of the clinical illness.

A3. **A.** The incubation period of hepatitis A is 15–50 days.

A4. **C.** HAV is 7.5-kb RNA, linear. All hepatitis viruses are RNA except HBV which is a DNA virus.

TAKE-HOME MESSAGE

- HAV is 7.5-kb RNA, linear. All hepatitis viruses are RNA except HBV which is a DNA virus.
- The onset of the disease is abrupt after an incubation period of approximately 28 days (range 15–50 days).
- The disease may be asymptomatic and unapparent in young children. Symptoms vary but are usually present in adults. The disease may be fulminant and fatal (not common).
- Symptoms of infection: These include fever, nausea, vomiting, loss of appetite, abdominal pain and dark urine, together with palpable and tender liver and spleen.
- There is loss of desire for cigarette smoking or alcohol.
- Serum ALT and serum AST are raised, in the range of 400–5000 units/L or more.
- Serum IgM anti-HAV antibodies are detected.
- Patients usually recover with no chronic liver disease or development of cirrhosis.
- Complications are more common in adults >50 years old and who have other comorbidities or liver disorders.
- Some patients (10%–15%) may have a relapse (up to 6 months after their recovery).
- Rare complications such as vasculitis, thrombocytopenia, autoimmune haemolytic anaemia, acute renal failure and Guillain–Barré syndrome may occur.
- The goals of management include the following: (i) provide supportive treatment and advise bed rest; (ii) ameliorate the patient's symptoms; (iii) minimise the transmission of infection (the patient should not return to work or school until fever and jaundice subside); and (iv) educate the patient.

FURTHER READINGS

Craig AS, Schaffner W. Prevention of hepatitis A with the hepatitis A vaccine. *N Engl J Med.* 2004;350(5): 476-481. Review.

Dienstag JL. Hepatitis B virus infection. *N Engl J Med.* 2008;359(14):1486-1500. Review.

Koff RS. Hepatitis A. *Lancet.* 1998;351(9116):1643-1649. Review.

Lemon SM, Ott JJ, Van Damme P, Shouval D. Type A viral hepatitis: a summary and update on the molecular virology, epidemiology, pathogenesis and prevention. *J Hepatol.* 2017 Sep 5. pii: S0168-8278(17)32278-X. Review.

Lucey MR, Mathurin P, Morgan TR. Alcoholic hepatitis. *N Engl J Med.* 2009;360(26):2758-2769.

Matheny SC, Kingery JE. Hepatitis A. *Am Fam Physician.* 2012;86(11):1027-1034; quiz 1010-1012. Review.

McCaughan G. Advances in viral hepatitis: 50 years of Australian gastroenterology. *J Gastroenterol Hepatol.* 2009;24(suppl 3):S132-S135. Review.

Rosen HR. Clinical practice. Chronic hepatitis C infection. *N Engl J Med.* 2011;364(25):2429-2438. Review.

CASE 1.7

'Not Feeling Well . . . '

Awad Amin, a 55-year-old businessman, is brought by an ambulance to a local hospital because he is suffering from persistent upper abdominal pain radiating to his back. He feels relieved on sitting up in bed and bending forward. He has nausea and vomited several times over the last few hours. He admits drinking alcohol particularly while travelling on business trips overseas. He is on hydrochlorothiazide for hypertension. On examination, his blood pressure is 110/70 mm Hg, pulse rate 110/min, temperature 37.8°C and respiratory rate 24/min. Abdominal examination reveals tenderness of the epigastrium. Murphy's sign is negative. Intestinal sounds are absent. Auscultation of the chest reveals crackles over the bases of both lungs. No murmurs or extracardiac sounds are present. Investigation results are as follows: ECG shows sinus tachycardia; chest X-ray shows nothing of significance; serum alanine aminotransferase is 160 units/L (normal: 3–36 units/L); white blood cell (WBC) count is 7.0 (normal 4.0–11.0 $\times$ 10^9/L); calcium, albumin, triglycerides and electrolyte levels are all normal; and serum amylase is 1045 (normal: <160 units/L).

CASE DISCUSSION

Q1. On the basis of Mr Amin's presentation, what is your diagnosis?

Q2. What is your differential diagnosis?

Q3. What are the key clinical features of this disease? What are the scientific bases for these features?

Q4. What is the pathophysiology underlying these changes?

Q5. What are your management goals and management options?

ANSWERS

1. The findings of persistent upper abdominal pain of acute onset, located in the epigastrium or periumbilical region and radiating to the back, together with nausea, vomiting, fever, hypotension, tenderness of the epigastrium, respiratory distress and elevation of serum amylase nearly 10 times the normal range are all consistent with the diagnosis of acute pancreatitis. The pain of acute pancreatitis, as it is described in this case, usually gets less when the patient gets up and leans forward. Also, the patient in this case has two risk factors for acute pancreatitis – drinking alcohol and being on hydrochlorothiazide.

2. The differential diagnosis of acute pancreatitis:
   - Acute myocardial infarction
   - Gastro-oesophageal reflux disease
   - Cholangitis
   - Acute cholecystitis
   - Perforated peptic ulcer
   - Gastric outlet obstruction
   - Gastric volvulus
   - Hepatitis
   - Pancreatic cancer
   - Diabetic ketoacidosis
   - Appendicitis
   - Tubo-ovarian abscess (in females)

   The following are essential for the diagnosis of acute pancreatitis:
   - Symptoms: Persistent upper abdominal pain of acute onset is present; the pain radiates to the back, chest, flanks or lower abdomen; the pain is relieved by bending forward; and nausea, vomiting, fever, respiratory distress and tenderness of the upper abdomen are present. Abdominal guarding and rigidity is usually absent because the inflammation is retroperitoneal.
   - Two physical signs may be present: (i) Cullen's sign: ecchymosis and oedema of subcutaneous tissues around the umbilicus and (ii) Grey Turner's sign: ecchymosis of the flank. These signs are features of severe pancreatitis and haemorrhage.
   - Raised serum amylase is more than three times the upper limit of normal in the setting of typical abdominal pain. Ultrasound or computed tomography (CT) scan shows evidence of pancreatic swelling.

3. Symptoms and signs:
   - Symptoms. Patients may present with sudden severe persistent upper abdominal pain (knife-like), which radiates to the back in 60%–65% of patients. Nausea, vomiting, fever and hypotension are common.
   - Signs: There is tenderness of the epigastrium but with no peritoneal signs (the pancreas is a retroperitoneal organ). Bowel sounds are absent (paralytic ileus). Hypovolaemia, hypotension, shock, hypoxia and oliguria may occur in severe cases.
   - Two physical signs may be present and they indicate haemorrhagic pancreatitis: (i) Cullen's sign: ecchymosis and oedema of subcutaneous tissues around the umbilicus and (ii) Grey Turner's sign: ecchymosis of the flank.
   - Risk factors for acute pancreatitis may be identified as follows: (i) excessive chronic alcohol use (more common in males as a cause), (ii) gallstones and (iii) intake of medications (such as azathioprine, thiazide and oestrogen), metabolic disorders (such as hypertriglyceridaemia >11.30 mmol/L) and duct obstruction (e.g. cancer of pancreas, pancreas divisum, abdominal trauma in children). About 20% of patients have no clearly defined risk factor.

- Laboratory tests: These include complete blood count, liver function tests including serum albumin, serum bilirubin, transaminases, serum alkaline phosphatase, prothrombin time, lactate dehydrogenase (LDH), blood glucose, blood urea and creatinine, blood calcium and arterial blood gases.
- Serum amylase levels that are more than three times the upper limit of normal in the presence of characteristic pain are diagnostic. Lipase levels are usually elevated and parallel those of serum amylase.
- Tests that are more specific but not widely available are (i) trypsinogen activation peptide and (ii) trypsinogen-2.
- Abdominal imaging: This includes CT scan, magnetic resonance imaging (MRI) or transabdominal ultrasound. These investigations have the following roles: (i) confirm the diagnosis of acute pancreatitis, (ii) rule out other causes/pathology, (iii) help in staging the severity of the disease and (iv) identify any complications (such as pancreatic pseudocyst).

4. Pathological features and pathogenesis:
   - The commonest causes of acute pancreatitis are excessive alcohol or an impacted stone in the common bile duct.
   - This results in damage of the pancreatic tissues and activation of pancreatic zymogen trypsinogen to trypsin → activation of other proenzymes → autodigestion of pancreatic tissues and inflammation.
   - The damage triggers the release of inflammatory mediators → released into the circulation → systemic inflammatory response syndrome.
   - The systemic inflammatory response syndrome → hypovolaemia and increased circulatory leakage of fluids into the third space, acute respiratory distress and acute kidney failure.
   - Patients at this stage are at a higher risk of developing sepsis and multiorgan dysfunction.

   Fig. 1.7.1 summarises the pathogenesis of acute pancreatitis.

5. Management goals:
   - Supportive therapy and pancreatic rest
   - Keeping the patient pain free
   - Treating the cause
   - Managing complications (e.g. pancreatic abscess)

BACK TO BASIC SCIENCES

Q1. What are the causes of acute pancreatitis?

- Excessive alcohol drinking and impacted biliary stones are the commonest causes. They are responsible for 80% of cases.
- Other causes of acute pancreatitis are as follows:
  - Hypertriglyceridaemia (>11.30 mmol/L)
  - Post-endoscopic retrograde cholangiopancreatography

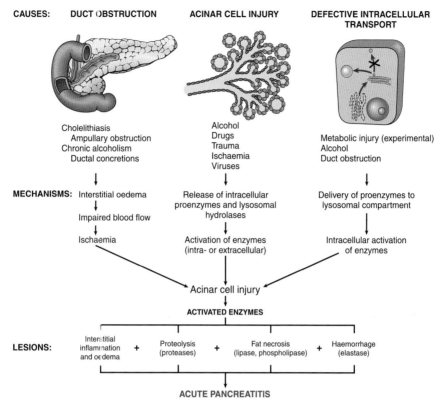

CAUSES: DUCT OBSTRUCTION   ACINAR CELL INJURY   DEFECTIVE INTRACELLULAR TRANSPORT

Cholelithiasis
   Ampullary obstruction
Chronic alcoholism
   Ductal concretions

Alcohol
Drugs
Trauma
Ischaemia
Viruses

Metabolic injury (experimental)
Alcohol
Duct obstruction

MECHANISMS: Interstitial oedema

Impaired blood flow

Ischaemia

Release of intracellular proenzymes and lysosomal hydrolases

Activation of enzymes (intra- or extracellular)

Delivery of proenzymes to lysosomal compartment

Intracellular activation of enzymes

Acinar cell injury

ACTIVATED ENZYMES

LESIONS: Interstitial inflammation and oedema   +   Proteolysis (proteases)   +   Fat necrosis (lipase, phospholipase)   +   Haemorrhage (elastase)

ACUTE PANCREATITIS

Figure 1.7.1 Pathogenesis of acute pancreatitis. *(Source: Kumar V, Abbas AK, Fausto N, Mitchell R. Robbins Basic Pathology. 8th ed. London, UK: Elsevier; 2007.)*

- Viral infections: Coxsackievirus, mumps virus, HIV and adenoviruses
- Autoimmune pancreatitis
- Pancreatic trauma
- Hypercalcaemia/hyperparathyroidism
- Obstruction of the pancreatic duct by pancreatic cancer, ascariasis or dysfunction of the sphincter of Oddi
- Hereditary pancreatitis
- Ischaemia: Coronary artery bypass, embolism, vasculitis and intra-abdominal surgery
- Scorpion venom and spider bite
- Drugs
- Idiopathic

Q2. List examples of drugs that may cause acute pancreatitis.
- Angiotensin-converting enzyme inhibitors
- Azathioprine

- 6-Mercaptopurine
- Frusemide
- Metronidazole
- Oestrogens
- Steroids
- Sulfonamides
- Tetracyclines

Q3. Briefly discuss the use of serum amylase and serum lipase measurements in the assessment of acute pancreatitis.

Table 1.7.1 summarises the use of serum amylase and serum lipase in the assessment of acute pancreatitis.

Table 1.7.1 Use of serum amylase and serum lipase in the assessment of acute pancreatitis

Item	Serum amylase	Serum lipase
Normal range	25–125 units/L	10–140 units/L
Serum rise in acute pancreatitis	Within 2–12 h of onset	Within 4–8 h of onset
Peak level	24–48 h	24 h
Remains detected in serum	3–7 days	8–14 days (remains raised for a longer duration)
Sensitivity	70%–80% (is only 60% if the cutoff is 1000 units/L)	94% (higher than that of serum amylase)
Specificity	88%–95%	>90% (higher than that of serum amylase)
Meaning of high levels	Serum levels higher than three times the upper normal limit are suggestive of acute pancreatitis. The greater rise does not mean severity but probably confirms acute pancreatitis If levels remain elevated for several weeks, it means possible pancreatic duct obstruction, peripancreatic inflammation or other local complications (CT scan is needed)	Serum levels higher than three times the upper normal limit are suggestive of acute pancreatitis It may be raised 7–11 times in acute pancreatitis Measurement is valuable when acute pancreatitis is suspected in the presence of another condition that causes an increase in S-type amylase
Falsely high levels	Chronic renal failure, acute appendicitis, mumps, salivary gland diseases, cholecystitis, diabetic ketoacidosis and tumours of testis, ovary, prostate, thyroid, lung	Chronic renal failure, acute appendicitis, diabetes mellitus
Falsely not raised	Alcohol-induced acute pancreatitis, hypertriglyceridaemia-induced acute pancreatitis	Serum lipase has a higher sensitivity in patients with alcohol-induced pancreatitis

Q4. How do patients with acute pancreatitis present?

- Severe upper abdominal pain
- Pain radiating to the back (in 40%–50% of patients)
- Nausea and vomiting
- Jaundice in patients with biliary obstruction
- Tachycardia and fever
- Signs of hypovolaemia (vomiting and loss of fluids in the third space)
- Small bowel ileus
- Grey Turner's sign (ecchymosis in the flanks)
- Cullen's sign (ecchymosis in the periumbilical area)

Q5. How would you identify patients with severe acute pancreatitis?

The scoring systems such as Ranson's criteria, Glasgow scores and APACHE-II scoring system are used in identifying patients with severe acute pancreatitis.

Patients who meet one of the following criteria can be classified as having severe acute pancreatitis:

- A score of 3 or more on Ranson's criteria
- A score of 3 or more on Glasgow criteria (within 48 hours)
- A score of 8 or more on APACHE-II
- A local complication such as pseudocyst, necrosis and pancreatic abscess
- Organ failure such as shock, gastrointestinal bleeding (>500 mL in 24 hours), pulmonary failure ($PaO_2 < 60$ mm Hg) and renal failure

Q6. Briefly discuss the Ranson's criteria and the Glasgow score systems used in predicting the severity of acute pancreatitis.

Table 1.7.2 summarises the Ranson's criteria and Glasgow score used in predicting the severity of acute pancreatitis.

Table 1.7.2 Ranson's criteria and Glasgow score used in predicting the severity of acute pancreatitis

Ranson's criteria (a total of 11 items)	Glasgow score (a total of 8 items)
On admission • Age >55 years • White blood count >16 × 10⁹ • Blood glucose >10 mmol/L • LDH >350 units/L • AST >250 units/L Within 48 h • Blood urea (increased) >1.8 mmol/L • PaO₂ <60 mm Hg • Serum calcium <2 mmol/L • Base deficit >4 mmol/L • Fluid sequestration >6 L • Packed cell volume (decreased) <10%	Within 48 h • Age >55 years • White blood count >15 × 10⁹ • Blood glucose >10 mmol/L • Serum urea >16 mmol/L • PaO₂ <60 mm Hg • Serum calcium <2 mmol/L • Serum albumin <32 g/L • LDH >600 units/L
Scoring: A score of 3 or more is consistent with the clinical diagnosis of severe acute pancreatitis.	*Scoring:* One score is given to each criterion if present. A score of 3 or more is consistent with the clinical diagnosis of severe acute pancreatitis.

Q7. What is the role of radiological imaging in the diagnosis of acute pancreatitis?

- Plain (erect) X-ray of the abdomen: It may show generalised or local ileus (sentinel loop) and a colon cutoff sign. Calcification of the pancreas or calcification of the gallbladder may be present.
- Plain X-ray of the chest: It may show pleural effusion or alveolar interstitial shadowing (usually seen in severe acute pancreatitis).
- Ultrasound of the abdomen: It should be carried out for all patients within the first 48 hours of presentation. It helps in detecting gallbladder stones as a potential cause and in ruling out acute cholecystitis.
- CT scan of the abdomen: It is recommended for all patients, and can help in staging the severity of acute pancreatitis. A contrast CT scan may be identified if there is diagnostic uncertainty and in severe cases to distinguish interstitial from necrotising pancreatitis and to diagnose local complications such as pancreatic pseudocyst.
- MRI: It is usually used in assessing the severity of acute pancreatitis.
- Magnetic resonance cholangiopancreatography (MRCP): It helps in detecting pancreatic duct disruption and choledocholithiasis. This investigation has reduced the need for Endoscopic Retrograde Cholangiopancreatography (ERCP).

REVIEW QUESTIONS

Q1. Which *one* of the following is correct about the Ranson's score?
A. Comprises 12 factors
B. Has a sensitivity of predicting poor outcomes of 90%
C. Predicts severity of pancreatitis and outcomes
D. Is based on CT severity index

Q2. Which of the following is *not part* of the Glasgow criteria for assessing acute pancreatitis?
A. Age >55 years
B. Prothrombin time 26 seconds
C. Albumin <32 g/L
D. Serum calcium <2 mmol/L
E. Urea >16 mmol/L (after rehydration)

Q3. All of the following are risk factors for acute pancreatitis *except*
A. Chronic use of alcohol.
B. Gallstones.
C. hypercholesterolaemia (>11.3 mmol/L).
D. Hydrochlorothiazide.
E. Scorpion bite.

Q4. Which *one* of the following clinical signs may indicate severe pancreatitis?
A. Epigastric tenderness
B. Epigastric guarding
C. Respiratory distress
D. Tachycardia
E. Cullen's sign

Q5. In severe acute pancreatitis with concern for pancreatic necrosis, which prophylactic antibacterial would you recommend?
A. Imipenem
B. Tetracycline
C. Metronidazole
D. Amoxicillin
E. Gentamicin

Q6. Which *one* of the following is associated with enteral nutrition in patients with acute pancreatitis?
A. Increased rate of infection
B. Increased surgical intervention
C. Increased costs of treatment
D. No different outcomes compared to those of parenteral nutrition
E. Reduced length of hospital stay

ANSWERS

A1. **C.** Ranson's criteria comprise 11 items (5 items on admission and 6 items during the initial 48 hours). The sensitivity of Ranson's criteria of predicting poor outcomes is only 70%. It is not based on CT severity index. However, the criteria help in predicting the severity and outcomes of acute pancreatitis.

A2. **B.** Prolonged prothrombin time is not an item of the Glasgow criteria for acute pancreatitis. The following are the eight items in the Glasgow criteria: age >55 years, PO_2 <8 kPa (60 mm Hg), WBC count >15 × 10^9/L, albumin <32 g/L, serum calcium <2 mmol/L, glucose >10 mmol/L, urea >16 mmol/L (after rehydration) and LDH >600 units/L.

A3. **C.** Hypertriglyceridaemia >11.3 mmol/L is a risk factor for acute pancreatitis and not hypercholesterolaemia. Other risk factors for acute pancreatitis are gallstones, excessive alcohol, post-ERCP and idiopathic. Rare causes are trauma, postsurgical procedures, hypercalcaemia, pancreas divisum, sphincter of Oddi dysfunction, infection (mumps virus, Coxsackievirus), medications (e.g. thiazide diuretics), severe hypothermia and scorpion bite.

A4. **D.** Cullen's sign and Grey Turner's sign usually indicate severe haemorrhagic pancreatitis.

A5. **A.** Several studies showed that imipenem reduced infectious complications including central line sepsis, pulmonary infection, urinary tract infection and infected pancreatic necrosis when used in acute pancreatitis.

A6. **E.** Meta-analysis of six randomised trials showed that enteral nutrition in acute pancreatitis decreased rate of infection, decreased surgical intervention, reduced length of hospital stay and reduced costs of management compared to total parenteral nutrition. Enteral nutrition is well tolerated in patients with ileus.

TAKE-HOME MESSAGE

- Acute pancreatitis is caused by two main causes: biliary calculi and alcohol abuse.
- Other causes of acute pancreatitis include abdominal trauma, post-ERCP, hypertriglyceridaemia, hyperparathyroidism, hypercalcaemia, autoimmune pancreatitis, viral infections, scorpion bites and idiopathic causes.
- The pathogenesis of acute pancreatitis is related to inappropriate activation of the pancreatic zymogen trypsin causing activation of other proenzymes and autodigestion of pancreatic tissues.
- Acute pancreatitis is associated with hyperdynamic circulation, hypovolaemia (loss of fluids in the third space), systemic inflammatory response syndrome, release of inflammatory mediators and multiple organ dysfunction.
- Several criteria systems are used in detecting the severity of acute pancreatitis. These include the following:
  - Ranson's criteria
  - Glasgow criteria
  - APACHE-II criteria
  - CT scan severity index
- Patients with acute pancreatitis present with severe upper abdominal pain that radiates to the back, nausea and vomiting, jaundice, fever, tachycardia, signs of hypovolaemia and small intestine ileus.
- Two clinical signs may be present in 5% of patients: Grey Turner's sign (ecchymosis in flanks) and Cullen's sign (ecchymosis in the periumbilical area). Both indicate severe pancreatitis.
- Acute pancreatitis is usually associated with complications including the following:
  1. Local complications: Pancreatic necrosis, pancreatic pseudocyst, pancreatic abscess, pancreatic haemorrhage and retroperitoneal necrosis
  2. Systemic complications: Shock, sepsis, pulmonary effusion, adult respiratory distress syndrome, paralytic ileus, acute renal failure, hypocalcaemia and disseminated intravascular coagulation

FURTHER READINGS

Carroll JK, Herrick B, Gipson T, Lee SP. Acute pancreatitis: diagnosis, prognosis, and treatment. *Am Fam Physician*. 2007;75(10):1513-1520. Review.

da Silva S, Rocha M, Pinto-de-Sousa J. Acute pancreatitis etiology investigation: a workup algorithm proposal. *GE Port J Gastroenterol*. 2017;24(3):129-136. Review.

Forsmark CE, Vege SS, Wilcox CM. Acute pancreatitis. *N Engl J Med*. 2016;375(20):1972-1981. Review.

Frossard JL, Steer ML, Pastor CM. Acute pancreatitis. *Lancet*. 2008;371(9607):143-152. Review.

Kingsnorth A, O'Reilly D. Acute pancreatitis. *BMJ*. 2006;332(7549):1072-1076. Review.

Lankisch PG, Apte M, Banks PA. Acute pancreatitis. *Lancet*. 2015;386(9988):85-96. Review.

Quinlan JD. Acute pancreatitis. *Am Fam Physician*. 2014;90(9):632-639.

Ranson JH. Diagnostic standards for acute pancreatitis. *World J Surg*. 1997;21(2):136-142.

Vaughn VM, Shuster D, Rogers MAM, et al. Early versus delayed feeding in patients with acute pancreatitis: a systematic review. *Ann Intern Med*. 2017;166(12):883-892.

Whitcomb DC. Clinical practice. Acute pancreatitis. *N Engl J Med*. 2006;354(20):2142-2150. Review.

CASE 1.8

'I Have the Runs . . . '

Amany Ali, a 45-year-old woman, comes in to see her general practitioner because of 5 days of diarrhoea. She says, 'I have the runs and my stools are grossly bloody.' She also has abdominal discomfort and, sometimes, abdominal cramps. She has had a fever for the last 2–3 days. Ms Ali gives no history of travel or contact with sick people. She has no past history of hospital admission and is not on any medications. She has always been fit.

CASE DISCUSSION

Q1. On the basis of Ms Ali's presentation, what is your diagnosis?

Q2. What is your differential diagnosis?

Q3. What are the key clinical features of this disease? What are the scientific bases for these features?

Q4. What is the pathophysiology underlying these changes?

Q5. What are your management goals and management options?

ANSWERS

1. The patient gives a history of loose bowel motions for 5 days with grossly bloody stools. She gives a history of abdominal discomfort and crampy abdominal pain, and she has had a fever for the last 2–3 days. She gives no history of travel or contact with sick patients. She has no significant past history or hospital admission and has always been fit. This presentation is consistent with bacterial colitis possibly caused by one of the Five bacterial enteropathogens known to cause bloody diarrhoea – *Shigella*, *Campylobacter*, *Salmonella*, nontyphoid *Salmonella* and Shiga toxin–producing *Escherichia coli*.

2. The differential diagnosis of acute bloody diarrhoea:
    *   *Shigella*
    *   *Campylobacter*
    *   Nontyphoid *Salmonella*
    *   Shiga toxin–producing *E. coli*
    *   *Aeromonas* species
    *   Noncholera *vibrio*
    *   *Yersinia enterocolitica*
    *   *Clostridium difficile*
    *   *Entamoeba histolytica*

The following are essential for the diagnosis:

- Symptoms: These include increased watery content, volume or frequency that lasts less than 14 days. Other symptoms that may be present are abdominal discomfort, crampy abdominal pain, nausea, vomiting, fever, loss of appetite and/or varying severity of toxic symptoms.
- Most cases do not require stool analysis or stool culture. However, very young patients and elderly patients (>65 years), patients with comorbidity or immunocompromised disease and hospital outbreaks need laboratory investigations.

3. Symptoms, history and clinical signs:
   - Symptoms: Loose bowel motions (onset, duration, severity, frequency), stool character (watery, bloody, mucus, purulent), symptoms suggestive of dehydration (decreased urine output, dark urine, thirst, dizziness, change in mental status), nausea, vomiting (usually suggestive of viral infection or presence of bacterial toxin), fever, tenesmus and grossly bloody stool (suggestive of bacterial infection)
   - History of food intake (food poisoning, if there are others who shared the same food and have the same symptoms) and travel history (traveller's diarrhoea)
   - Children in day care, nursing house residents or persons in contact with patients who have been admitted to hospital
   - Sexual practices that include anal/or oral–anal contact
   - History of immunodeficiency virus infection, long use of corticosteroids, chemotherapy and immunoglobulin A deficiency

   Table 1.8.1 summarises the clinical characteristics of bacterial infectious diarrhoea.
   - Physical signs: These are the following: (i) degree of dehydration (dry mucous membrane, delayed capillary refill time, increased heart rate and abnormal orthostatic changes of blood pressure), (ii) fever together with bloody diarrhoea (suggestive of inflammatory bacterial infection), (iii) abdominal tenderness and abdominal guarding (site), (iv) urine output and (v) rectal examination (presence of blood, anal/rectal tenderness, stool consistency).
   - Laboratory findings: (i) Patients presenting with watery diarrhoea and no fever are usually managed on the basis of clinical findings. (ii) Laboratory investigations are needed in patients presenting with severe bloody diarrhoea, fever and systematic symptoms, with evidence of dehydration, having comorbidity, being immunocompromised or being of extreme age (<3 months or >65 years).
   - Stool examination for occult blood is done (the test has a sensitivity of 70% and specificity of 80% and when positive, it suggests bloody diarrhoea).
   - Stool leukocytes and lactoferrin: Both tests are used to assess whether there are excessive leukocytes in stools. Increased leukocytes suggest inflammatory diarrhoea. Increased lactoferrin is more sensitive as the test measures lactoferrin from the damaged leukocytes.
   - Stool microscopy for ova and parasites is done.

Table 1.8.1 Clinical characteristics of bacterial infectious diarrhoea

Pathogen	Incubation period	Duration	Diarrhoea	Vomiting	Abdominal cramps	Fever
			Symptoms			
Salmonella	6 h to 2 days	48 h to 7 days	Watery	+	+	+
Campylobacter	2–11 days	3 days to 3 weeks	Bloody	−	+	+
Shigella	1–4 days	2–3 days	Bloody	−	+	+
Vibrio cholerae	2–3 days	Up to 7 days	Watery	+	+	−
Clostridium perfringens	8 h to 1 day	12 h to 1 day	Watery	−	+	−
Bacillus cereus	8–12 h	12 h to 2 days	Watery	−	+	−
Diarrhoeal Emetic	15 min to 4 h	12 h to 1 day	Watery	+	+	−
Yersinia enterocolitica	4–7 days	1–2 weeks	Bloody	−	+	+
Enteropathogenic *E. coli* (EPEC)	1–2 days	Days to weeks	Watery	+	+	+
Enterotoxigenic *E. coli* (ETEC)	1–7 days	2–6 days	Watery	+	+	−
Enterohaemorrhagic *E. coli* (EHEC)	3–4 days	5–10 days	Bloody	+	+	−
Enteroinvasive *E. coli* (EIEC)	1–3 days	7–10 days	Bloody	+	+	+

Source: Goering R, Dockrell N, Zuckerman M, Wakelin D, Roitt I, Mims C, Chiodini P. Mims' Medical Microbiology, 4th Edition. Lodon, UK: Elsevier; 2007.

- Stool cultures: Stool cultures are expensive and are positive in only 2%–6% of cases. This percentage is increased up to 30% when patients have bloody diarrhoea and the stools are positive for leukocytes. Stool cultures are indicated when there are nosocomial outbreaks, patients are immunocompromised, patients have comorbidity (end-stage liver failure, renal failure, etc.), patients have inflammatory bowel disease or patients are older than 65 years.
- *C. difficile* testing is done for toxins A and B.
- Complete blood count, blood electrolytes, urea and creatinine are measured.

4. Pathological features:

   In noninflammatory diarrhoea, there are no or minimal mucosal changes; in inflammatory diarrhoea, the mucous membrane shows signs of inflammation, necrosis and cellular infiltration.

5. Management goals:
   - Assess the severity of diarrhoea, degree of dehydration, any haemodynamic changes and any comorbidity or immunocompromised state.
   - Correct dehydration and any electrolyte imbalance.

- Monitor vital signs; measure fluid input and urinary output.
- Provide supportive treatment. Decide whether antibiotics are needed.
- Educate the patient.

If the results for *Shigella* toxin are positive, the patient should receive supportive treatment with no antibiotic therapy. Antibiotic treatment should be carefully selected if Shiga toxin–producing *E. coli* are present (to avoid haemolytic–uraemic syndrome). Other indications for antibiotic treatment are prolonged severe illness, fever, bloody diarrhoea and patients with immunocompromised state.

BACK TO BASIC SCIENCES

Q1. How would you differentiate between noninflammatory and inflammatory acute diarrhoea?

Table 1.8.2 summarises the differences between noninflammatory and inflammatory acute diarrhoea.

Table 1.8.2 Differences between noninflammatory and inflammatory acute diarrhoea

Item	Noninflammatory	Inflammatory
Causative agent	Usually viral infection, sometimes bacteria or parasites	Toxin-producing bacteria or parasites
Examples of pathogens	Rotavirus *Vibrio cholerae* Enterotoxigenic *Escherichia coli* (ETEC) *Bacillus cereus* *Giardia* *Cryptosporidium*	*Salmonella* (nontyphoidal) *Shigella* *Campylobacter* Shiga toxin–producing *E. coli* *Clostridium difficile* *Entamoeba histolytica* *Yersinia enterocolitica*
Clinical picture	Usually mild disease Nausea, vomiting, abdominal pain, nonbloody watery stool	Usually more severe disease Inflammatory changes: Fever, sweating, tenesmus, mucus and bloody stool
Pathology and stool analysis	No pathological changes in intestinal mucosa Functional changes (increased secretion) No faecal leukocytes	Inflammatory changes, tissue invasion, necrosis, cellular infiltration of the mucosa of the intestine Faecal leukocytes +++, faecal red blood cells +++, necrotic tissues ++/+++

Q2. What are the common causes for acute bloody diarrhoea?

- *Shigella*
- *Campylobacter*
- Nontyphoidal *Salmonella*
- Shiga toxin–producing *E. coli*
- Noncholera *vibrio*

- *Y. enterocolitica*
- *E. histolytica*
- Salmonella

Q3. What do you know about Shiga toxin–producing *E. coli* infection?

- It causes watery diarrhoea that becomes bloody in 1–5 days.
- Infection is characterised by severe crampy abdominal pain and passage of five or more unformed stool.
- Infection in children is the main cause of renal failure. The Shiga toxin released enters the bloodstream and reaches the renal endothelium causing haemolytic–uraemicsyndrome (patients require dialysis) and is associated with mortality in approximately 5% of patients.
- The Shiga toxin also causes haemorrhagic colitis but ischaemic colitis may occur.
- Shiga toxin 2 is more important in the pathogenesis of haemolytic–uraemic syndrome than Shiga toxin 1.
- Approximately 40% of Shiga toxin–producing *E. coli* infections are non-O157 strains. However, both non-O157 strains and O157:H7 strains cause the same spectrum of disease (they are differentiated microbiologically via sorbitol fermentation).

Q4. Briefly discuss examples of enteric infections related to food poisoning indicating incubation period and food mostly related to each enteropathogen.

Table 1.8.3 summarises enteric infections related to food poisoning.

Table 1.8.3 Enteric infections related to food poisoning

Enteropathogens	Clinical picture	Incubation period	Related food
Staphylococcus aureus	Vomiting	2–7 h	Improperly cooked stored food containing a heat-stable toxin
Clostridium perfringens	Watery diarrhoea	8–14 h	Contaminated meat, vegetables, poultry
Bacillus cereus	Vomiting[a] Diarrhoea	30 min to 6 h 6–15 h	Fried rice, vegetables

[a]Depending on the presence of one or two toxins, the clinical picture may show early vomiting (in 30 minutes to 6 hours) and/or diarrhoea (in 6–15 hours).

Q5. What is the most common pathogen causing traveller's diarrhoea?

- In more than 50% of cases, it is caused by enterotoxigenic *E. coli* (particularly in Latin America and Africa).
- Other organisms responsible are *Shigella, Salmonella, Campylobacter* and noncholera *vibrio.*
- In Asia and South East Asia, the invasive organisms commonly responsible are *Campylobacter, Shigella* and *Salmonella.*

Q6. What investigations are needed for managing a healthy patient presenting with traveller's diarrhoea?

- Healthy patients with no systematic symptoms and presenting with mild illness should be treated empirically with antibiotics without stool examination.
- Patients presenting with severe symptoms, patients having comorbidity or immuno-compromised patients should be investigated (complete blood count, urea, creatinine and electrolytes, stool analysis, stool culture).

Q7. Briefly discuss nosocomial diarrhoea.

- These patients have diarrhoea while admitted in hospital. They usually have existing pathological conditions, are on medications and are exposed to *C. difficile* spores.
- *C. difficile* is important, though not common, and should be considered in patients with significant diarrhoea, toxic dilatation of the colon or unexplained leukocytosis.
- The diarrhoea caused by *C. difficile* is usually watery diarrhoea but may become bloody diarrhoea.
- *C. difficile* diarrhoea may be seen in an outpatient setting, particularly in old patients. It should be considered in the differential diagnosis because it is a known cause of mortality.

Q8. What considerations should be taken in managing patients with diarrhoea caused by nontyphoidal *Salmonella*?

Bacteraemia complicates the infection causing fever and systematic and toxic effects; systematic *Salmonella* infection may particularly occur in very young patients (<3 months) and elderly patients (>65 years). Other groups of patients at risk are immunocompromised patients, those on corticosteroids, patients with sickle cell disease, patients with prosthetic heart valves and patients with aortic abdominal aneurysm.

Q9. Which antibiotic is recommended in patients with Shiga toxin–producing *E. coli* diarrhoea?

Antibiotics recommended in treating these patients are the following:

- Fosfomycin
- Azithromycin

These antibiotics inhibit the bacterial cell wall by inactivating the enzyme UDP-N-acetylglucosamine-3-enolpyruvyltransferase. Thus, these antibiotics appear to inhibit the production of Shiga toxin. Other antibiotics may carry the risk of aggravating haemolysis.

REVIEW QUESTIONS

Q1. Shiga toxin–producing *E. coli* is the main cause of which *one* of the following?
A. Renal failure in children
B. Nonbloody diarrhoea

C. Traveller's diarrhoea
D. Food poisoning

Q2. All of the following enteropathogens cause bloody diarrhoea *except*
A. *Shigella.*
B. Nontyphoid *Salmonella.*
C. Shiga toxin–producing *E. coli.*
D. *Staphylococcus aureus.*

Q3. Microbiological studies may *not* be needed and management is usually based on clinical presentation in all of the following cases *except*
A. Food poisoning.
B. Traveller's diarrhoea.
C. Mild watery diarrhoea in a febrile healthy patient.
D. Nosocomial outbreak.

Q4. Which *one* of the following pathogens is the most common cause of traveller's diarrhoea?
A. Nontyphoid *Salmonella*
B. Enterotoxigenic *E. coli*
C. *Shigella dysenteriae*
D. *Vibrio cholerae*

Q5. A 35-year-old patient, who presented with acute diarrhoea caused by nontyphoid salmonellosis, is found to have mild fever and systematic toxic effects. Which *one* of the following is an indication for antibiotic treatment?
A. Watery diarrhoea
B. Being hypertensive
C. Having a prosthetic heart valve
D. Abdominal pain

Q6. Which *one* of the following antibiotics is recommended in a 12-year-old child presenting with acute diarrhoea caused by Shiga toxin–producing *E. coli*?
A. Azithromycin
B. Tetracycline
C. Fluoroquinolones
D. Trimethoprim–sulfamethoxazole

ANSWERS

A1. **A.** Shiga toxin–producing *E. coli* causes haemolytic–uraemic syndrome in children.

A2. **D.** *S. aureus* causes acute diarrhoea. The stool is usually watery, unformed stool.

A3. **D.** Nosocomial outbreaks should be investigated and a number of microbiological and blood studies are indicated.

A4. **B.** In more than 50% of cases, it is caused by enterotoxigenic *E. coli* (particularly in Latin America and Africa).

A5. **C.** Bacteraemia complicates the infection causing fever and systematic and toxic effects; systematic *Salmonella* infection may particularly occur in very young patients (<3 months) and elderly patients (>65 years). Other groups of patients at risk are immunocompromised patients, those on corticosteroids, patients with sickle cell disease, patients with prosthetic heart valves and patients with aortic abdominal aneurysm.

A6. **A.** Antibiotics recommended in treating these patients are the following: (i) fosfomycin or (ii) azithromycin. These antibiotics inhibit the bacterial cell wall by inactivating the enzyme UDP-*N*-acetylglucosamine-3-enolpyruvyltransferase. Thus, these antibiotics appear to inhibit the production of Shiga toxin. Other antibiotics may carry the risk of aggravating haemolysis.

TAKE-HOME MESSAGE

- The differential diagnosis of acute bloody diarrhoea includes *Shigella*, *Campylobacter*, nontyphoid *Salmonella*, Shiga toxin–producing *E. coli*, *Aeromonas* species, noncholera *vibrio*, *Y. enterocolitica*, *C. difficile* or *E. histolytica*.
- The presenting symptoms include loose bowel motions (onset, duration, severity, frequency), stool character (watery, bloody, mucus, purulent), symptoms suggestive of dehydration (decreased urine output, dark urine, thirst, dizziness, change in mental status), nausea, vomiting (usually suggestive of viral infection or presence of bacterial toxin), fever, tenesmus and grossly bloody stool (suggestive of bacterial infection).
- Physical signs include the following: (i) degree of dehydration (dry mucous membrane, delayed capillary refill time, increased heart rate and abnormal orthostatic changes of blood pressure), (ii) fever together with bloody diarrhoea (suggestive of inflammatory bacterial infection), (iii) abdominal tenderness and abdominal guarding (site), (iv) urine output and (v) rectal examination (presence of blood, anal/rectal tenderness, stool consistency).
- In noninflammatory diarrhoea, there are no or minimal mucosal changes; in inflammatory diarrhoea, the mucous membrane shows signs of inflammation, necrosis and cellular infiltration.
- Investigations include the following: (i) full blood count, (ii) stool examination for occult blood, (iii) stool leukocytes and lactoferrin, (iv) stool microscopy, (v) stool cultures and (vi) *C. difficile* testing for toxins A and B.
- The goals of management: (i) assess the severity of diarrhoea, degree of dehydration, any haemodynamic changes and any comorbidity or immunocompromised state; (ii) correct dehydration and any electrolyte imbalance; (iii) monitor vital signs, and measure fluid input and urinary output; (iv) provide supportive treatment and decide whether antibiotics are needed; and (v) educate the patient.

FURTHER READINGS

Al-Abri SS, Beeching NJ, Nye FJ. Traveller's diarrhoea. *Lancet Infect Dis.* 2005;5(6):349–360. Review.

Bartlett JG. Clinical practice. Antibiotic-associated diarrhea. *N Engl J Med.* 2002;346(5):334–339. Review.

Das JK, Bhutta ZA. Global challenges in acute diarrhea. *Curr Opin Gastroenterol.* 2016;32(1):18–23. Review.

de Bruyn G. Diarrhoea in adults (acute). *BMJ Clin Evid.* 2008;2008:0901. Review.

DuPont HL. Acute infectious diarrhea in immunocompetent adults. *N Engl J Med.* 2014;370(16): 1532–1540. Review.

DuPont HL. Clinical practice. Bacterial diarrhea. *N Engl J Med.* 2009;361(16):1560–1569. Review.

Gottlieb T, Heather CS. Diarrhoea in adults (acute). *BMJ Clin Evid.* 2011;2011:0901. Review.

Razzaq S. Hemolytic uremic syndrome: an emerging health risk. *Am Fam Physician.* 2006;74(6):991–996. Review.

Schroeder MS. Clostridium difficile—associated diarrhea. *Am Fam Physician.* 2005;71(5):921–928. Review.

Thielman NM, Guerrant RL. Clinical practice. Acute infectious diarrhea. *N Engl J Med.* 2004;350(1): 38–47. Review.

CASE 1.9

'Nothing Is Working for Me . . . '

Miranda Clark, a 30-year-old administrator, presents to her general practitioner because she is suffering from cramps in her left lower quadrant abdomen, bloating and loose bowel motions for the last 2 weeks. The pain is recurrent, and she has had similar pain since childhood. The pain frequently occurs after meals. It is sometimes relieved by defecation, and at other times, passing stools makes it worse. She admits that she gets anxious and is always worried about minor issues at work or home. Mrs Clark has no family history of coeliac disease or colon cancer. She gives no history of anaemia, weight loss, loss of appetite, fever, bleeding per rectum or vomiting. On examination, her vital sign readings are within normal range. Abdominal examination showed tenderness of the left lower quadrant but no guarding or rigidity. Per rectum examination was normal.

CASE DISCUSSION

Q1. On the basis of Mrs Clark's presentation, what is your diagnosis?

Q2. What is your differential diagnosis?

Q3. What are the key clinical features of this disease? What are the scientific bases for these features?

Q4. What is the pathophysiology underlying these changes?

Q5. What are your management goals and management options?

ANSWERS

1. The findings of a long history of recurrent abdominal pain since childhood together with loose bowel motions, bloating, anxiety and the absence of warning signs such as anaemia, weight loss, fever, bleeding per rectum, loss of appetite and vomiting as well as the absence of family history of coeliac disease and colon cancer are suggestive of the diagnosis of irritable bowel syndrome (IBS).
2. The differential diagnosis of IBS:
   - Coeliac disease
   - Microscopic colitis
   - Collagen colitis
   - Crohn disease
   - Amoebic dysentery
   - Chronic diarrhoea

The following are essential for the diagnosis of IBS:

- The Roma IV criteria for IBS are currently the basis for the diagnosis. These criteria comprise the following:
  - The patient has recurrent abdominal pain >1 day per week, on average, in the previous 3 months with an onset of >6 months before diagnosis.
  - The abdominal pain is associated with at least two of the following three symptoms: (i) pain related to defecation, (ii) change in the frequency of stool and (iii) change in the form or appearance of stool.
  - The patient has none of the warning signs or 'alarm features', e.g. anaemia, nocturnal pain or nocturnal symptoms, weight loss and family history of colorectal cancer, ovarian cancer or inflammatory bowel disease (the whole list is discussed later).

3. Symptoms and signs:
   - Abdominal pain caused by defecation is present.
   - Bloating occurs.
   - There occur changes in bowel habits.
   - There occur changes in the form of stools.
   - The warning signs or 'alarm features' are absent.
   - The diagnosis is usually based on the clinical presentation and not on biochemical or histological examination.
   - The diagnosis is based on the Roma IV criteria and is not reached by exclusion.
   - However, in the primary care, the doctor may need to order basic tests to exclude other related conditions (e.g. coeliac disease, tropical sprue, inflammatory bowel disease).
   - Four types (categories) of IBS have been identified: (i) Constipation-predominant (IBS-C), (ii) diarrhoea-predominant (IBS-D), (iii) mixed bowel pattern (IBS-M) and (iv) unclassified (IBS-U).
   - On making the diagnosis, the 'alarm features' should be excluded. The presence of any of the following features makes the diagnosis of IBS unlikely:
     (1) Anaemia
     (2) Rectal bleeding
     (3) Unintentional and unexplained weight loss
     (4) Abdominal mass
     (5) Rectal mass
     (6) Presence of inflammatory markers for inflammatory bowel disease
     (7) A family history of colorectal cancer, ovarian cancer or inflammatory bowel disease
     (8) Nocturnal symptoms
     (9) Appearance of symptoms of changes in bowel habits for the first time in a male over the age of 50

4. Investigations:
   - Full blood count and blood film
   - C-reactive protein or erythrocyte sedimentation rate

- Blood urea/creatinine and electrolytes
- Coeliac antibodies
- Faecal calprotectin

More investigations are needed in patients who have 'alarm features' to make a final diagnosis. These investigations may include the following:

- Sigmoidoscopy
- Colonoscopy/barium enema
- Microscopic examination of stools for ova and parasite test
- Thyroid function tests

Pathology and pathogenesis:

In IBS, biochemical tests are expected to be normal. The exact pathophysiology of IBS is not known. The key pathophysiological processes underlying IBS can be summarised as follows:

(1) Gut dysmotility: This includes delayed gastric emptying, increased small bowel mobility and increased colonic motility in response to a meal.

(2) Intestinal hypersensitivity: It is responsible for the chronic abdominal discomfort and pain. Tissue damage and inflammation → release of inflammatory mediators → sensitivity and excitability of nociceptor terminals → perceived as hyperalgesia or discomfort.

(3) Postinfectious gastrointestinal IBS: Acute gastroenteritis could trigger ongoing inflammation and the development of IBS symptoms. This is not related to a particular organism but *Shigella*, *Campylobacter* and *Salmonella* infections have been reported.

Postinfectious IBS could be related to inflammatory changes, release of inflammatory mediators, changes in or increased permeability from weak tight junctions and alterations in ion channels (sodium and type 2 chloride channels).

(4) Stress response and IBS: Patients with IBS report more negative life events than do matching controls. Stress is mediated via the hypothalamic–pituitary–adrenal axis → release of corticotrophin-releasing factor (CRF) from the hypothalamus → stimulates the release of adrenocorticotrophic hormone (ACTH) from the anterior pituitary → cortisol release from the adrenal gland. Both the stimulation of the autonomic nervous system and the increased secretion of cortisol are responsible for the changes and symptoms of IBS.

5. Management goals:

- Support and reassurance
- Ameliorating the patient's symptoms
- Improvement of the quality of life
- Educating the patient

However, the management of IBS is challenging and the patient's symptoms are often recurrent and resistant to therapy.

Therapeutic options include exercise, dietary changes, antispasmodics, increased fibre in diet, laxatives (IBS-C), antidiarrhoeals (IBS-D), serotonin agonists (5-HT4) and serotonin antagonists (5-HT3), antibiotics, probiotics and the use of guanylate cyclase C agonists.

BACK TO BASIC SCIENCES

Q1. Briefly discuss the role of psychological factors in the pathogenesis of IBS.

- A range of disturbances may be present in patients with IBS including anxiety, depression, neurosis and panic attacks.
- Patients may also have reduced coping abilities, increased stress, past exposure to childhood abuse or psychological difficulties.
- The mechanism related to stress and IBS could be explained on the basis of stimulation of the hypothalamic–pituitary–adrenal axis and stimulation of the autonomic nervous system (review earlier discussion).
- This relationship and the role of CRF from the hypothalamus could explain the role of corticotrophin-releasing factor-1 receptor (CRF-1) antagonist in the treatment of IBS.

Q2. What are the essential laboratory tests that you may order in a patient with IBS?

Usually the diagnosis of IBS is based on the clinical presentation and the application of Roma IV criteria. However, some basic tests may be ordered to exclude coeliac disease and inflammatory bowel disease. These tests are (i) full blood count and blood film; (ii) C-reactive protein or erythrocyte sedimentation rate; (iii) blood urea, creatinine and electrolytes; (iv) coeliac disease; and (v) faecal calprotectin.

Q3. What are the 'alarm features' in IBS?

1. Anaemia
2. Rectal bleeding
3. Unintentional and unexplained weight loss
4. Abdominal mass
5. Rectal mass
6. Presence of inflammatory markers for inflammatory bowel disease
7. A family history of colorectal cancer, ovarian cancer or inflammatory bowel disease
8. Nocturnal symptoms
9. Appearance of symptoms of changes in bowel habits for the first time in a male over the age of 50

Q4. What is the role of guanylate cyclase C agonists in the management of IBS?

Guanylate cyclase C agonists (e.g. linaclotide) are recommended in managing IBS-C. The therapy comprises a minimally absorbed 14–amino acid peptide → activation of guanylate C → stimulation of the production of cyclic guanosine monophosphate

→ stimulation of bicarbonate and chloride secretion via the cystic fibrosis transmembrane conductance regulator → increased intestinal motility and stool softness.

REVIEW QUESTIONS

Q1. Which *one* of the following symptoms is not consistent with the diagnosis of IBS?
A. Abdominal pain is related to defecation.
B. Abdominal pain is associated with changes in the frequency of stool.
C. Abdominal pain is associated with a change in the form of stool.
D. Abdominal pain awakens the patient from sleep.

Q2. Which *one* of the following laboratory tests may you order for a patient presenting with IBS–D or IBS–M?
A. Hydrogen breath test
B. Coeliac antibodies
C. Serum albumin
D. Faecal calprotectin

Q3. Which *one* of the following is recommended in the management of IBS?
A. Test for food allergy.
B. Ask the patient to have a food diary.
C. Increase soluble fibre in diet.
D. Prescribe polyethylene glycol to relieve abdominal pain.

Q4. Which *one* of the following does not reduce abdominal pain in IBS?
A. Rifaximin
B. Antispasmodics
C. Probiotics
D. Loperamide
E. Antidepressants

ANSWERS

A1. **D.** The abdominal pain in IBS does not awaken the patient from sleep. This finding in the history should direct the attention to the possibility of other organic disorders. Also, abdominal pain associated with anorexia, weight loss or bleeding per rectum is not consistent with IBS.

A2. **B.** Routine testing for coeliac disease in patients with IBS–D or IBS–M should always be considered. Coeliac antibody test is recommended in these patients.

A3. **B.** There is no evidence that testing for food allergies will help in the management of IBS. Also there is no evidence that increasing soluble or insoluble fibre in diet in patients with IBS has a beneficial effect over placebo for improving pain or other symptoms (for further reading, check Ruepert et al., 2011). Polyethylene glycol is prescribed for patients with constipation, not IBS. There is no solid evidence that its use helps in reducing symptoms in IBS (for further reading, check Khoshoo et al., 2006). However, there is evidence that the use of a food diary can help the patient to identify food that could trigger his/her symptoms.

A4. **D.** Loperamide, a synthetic opioid, is used as an antidiarrhoeal. Studies showed that it is effective in decreasing stool frequency and enhancing stool consistency. However, it did not improve abdominal pain (Lesbros-Pantoflickova et al., 2004). Antibiotics such as rifaximin or neomycin for 2 weeks were found to improve bloating, abdominal pain and stool consistency in IBS (Pimentel et al., 2011). Antispasmodics were effective in reducing abdominal pain. Antidepressants also reduced abdominal pain in IBS. Probiotics reduced IBS symptoms including abdominal pain and flatulence (Moayyedi et al., 2010).

TAKE-HOME MESSAGE

- The diagnosis of IBS is based on the Roma IV criteria.
- Diagnosis is based on the finding of recurrent abdominal pain related to defecation or in association with a change in stool frequency or form. Bloating is common.
- Symptoms are chronic such as abdominal pain at least once per week, on average, in the previous 3 months, or altered bowel habits for at least 6 months as per Roma IV criteria.
- No obvious structural or biochemical abnormalities are found in IBS (no fever, no raised C-reactive protein or erythrocyte sedimentation rate, normal haemoglobin, normal serum albumin, negative tests for coeliac disease, etc.).
- The 'alarm features' include anaemia, unexplained loss of body weight, bleeding per rectum, abdominal mass, rectal mass, family history of colorectal cancer, ovarian cancer, inflammatory bowel disease and presence of markers for inflammatory bowel disease; development of symptoms in a male patient after the age of 50 should be carefully considered before making a final diagnosis. These features indicate that IBS is less likely.
- Coeliac antibody test and faecal calprotectin, full blood count and C-reactive protein may be needed.
- The pathogenesis of IBS is explained on the following bases: (i) gut dysmotility, (ii) intestinal hypersensitivity, (iii) postinfectious IBS and (iv) stress response in IBS.
- The management of IBS aims at the following: (i) support and reassurance, (ii) ameliorating the patient's symptoms, (iii) improvement of the quality of life and (iv) patient education.

FURTHER READINGS

Dimidi E, Rossi M, Whelan K. Irritable bowel syndrome and diet: where are we in 2018? *Curr Opin Clin Nutr Metab Care*. 2017;20(6):456-463.

Ford AC, Lacy BE, Talley NJ. Irritable bowel syndrome. *N Engl J Med*. 2017;376(26):2566-2578. Review.

Khoshoo V, Armstead C, Landry L. Effect of a laxative with and without tegaserod in adolescents with constipation predominant irritable bowel syndrome. *Aliment Pharmacol Ther.* 2006;23(1):191-196.

Lesbros-Pantoflickova D, Michetti P, Fried M, Beglinger C, Blum AL. Meta-analysis: the treatment of irritable bowel syndrome. *Aliment Pharmacol Ther.* 2004;20(11-12):1253-1269.

Moayyedi P, Ford AC, Talley NJ, et al. The efficacy of probiotics in the treatment of irritable bowel syndrome: a systematic review. *Gut.* 2010;59(3):325-332. Review.

Pimentel M, Morales W, Chua K, et al. Effects of rifaximin treatment and retreatment in nonconstipated IBS subjects. *Dig Dis Sci.* 2011;56(7): 2067-2072.

Ruepert L, Quartero AO, de Wit NJ, van der Heijden GJ, Rubin G, Muris JW. Bulking agents, antispasmodics and antidepressants for the treatment of irritable bowel syndrome. *Cochrane Database Syst Rev.* 2011;(8):CD003460.

Simrén M, Törnblom H, Palsson OS, Whitehead WE. Management of the multiple symptoms of irritable bowel syndrome. *Lancet Gastroenterol Hepatol.* 2017;2(2):112-122.

Sultan S, Malhotra A. Irritable bowel syndrome. *Ann Intern Med.* 2017;166(11):ITC81-ITC96. Review.

Cardiovascular and Respiratory Systems

CASE 2.1

'Short of Breath . . . '

Allan Goldman, an 18-year-old factory paint worker, comes in to see his general practitioner because he is suffering from bouts of shortness of breath, cough, recurrent respiratory infections and at times chest tightness particularly after exercise. The episodes of shortness of breath started 5–6 years ago but gradually progressed. Recently, he noticed that he wakes up at night because of cough, shortness of breath and wheezing. He usually feels unwell after returning to work from holidays. He also gives a history of watery nose and sneezing with a sense of itching. He has smoked 10 cigarettes per day for the past 5 years. On examination, his pulse is 98/min regular, blood pressure 118/75 mm Hg (supine), temperature 37.0°C and respiratory rate 20/min. Heart sounds are normal and regular, and there are no murmurs or added sounds. Auscultation of the lungs is normal. There is no oedema of the lower limbs. Full blood count, blood urea, creatinine and liver function tests are all normal. The echocardiogram shows normally functioning valves and heart muscles with an ejection fraction of 75%. A 12-lead ECG is normal. A chest X-ray is normal. A spirometry shows a forced expiratory volume of 1 second (FEV_1) of 3.05 L/min (72% of predicted volume). Fifteen minutes after inhalation of salbutamol, the spirometry volume is FEV_1 is 3.80 L/min.

CASE DISCUSSION

Q1. On the basis of Allan's presentation, what is your diagnosis?

Q2. What is your differential diagnosis?

Q3. What are the key clinical features of this disease? What are the scientific bases for these features?

Q4. What is the pathophysiology underlying these changes?

Q5. What are your management goals and management options?

ANSWERS

1. The presentation of this patient is suggestive of bronchial asthma and allergic rhinitis. The supportive evidence for the diagnosis is history of progressive shortness of breath, cough, recurrent respiratory infections and chest tightness. The symptoms wake the patient up at night and are particularly present when he returns back to work (paint factory) from holidays. History of running nose, itching and sneezing is suggestive of allergic rhinitis. The improvement in the FEV_1 after the inhalation of salbutamol is suggestive of the reversibility of the bronchospasm after the inhalation

of a short-acting β-agonist and is supportive of the diagnosis of bronchial asthma. This simple test is usually used to differentiate between bronchial asthma (reversible condition) and chronic obstructive pulmonary disease (COPD; irreversible condition). An increase of about 12% is a cutoff point for a positive result according to the Global Institute for Asthma (GINA) guidelines (Global Strategy for Asthma Management and Prevention, 2016 update).

2. The differential diagnosis of bronchial asthma can be discussed under four headings:

First: Upper respiratory tract disorders
- Foreign body aspiration
- Vocal cord problems
- Laryngotracheal mass
- Tracheal stenosis
- Tracheomalacia
- Angio-oedema
- Airway oedema

Second: Lower respiratory tract disorders
- COPD
- Cystic fibrosis (CF)
- Bronchiectasis
- Allergic bronchopulmonary aspergillosis
- Pneumonia
- Pneumothorax
- Eosinophilic pneumonia

Third: Cardiac conditions and others
- Left-sided heart failure
- Pulmonary oedema
- Pulmonary embolism

Fourth: Differential diagnosis of exercise-induced bronchial asthma
- Anxiety
- Hyperventilation syndrome
- Myopathies
- Vocal cord dysfunction
- Coronary artery disease
- Hypertrophic cardiomyopathy
- Arrhythmias
- Congestive heart failure
- Valvular malfunctions/abnormalities

3. The following are essential for the diagnosis of bronchial asthma:
- Symptoms: Shortness of breath, wheezing, cough and chest tightness. Wheezing may be present with normal breathing. Cough is present at night, and generally symptoms are worse at night.
- There is a history of exposure to allergens such as dust mites, cockroaches, pollen, cats, other animals and chemicals. There is an exposure to mould growth following water damage to a home or building.

- Other factors that may precipitate an asthmatic attack are exercise, rhinitis, sinusitis, cold weather, intake of aspirin and NSAIDs, viral upper respiratory tract infection, postnasal drip, gastro-oesophageal reflux, change in weather, stress, tobacco smoking and passive smoking.
- Symptoms fluctuate over the course of 1 day, from day to day and from month to month.
- Asthma usually displays a diurnal pattern and the lung functions are usually worse in the early morning.
- Clinical signs:
  (a) Physical examination may be normal or show some wheezing.
  (b) Rhinitis or nasal polyps may be present.
  (c) In acute exacerbation, the patient has difficulty in talking and is usually using accessory muscles of inspiration.
  (d) Pulsus paradoxus may be present.
  (e) Changes in the mental status may be present. These changes necessitate immediate aggressive treatment.

4. Laboratory findings: According to the GINA, the diagnosis of asthma is based on the medical history and clinical examination and lung function tests. These tests are as follows:
  (i) FEV_1 ≥12% increase following administration of a bronchodilator of corticosteroids
  (ii) Diurnal variation in Peak expiratory flow (PEF) >20% on more than 3 days in a week for 2 weeks
  (iii) FEV_1 ≥15% decrease after 6 minutes of exercise
  - A diurnal variation in PEF (lowest in the morning) and a variation of ≥20% are consistent with the diagnosis of bronchial asthma. The magnitude of variability may reflect some degree of disease severity.
  - A trial of corticosteroids (30 mg daily over 2 weeks) with documented improvement in FEV_1 or PEF also can confirm the diagnosis of asthma.
  - In patients with a normal lung function test, a challenge test by administering sequentially increasing concentration of histamine or methacholine, a decrease of FEV_1 of 20% is diagnostic of asthma (Table 2.1.1).

5. Pathophysiological changes in asthma:
- Inflammation of the bronchi and small airways (mucosal, submucosal and adventitial oedema)
- Airway smooth muscle constriction
- Narrowing and closure of airways
- Mucous plugs
- Excessive increase in airway smooth muscle mass (hyperplasia)
- Cellular infiltrates of airways (eosinophils, neutrophils, helper T-helper lymphocytes and mast cells)
- Increased airway secretion
- Increased secretion of mucus in airways
- Increased desquamation of airway lining cells
- Capillary enlargement
- Goblet cells hyperplasia

Table 2.1.1 Diagnostic studies in asthma

Routine pulmonary function test Special pulmonary function test	Decreased FEV_1; hyperinflation; improvement with bronchodilator
Methacholine or cold air challenge	Indicates the presence of nonspecific bronchial hyper-reactivity; bronchoconstriction occurs at lower doses in asthma
Challenge with specific agents: occupational, drugs	Occasionally performed
Chest radiograph	Fleeting infiltrates and central bronchiectasis in ABPA
Skin tests	Demonstrate atopy; little value except prick test to *Aspergillus fumigatus* positive in ABPA
Blood tests	Eosinophils and IgE are usually increased in atopy; levels may be very high in ABPA; *Aspergillus precipitins* increased in many, but not all, patients with ABPA

ABPA, allergic bronchopulmonary aspergillosis; FEV_1, forced expiratory volume in 1 second; IgE, immunoglobulin E.
(Source: Andreoli TE, Benjamin IJ, Griggs RC, Wing EJ. Andreoli and Carpenter's Cecil Essentials of Medicine. 8th ed. Philadelphia, PA: Elsevier; 2010.)

Factors precipitating asthma:
* Cold air
* Tobacco smoke
* Dust, acid fumes and mites
* Emotional distress and anxiety
* Respiratory infection (viral/bacterial)
* Exercise
* Environmental pollution
* Sand storms
* Drugs (NSAIDs, β-blockers, aspirin)
* Chemicals, e.g. sulphur dioxide
* Allergens (e.g. fish, nuts, strawberries, dust, pollens, house dust mites, food additives, wood dust)

6. Management:
The goals of management of asthma:
* Patient education
* Treatment of infection
* Avoidance of allergens and other precipitating factors
* Drug treatment – quick relief: β-Adrenergic agonists by inhalation
* Long-term control, e.g. inhaled corticosteroids
* Management of acute severe asthma (high-concentration oxygen, high dose of β$_2$-agonists by nebuliser, systemic corticosteroids, ipratropium bromide by nebuliser or IV aminophylline 250 mg over 20 minutes, monitoring treatment, pulse oximeter, assisted ventilation when needed).

The drugs used in the treatment of asthma are summarised in Table 2.1.2.

Table 2.1.2 Drugs used in treatment of asthma

Drug group	Examples (brand name)	Mechanisms of action	Advantages	Side effects
Short-acting β-adrenergic agonists	Albuterol (Ventolin) Levalbuterol (Xopenex)	A β_2-adrenergic agonist; its binding to β_2 receptors in the lungs → relaxation of bronchial smooth muscles. It increases cAMP production by activating adenylate cyclase → increases the activity of cAMP-dependent protein kinase A, which inhibits the phosphorylation of myosin and lowers intracellular calcium concentrations. A lowered intracellular calcium concentration leads to a smooth muscle relaxation and bronchodilation. In addition, salbutamol inhibits the release of bronchoconstrictor agents from mast cells and inhibits microvascular leakage.	Selective β_2-adrenergic receptor agonist used in treatment of asthma, bronchospasm and chronic obstructive pulmonary disease (COPD). It is used in acute episodes and prophylactically for exercise-induced asthma.	Palpitation, restlessness, nervousness, throat irritation, ankle oedema.
Methylxanthines	Theophylline Aminophylline	These drugs cause inhibition of cyclic nucleotide phosphodiesterase → prevent the conversion of cAMP and cGMP to 5'-AMP and 5'-GMP, respectively. Inhibition of cyclic nucleotide phosphodiesterase → increase of intracellular cAMP and cGMP → bronchodilation, vasodilation and cardiac stimulation.	Used in treatment of asthma, bronchospasm and COPD.	Palpitation, restlessness, vomiting, tremor, agitation, flushing, increased muscle tone, convulsions. Cardiac and nervous system stimulation. If given IV rapidly → syncope and death.
Anticholinergics (muscarinic receptor antagonist)	Ipratropium bromide	These drugs block acetylcholine (anticholinergics) → bronchodilatation and decreased respiratory secretion. Their effect is less than sympathomimetics.	Used in acute asthma and in COPD. Tiotropium has a longer action compared to ipratropium.	Dry mouth, epigastric upset, vomiting, muscle pain, chest discomfort.

Continued

Table 2.1.2 Drugs used in treatment of asthma—cont'd

Drug group	Examples (brand name)	Mechanisms of action	Advantages	Side effects
Inhaled corticosteroids	Beclomethasone (Qvar) Budesonide (Pulmicort) Ciclesonide (Alvesco) Triamcinolone (Azmacort) Flunisolide (Aerobid)	Unbound corticosteroids → cross the cell membranes → bind with specific cytoplasmic receptors → inhibition of leukocyte infiltration at the inflammation area + interference with released inflammatory mediators (anti-inflammatory effects).	Maintenance treatment of asthma as prophylactic therapy.	Mild side effects. However, chronic use could result in suppression of the hypothalamic–pituitary–adrenal axis, resulting in adrenal suppression.
Mast cell stabilisers	Sodium cromoglycate, ketotifen	Ketotifen is a selective, noncompetitive histamine antagonist (H1-receptor) and acts as mast cell stabiliser. It inhibits the release of mediators from mast cells involved in hypersensitivity reactions. Also it decreases chemotaxis and activation of eosinophils. Ketotifen also inhibits cAMP phosphodiesterase and has antiallergic activity. It inhibits the development of airway hyper-reactivity and inhibits platelet-activating factor (PAF)–induced accumulation of eosinophils and platelets in the airways. Ketotifen inhibits the release of allergic mediators such as histamine, leukotrienes C_4 and PAF Sodium cromoglycate inhibits the release of anaphylactic mediators from the mast cells.	Used as add-on or prophylactic therapy in mild atopic asthmatic children.	Headaches, rhinitis, conjunctivitis.

Long-acting inhaled β–agonist	Arformoterol (Brovana) Salmeterol (Serevent)	It stimulates intracellular Adenylyl cyclase, also known as adenylate cyclase, the enzyme that catalyses the conversion of adenosine triphosphate (ATP) to cyclic 3′,5′-adenosine monophosphate (cyclic AMP). Increased intracellular cyclic AMP levels cause relaxation of bronchial smooth muscle and inhibition of release of proinflammatory mediators from cells, especially from mast cells.	Used as bronchodilator for symptomatic treatment of bronchoconstriction in patients with COPD and asthma.	Cardiac and nervous system stimulation and related changes/symptoms.
Leukotriene modifiers	Montelukast (Singulair)	Montelukast selectively antagonises leukotriene D_4 (LTD_4) at the cysteinyl leukotriene receptor, $CysLT_1$, in the human airway. It also prevents airway oedema, smooth muscle contraction and secretion of thick mucus.	Treatment of asthma.	Skin rash, bruising, tingling, numbness, pains, tremors.
Anti-IgE antibody	Omalizumab (Xolair)	Xolair binds to IgE, which prevents their binding to mast cells and basophils.	Used in treatment of asthma caused by allergies.	Fever, muscle aches, rashes, allergic reactions.

BACK TO BASIC SCIENCES

Q1. Discuss the pathogenesis of exercise-induced bronchoconstriction.

- Approximately 90% of patients previously diagnosed with asthma have exercise-induced bronchoconstriction.
- In these patients, the exercise-induced bronchoconstriction is related to exacerbation of the underlying inflammation and airway hyper-reactivity, e.g. environmental irritants such as exposure to sand storms and chlorine gas in swimming pools.
- Only 10% of the general population has exercise-induced bronchoconstriction without underlying asthma. In these patients, the pathophysiology of bronchoconstriction may be related to rapid breathing of cold, dry air over prolonged time. With the end of exercise, the airway responds with vasodilatation to warm the airway, resulting in water loss and engorgement of the airway. These changes stimulate the release of proinflammatory mediators and the development of bronchoconstriction.

Q2. What are the indications to refer a patient with bronchial asthma to hospital?

- Diagnosis difficult to confirm (additional diagnostic tests are required)
- Suspect allergic bronchopulmonary aspergillosis
- Suboptimal response to therapy
- Life-threatening asthma execration requiring hospitalisation

Q3. List the cells involved in the pathogenesis of asthma.

- Macrophages
- Neutrophils
- Mast cells
- B-Lymphocytes
- T-helper lymphocytes
- Eosinophils
- Endothelial cells

REVIEW QUESTIONS

Q1. Airway hyper-reactivity (AHR) challenge test may be positive in all of the following conditions *except*

A. Chronic obstructive pulmonary disease (COPD)

B. Bronchiectasis

C. Cystic fibrosis (CF).

D. Bronchial asthma

E. Normal people

Q2. Which *one* of the following is *not* diagnostic of bronchial asthma?
A. An increase of $\geq$12% in FEV_1 after bronchodilator inhalation
B. A decrease of $\geq$15% in FEV_1 after exercise
C. Diurnal variation $\geq$20% on PEF
D. Hypoinflation on chest X-ray

Q3. Which *one* of the following is *not part* of the pathogenesis of bronchial asthma?
A. Neurogenic mechanisms
B. Airway hyper-reactivity (AHR)
C. Elevated serum-specific IgE
D. Inhibition of cysteinyl leukotrienes

Q4. Which *one* of the following is *less helpful* in the diagnosis of bronchial asthma?
A. Increased eosinophil count in sputum >2%
B. Exhaled breath nitric oxide concentration
C. Total and allergen-specific IgE
D. Diurnal variation of PEF of >20%

Q5. Which *one* of the following is *not correct* about exercise-induced bronchoconstriction?
A. Symptoms peak after exercise.
B. Ninety percent of patients have underlying asthma.
C. Symptoms alone can diagnose majority of patients.
D. Resting spirometry is usually normal.
E. Bronchial provocation tests may be needed.

Q6. Which *one* of the following chest X-ray changes is less likely to be related to bronchial asthma?
A. Hyperinflation of the lung fields
B. Bronchial wall thickening
C. Diminished pulmonary lung vascular shadows
D. Enlarged hilar lymph nodes

ANSWERS

A1. **E.** Patients stated in items A–D have their AHR challenge test positive. Normal individuals have this test not positive.

A2. **D.** Hyperinflation of the lungs is noted in bronchial asthma.

A3. **D.** Increased production of cysteinyl leukotriene is part of the pathogenesis of aspirin-associated asthma.

A4. **B.** Exhaled breath nitric oxide concentration is not well developed to be used in clinical assessment.

A5. **C.** Symptoms alone should not be used to diagnose exercise-induced asthma.

A6. **D.** Enlarged hilar lymph nodes are not consistent with the diagnosis of bronchial asthma.

TAKE-HOME MESSAGE

- Patients with bronchial asthma present with shortness of breath, wheezing, cough and chest tightness.
- Cough is usually at night and generally symptoms are worse at night.
- There is a history of exposure to allergens such as dust mites, cockroaches, pollen, cats and other animals and chemicals.
- Other precipitating factors are exercise, rhinitis, sinusitis, cold weather, intake of aspirin and viral upper respiratory tract infection.
- Symptoms fluctuate over the course of 1 day.
- The patient in severe attack is unable to talk and uses the accessory muscles of inspiration.
- The pathological process is reversible after the use of bronchodilators (this differentiates bronchial asthma from COPD).
- Treatment includes patient education, bronchodilators (β-adrenergic agonists by inhalation) and avoidance of allergens. Corticosteroids may be needed in severe attacks.

FURTHER READINGS

Beasley R, Semprini A, Mitchell EA. Risk factors for asthma: is prevention possible? *Lancet.* 2015;386(9998):1075-1085. Review.

Chung KF. New treatments for severe treatment-resistant asthma: targeting the right patient. *Lancet Respir Med.* 2013;1(8):639-652.

Dennis RJ, Solarte I, Rodrigo G. Asthma in adults. *BMJ Clin Evid.* 2011;2011:1512. Review.

Global Strategy for Asthma Management and Prevention (2016 update). *Global Institute for Asthma.* 2016. Available at: http://ginasthma.org/wp-content/uploads/2016/04/GINA-2016-main-report_tracked.pdf

Jolliffe DA, Greenberg L, Hooper RL, et al. Vitamin D supplementation to prevent asthma exacerbations: a systematic review and meta-analysis of individual participant data. *Lancet Respir Med.* 2017;5(11): 881-890.

Martinez FD, Vercelli D. Asthma. *Lancet.* 2013;382(9901):1360-1372. Review.

Olin JT, Wechsler ME. Asthma: pathogenesis and novel drugs for treatment. *BMJ.* 2014;349:g5517. Review.

Papi A, Brightling C, Pedersen SE, Reddel HK. Asthma. *Lancet.* 2018;391(10122):783-800. Review.

Pavord ID, Bush A, Holgate S. Asthma diagnosis: addressing the challenges. *Lancet Respir Med.* 2015;3(5): 339-341. Review.

Rodrigo G. Asthma in adults (acute). *BMJ Clin Evid.* 2011;2011:1513. Review.

CASE 2.2

'Still Coughing . . .'

Othman Majeed, a 27-year-old information technology officer, comes in to see his general practitioner because he is suffering from cough, expectoration, nocturnal sweating and loss of appetite. He was seen by another general practitioner about 2 weeks earlier for the same problem and was treated with amoxicillin capsules. Although Othman has completed the course of amoxicillin as advised, his cough has progressively increased. Today he noticed blood in his phlegm. On examination, his body temperature is 38°C, pulse rate 110/min, blood pressure 120/80 mm Hg, respiratory rate 25/min and oxygen saturation 98% on room air. He looks ill and depressed. No cyanosis or palpable cervical lymph nodes are present. On chest auscultation, crepitations are heard over the upper left lung zone. Heart is regular S1 + S2, and there are no murmurs or added sounds. On abdominal examination, the abdomen is found to be soft and not tender. There is no organomegaly. There is no peripheral oedema. Chest X-ray shows infiltration of the left upper zone 1.5 × 1.6 cm with signs of cavitation. Sputum Gram stain did not identify any organisms. On performing blood culture (5 days), no growth is found. Many acid-fast (A/F) bacilli (AFB) are found on performing the sputum AFB test. Sputum polymerase chain reaction (PCR) is positive for *Mycobacterium tuberculosis*. Sputum was sent for AFB culture.

CASE DISCUSSION

Q1. On the basis of Othman's presentation, what is your diagnosis?

Q2. What is your differential diagnosis?

Q3. What are the key clinical features of this disease? What are the scientific bases for these features?

Q4. What is the pathophysiology underlying these changes?

Q5. What are your management goals and management options?

ANSWERS

1. The clinical presentation of this patient is suggestive of pulmonary tuberculosis (TB). The supportive evidence for the diagnosis is history of cough and expectoration not responding to broad-spectrum antibiotics, nocturnal sweating, loss of appetite and the presence of blood in his phlegm. The clinical examination shows that he is feverish, has increased respiratory rate and looks ill and depressed. Chest examination shows

crepitations over the upper left lung zone. The chest X-ray confirms the presence of cavitation and infiltration of the left upper lung zone. Gram stain of sputum is negative but A/F stain confirms the presence of many AFB. PCR test is positive for *M. tuberculosis*.

2. The differential diagnosis of pulmonary TB includes the following:
   - Lung abscess
   - Bronchiectasis
   - Aspergillosis – aspergilloma
   - Fungal pneumonia
   - Lung cancer
   - Histoplasmosis
   - Actinomycosis
   - Community-acquired pneumonia
   - Consolidation

3. The clinical picture:
   - Symptoms and signs:
     - Cough
     - Fever
     - Weight loss
     - Sputum production (initially usually dry cough but with time the sputum becomes purulent)
     - Haemoptysis
     - Possibility of presence of pleuritic chest pain
     - Shortness of breath (usually is noted later as the disease progresses)
     - Tiredness, fatigue and progressive wasting
     - Also, patients may present with signs and symptoms suggestive of involvement of other body systems:
       - Central nervous system:
         - Headache
         - Neurological deficit
         - Confusion
         - Coma
       - Genitourinary system:
         - Flank pain
         - Dysuria
         - Frequent micturition
         - Scrotal mass
         - Epididymitis
         - Orchitis
         - Prostatitis (in males)
         - Pelvic inflammatory disease (in females)
       - Gastrointestinal system:
         - Difficulty in swallowing

- Abdominal pain
- Peptic ulcer–like symptoms
- Malabsorption
- Diarrhoea
- Haematochezia

4. Laboratory findings:
   - Sputum smears: Ziehl–Neelsen staining (three sputum samples obtained from the patient early in the morning) must be examined. Finding AFB in the sputum has a 98% positive productive value for culture-positive TB.
   - Auramine fluorescence microscopy is taking over Ziehl–Neelsen staining.
   - AFB culture: This is the most specific test for TB and must be considered even if AFB test was negative.
   - Human immunodeficiency virus (HIV) serology is performed in all patients with positive tests for TB.
   - Blood culture is performed.
   - Nucleic acid amplification test (PCR) is performed.
   - Specific enzyme-linked immunospot (ELISpot) is performed.
   - For patients with rifampicin resistance, the Xpert MTB/RIF is currently promoted by the WHO as a more accurate test for pulmonary TB and detection of rifampicin resistance. The test uses PCR to identify TB DNA and the gene sequences that code the rifampicin resistance. Results can be obtained within 2 hours.
   - Chest X-ray is sensitive but not specific for the diagnosis of active TB. Typical changes that may be found in pulmonary TB may include the following:
     - Consolidation
     - Tracheal deviation
     - Elevation of the hemi-diaphragm
     - Cavities
     - Probably pneumothorax associated with lung changes

5. Pathology and pathogenesis:
   - The disease is spread by inhalation of aerosolised droplet nuclei from other infected patients.
   - Inhaled organisms lodge in the alveoli and trigger macrophages and lymphocytes.
   - Macrophages transform into epithelioid and Langhans giant cells which aggregate with the lymphocytes and form tuberculous granuloma.
   - The typical lesion is an epithelioid granuloma with central caseous necrosis.
   - The primary TB lesion and numerous granulomas aggregate to form the 'Ghon focus' in the periphery of the lung (subpleural lesion).
   - The organisms spread to hilar lymph nodes; the combination of a primary lesion and regional lymph nodes is referred to as the 'primary complex of Ranke'.
   - The tubercles are characterised with the following features (Fig. 2.2.1):
     - A central area of caseation necrosis

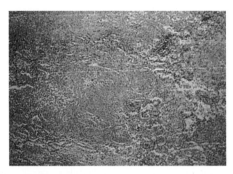

Figure 2.2.1 Histopathological inflammatory changes and formation of caseous necrosis in pulmonary tuberculosis. *(Source: Goering R, Dockrell N, Zuckerman M, Wakelin D, Roitt I, Mims C, Chiodini P. Mims' Medical Microbiology. 4th ed. Lodon, UK: Elsevier; 2007.)*

- An inner cellular zone with dominant presence of Langhans giant cells and epithelioid macrophages
- An outer cellular zone of plasma cells, lymphocytes and some macrophages
- Fibrosis and calcification may occur.
- Blood spread and lymphatic spread may occur before immunity is established resulting in secondary foci in other body organs.
- TB is associated with immunosuppression such as HIV, high doses of corticosteroids, cytotoxic drugs, malignancy, type 1 diabetes, chronic renal failure, silicosis, malnutrition and deficiency of vitamins A and D.

6. Management goals:
   - Chemotherapy – start with quadruple therapy.
   - Treatment continues for 9–12 months.
   - Ameliorate the patient's symptoms.
   - Minimise the transmission of infection (isolation in active disease, report new cases).
   - Educate the patient.
   - Test whether the patient has HIV as well or is immunosuppressed.
   - Provide continuous support, monitor improvement and watch for complications.
   - Improve the nutritional status, prescribe pyridoxine and vitamin supplementation.

Chemotherapy should be initiated immediately in patients with confirmed positive tests. Start with quadruple therapy (rifampicin, isoniazid, pyrazinamide for 2 months), followed by rifampicin and isoniazid for 4 months.

Six-month therapy is appropriate. If the patient is HIV-positive, the treatment should continue to 9–12 months.

Meningitis should be treated to a minimum of 12 months.

Pyridoxine should be prescribed with chemotherapy (to minimise the risk of peripheral neuropathy in patients on isoniazid).

BACK TO BASIC SCIENCES

Q1. Discuss some of the factors that may play a role in increasing the incidence of TB.

- Reactivation of infection acquired in the remote past
- Homeless, drug addicts and imprisoned persons
- Vitamin D and/or vitamin A deficiency, and other nutritional deficiencies
- HIV infection and immunosuppression
- Elderly
- Increased risk of close contact with TB in homeless
- Anti-tuberculous treatment rendered ineffective by antituberculous drug resistance (patients may be semi-infectious for prolonged periods [only 10%–15% of patients are tested for drug resistance])
- Patients with 'latent TB' (approximately 10% of these patients will develop clinical TB in their lifetime [immunosuppression, untreated HIV])

Q2. How would you manage a patient suspected clinically to have pulmonary TB but all three sputum samples for AFB are negative?

- Your aim should be to microbiologically confirm the patient's infection with TB with typing and culture and drug sensitivity testing.
- You should prepare the patient for a bronchoscopy with lavage. This will help to distinguish between TB and other conditions such as bacterial (pneumonia) or tumour.

Q3. Discuss the clinical features of TB in HIV patients.

- It is difficult to diagnose pulmonary TB in HIV and immunosuppressed patients.
- Patients are usually very sick and may die.
- Sputum smears are usually negative for AFB.
- The chest X-rays do not show typical pulmonary TB pattern, have less preference for upper lobe lesion and show fewer or no cavities.
- Extrapulmonary TB is more common and is usually multifocal.
- TB in these patients is treated with standard antituberculous agents.
- Drug interaction: Rifampicin induces the activity of cytochrome P450 CYP3A resulting in a *reduction* in the plasma concentration of protease inhibitors and non-nucleoside reverse transcriptase inhibitors (used in HIV treatment).

Q4. What is a Mantoux test? How would you interpret the results?

Mantoux test, also known as tuberculin test, is a screening test for TB, in which a purified protein derivative is injected intradermally in the forearm and the reaction is read 48–72 hours later. The reading involves measuring in millimetres the diameter of induration (not erythema) developed around the injection. Several factors could affect the interpretation of the results such as HIV infection, recent vaccination and exposure to TB patients and others.

REVIEW QUESTIONS

Q1. One of the main causes for the increasing rates of TB in many cities in developing countries is
A. Drug resistance.
B. Migration from endemic areas.
C. Lack of facilities to diagnose TB.
D. Vitamin D deficiency.
E. Malnutrition.

Q2. Which country/area in the world has the highest percentage of patients with TB coinfected with HIV?
A. The United Kingdom
B. Australia
C. The United States
D. Sub-Saharan Africa
E. South Africa

Q3. Which one of the following is *not* among the clinical features of TB coinfected with HIV?
A. Patients are often sicker.
B. Chest X-ray is less characteristic.
C. The disease is more often extrapulmonary.
D. Sputum is more frequently positive for AFB.

Q4. Which test would you do next in a patient presenting with a clinical picture suggestive of pulmonary TB for more than 4 weeks and three negative sputum samples for AFB?
A. Blood culture
B. Sputum culture
C. Erythrocyte sedimentation rate
D. C-reactive protein
E. Bronchoscopy with lavage

Q5. Which patient with pulmonary TB is more likely to develop aspergilloma?
A. A patient with a smear positive for AFB
B. A patient with haemoptysis
C. A patient with healed fibrocavitary scarring
D. A patient with extrapulmonary TB

ANSWERS

A1. **B.** Migration from endemic areas is the main cause for the increased rates of TB in large cities in developing countries.

A2. **D.** Approximately 74% of patients with TB and coinfection with HIV are in Sub-saharan Africa.

A3. **D.** The sputum is more frequently negative for AFB in these patients.

A4. **E.** Bronchoscopy with lavage will help in obtaining better samples for further analysis.

A5. **C.** An aspergilloma is relatively common in patients with healed TB and a fibro-cavitary scarring formation.

TAKE-HOME MESSAGE

- The disease is spread by inhalation of aerosolised droplet nuclei from other infected patients.
- Inhaled organisms lodge in the alveoli and trigger macrophages and lymphocytes.
- Macrophages transform into epithelioid and Langhans giant cells which aggregate with the lymphocytes and form tuberculous granuloma.
- The typical lesion is an epithelioid granuloma with central caseous necrosis.
- The primary TB lesion and numerous granulomas aggregate to form the 'Ghon focus' in the periphery of the lung (subpleural lesion).
- The organisms spread to hilar lymph nodes; the combination of a primary lesion and regional lymph nodes is referred to as the 'primary complex of Ranke'.
- The tubercles are characterised by the following features: (i) a central area of caseation necrosis; (ii) an inner cellular zone with dominant presence of Langhans giant cells and epithelioid macrophages; and (iii) an outer cellular zone of plasma cells, lymphocytes and some macrophages.
- Symptoms and signs: These include cough, fever, weight loss, sputum production (initially usually dry cough but with time the sputum becomes purulent), haemoptysis, pleuritic chest pain (may be present), shortness of breath (usually is noted later as the disease progress), tiredness, fatigue, progressive wasting and symptoms related to infection of other body organs.
- Investigations include the following: (i) sputum smears – Ziehl–Neelsen staining (three sputum samples obtained from the patient early in the morning); (ii) auramine fluorescence microscopy, which is taking over Ziehl–Neelsen staining; (iii) AFB culture: this is the most specific test for TB and must be considered even if AFB test was negative; (iv) HIV serology in all patients with positive tests for TB; (v) blood culture; (vi) nucleic acid amplification test (PCR); (vii) specific ELISpot; and (viii) chest X-ray, which is sensitive but not specific for the diagnosis of active TB.
- The management goals include the following: (i) chemotherapy – start with quadruple therapy; (ii) treatment continues for 9–12 months; (iii) ameliorate the patient's symptoms; (iv) minimise the transmission of infection (isolation in active disease, report new cases); (v) educate the patient; (vi) test whether the patient has HIV as

well or is immunosuppressed; (vii) provide continuous support, monitor improvement and watch for complications; and (viii) improve the nutritional status, and provide pyridoxine and vitamin supplementation.

FURTHER READINGS

Barnes PF, Cave MD. Molecular epidemiology of tuberculosis. *N Engl J Med*. 2003;349(12):1149-1156. Review.

Detjen AK, DiNardo AR, Leyden J, et al. Xpert MTB/RIF assay for the diagnosis of pulmonary tuberculosis in children: a systematic review and meta-analysis. *Lancet Respir Med*. 2015;3(6):451-461. Review.

Golden MP, Vikram HR. Extrapulmonary tuberculosis: an overview. *Am Fam Physician*. 2005;72(9):1761-1768. Review.

Harries AD, Zachariah R, Corbett EL, et al. The HIV-associated tuberculosis epidemic—when will we act? *Lancet*. 2010;375(9729):1906-1919. Review.

Jasmer RM, Nahid P, Hopewell PC. Clinical practice. Latent tuberculosis infection. *N Engl J Med*. 2002;347(23):1860-1866. Review.

Lawn SD, Zumla AI. Tuberculosis. *Lancet*. 2011;378(9785):57-72. Review.

Potter B, Rindfleisch K, Kraus CK. Management of active tuberculosis. *Am Fam Physician*. 2005;72(11):2225-2232. Review.

Sharma SK, Mohan A, Sharma A, Mitra DK. Miliary tuberculosis: new insights into an old disease. *Lancet Infect Dis*. 2005;5(7):415-430. Review.

Small PM, Fujiwara PI. Management of tuberculosis in the United States. *N Engl J Med*. 2001;345(3):189-200. Review.

Steingart KR, Henry M, Ng V, et al. Fluorescence versus conventional sputum smear microscopy for tuberculosis: a systematic review. *Lancet Infect Dis*. 2006;6(9):570-581. Review.

Ziganshina LE, Eisenhut M. Tuberculosis (HIV-negative people). *BMJ Clin Evid*. 2011;2011:0904. Review.

Zumla A, Raviglione M, Hafner R, von Reyn CF. Tuberculosis. *N Engl J Med*. 2013;368(8):745-755.

CASE 2.3

'I Was Admitted to Hospital . . .'

Mark Aldren, a 68-year-old retired policeman, is brought to the emergency department because he is suffering from productive cough, fever and shaking chills. He has been feeling unwell for the past 3–4 days but over the past 12 hours his cough has become productive of thick yellowish sputum, he has developed shaking chills and fever and he has lost appetite. He has smoked two packs of cigarettes daily for the past 10 years. On examination, he looks unwell, coughs continuously and is semisitting on the bed. His pulse rate is 110/min, temperature 39.3°C, respiratory rate 23/min, blood pressure 140/88 mm Hg and pulse oximetry 93%. Both lungs are resonant to percussion with the exception of the right mid-anterior field which is dull. Auscultation reveals diminished vesicular breathing sound and inspiratory crackles over the right mid-anterior lung field. The remaining lung is normal on auscultation. The patient has no clubbing of fingers. White blood cell count is 17,000/μL, neutrophils 70%, bands 15% and lymphocytes 15%. Chest X-ray supports focal consolidation of the right middle and lower lobes. The patient was admitted to hospital for further investigation and management.

CASE DISCUSSION

Q1. On the basis of Mark's presentation, what is your diagnosis?

Q2. What is your differential diagnosis?

Q3. What are the key clinical features of this disease? What are the scientific bases for these features?

Q4. What is the pathophysiology underlying these changes?

Q5. What are your management goals and management options?

ANSWERS

1. The presentation of this patient is suggestive of community-acquired bacterial pneumonia. The supportive evidence for the diagnosis includes fever and chills, cough with purulent sputum, tachycardia, increased respiratory rate and decreased oxygen saturation. Crackles are heard over the right middle lobe, white blood cells are increased (17,000/μL) and the chest X-ray supports consolidation of the right middle and lower lobes.
2. The differential diagnosis of pneumonia includes the following:
   - Bacterial pneumonia
   - Viral pneumonia

- Aspiration pneumonia
- Bronchitis
- Pulmonary tuberculosis
- Lung abscess
- Pulmonary embolism
- Heart failure
- Lung cancer
- Drug reaction
- Sarcoidosis
- Atelectasis

3. The following are essential for the diagnosis of pneumonia:
   - Symptoms: Acute onset of fever, cough, expectoration (cough and expectoration may be absent), acute severe malaise, chills and pleuritic chest pain (if there is pleurisy); sputum may show streaks of blood, and some patients may have diarrhoea.
   - Elderly patients may present with disorientation, confusion and fatigue.
   - Clinical signs: The patient usually looks ill, with respiratory rate >20/min, oxygen saturation <92% (indicates low partial pressure of oxygen and a low saturation) and tachycardia (the presence of tachycardia and oxygen saturation <90% indicates respiratory distress). There is dullness to percussion of the affected area (this sign may be positive in 50%–60% of patients), bronchial breathing is heard over the lesion and crackles and rales may be also heard.
   - Increased tactile fremitus: This test distinguishes pneumonia from a pleuritic effusion (tactile fremitus is diminished or absent over a pleuritic effusion).
   - Because of the low sensitivity and specificity of clinical signs, radiological images of the chest are of great help.

4. Pathological features:
   - *Streptococcus pneumoniae* is the commonest pathogen in community-acquired pneumonia (CAP) even in patients with chronic obstructive pulmonary disease (COPD).
   - *Haemophilus influenzae* is the second commonest, particularly in older people.
   - Other organisms include atypical organisms in younger people and *Staphylococcus aureus*, *Moraxella catarrhalis* and influenza viruses A and B in older people (Table 2.3.1).
   - Gram-negative bacteria and anaerobic bacteria are usually associated with aspiration.
   - The pathology typically is lobar consolidation and herpetic cold sores are common.
   - The severity of pneumonia can be determined by using CURB-65 score, where:
     C: Confusion
     U: Urea >7 mmol/L
     R: Respiratory rate >30/min
     B: Blood pressure <90 mm Hg or diastolic <60 mm Hg
     65: age >65
   - Other parameters in assessing severity of pneumonia include the following:
     Albumin <30 g/L

Table 2.3.1 Organisms causing community-acquired pneumonia

Bacteria

• *Streptococcus pneumoniae* • *Mycoplasma pneumoniae* • *Legionella pneumophila* • *Chlamydia pneumoniae* • *Haemophilus influenzae*	• *Staphylococcus aureus* • *Chlamydia psittaci* • *Coxiella burnetii* (Q fever) • *Klebsiella pneumoniae* (Freidländer's bacillus)

Viruses

• Influenza virus, parainfluenza virus • Measles virus • Herpes simplex virus • Varicella virus	• Adenovirus • Cytomegalovirus • Coronaviruses (SARS-CoV and MERS-CoV)

MERS, Middle East respiratory syndrome; SARS, severe acute respiratory syndrome.
(Source: Ralston S, Penman I, Strachan M, Hobson R. Davidson's Principles & Practice of Medicine. 23rd ed. UK: Elsevier; 2018.)

White blood cells <4 or >20 × 10^9/L

Severe hypoxia

Bilateral disease or a disease affecting several lobules

- Pathological stages:
    - **(i)** Stage of congestion
    - **(ii)** Stage of red hepatisation
    - **(iii)** Stage of grey hepatisation
    - **(iv)** Stage of resolution
- Possible complications of pneumonia include respiratory failure, pleural effusion, empyema (less common), lung abscess (rare), cavitation and lung fibrosis.

5. Management goals:
    - Support
    - Ameliorating the patient's symptoms
    - Appropriate antibiotic treatment for 1–2 weeks
    - Monitoring and assessing for complications
    - Ventilatory support when needed
    - Educating the patient
    - Prevention by pneumococcal vaccine

BACK TO BASIC SCIENCES

Q1. What is the definition of pneumonia?

- It is an infection of the lung parenchyma causing a lower respiratory and pulmonary infiltrate detected on a chest radiograph.
- Patients usually present with cough, acute onset of fever, expectoration, malaise and chills, and may have pleuritic chest pain. In elderly patients, disorientation, confusion and fatigue may occur.

- Viral pneumonia may present with rhinorrhoea and sore throat.
- Pneumonia may be classified into CAP, hospital-acquired pneumonia (HAP), ventilation-associated pneumonia (VAP), typical and atypical pneumonia and aspiration pneumonia.

Q2. Discuss the predisposing factors for pneumonia.
- Cigarette smoking
- Excessive intake of alcohol
- Malnutrition
- Hepatic and renal diseases
- Diabetes mellitus
- Immunoglobulin deficiencies
- AIDS (100-fold increases in bacterial pneumonia)
- Physical exhaustion and stress
- COPD
- Cystic fibrosis, bronchitis or other structural damages of the lungs
- Patients on corticosteroids
- Immunocompromised patients
- Pregnancy (increases the risk)
- Old age (diminished gag and cough reflexes, poor glottal function, changes in immune system responses, diminished toll-like receptor responses)
- Patients with epilepsy/seizure
- People with neurological disorders affecting swallowing involving the cranial nerves 7, 9 and 10

Q3. What are the types of pneumonia?
- CAP: It occurs outside the hospital or within 48 hours of hospital admission.
- HAP: It occurs within 48 hours after admission to hospital or other health facilities.
- VAP: It develops 48 hours after placing patients on a mechanical ventilator/endotracheal intubation.
- Typical bacterial pneumonia: It is usually caused by *S. pneumoniae*, *H. influenzae* and *Klebsiella pneumoniae*.
- Atypical pneumonia: It is usually caused by *Mycoplasma pneumoniae*.
- Aspiration pneumonia: It occurs in alcoholics, patients with seizures and those with neurological lesions affecting swallowing (gag reflex). Aspiration of mixed micro-aerophilic and anaerobic organisms of the mouth and upper respiratory tract is responsible.

Q4. To whom would you recommend pneumococcal vaccination?
(i) Those older than 65 years; (ii) asplenic patients; (iii) splenic dysfunction (e.g. celiac disease); (iv) chronic respiratory, heart, renal or liver conditions; (v) immunosuppressed patients; and (vi) patients with cerebrospinal fluid leak.

REVIEW QUESTIONS

Q1. Which *one* of the following is the most likely cause of pneumonia in a patient using intravenous drugs?
A. *H. influenzae*
B. *M. catarrhalis*
C. *Pseudomonas aeruginosa*
D. *S. aureus*

Q2. Which *one* of the following is the most likely cause of pneumonia in a patient giving a history of exposure to birds?
A. *Chlamydophila psittaci*
B. *S. pneumoniae*
C. *H. influenzae*
D. *S. aureus*

Q3. Which *one* of the following describes the mechanism by which *M. pneumoniae* causes pneumonia?
A. Replicates within epithelium cell lining airways
B. Adheres to the cell surface and impairs ciliary activity
C. Stimulates secondary bacterial infection
D. Adversely affects phagocytic cells
E. Adheres to specific cellular receptors and replicates within cells

Q4. In a patient with pneumonia, which *one* of the following clinical findings raises concerns of impending respiratory distress?
A. Tachycardia plus oxygen saturation (SaO_2) <90%
B. Increased respiratory rate to 20/min
C. Oxygen saturation (SaO_2) <92%
D. Tachycardia 120/min

Q5. On a chest X-ray of a patient with pneumonia, which organism is responsible for radiological changes showing a mass within a cavity with no fluid level?
A. *H. influenzae*
B. *Aspergillus*
C. *Mycoplasma*
D. *Pneumocystis jirovecii*

Q6. In an elderly patient with pneumonia, which *one* of the following biochemical tests can differentiate between bacterial and nonbacterial infections?
A. Serum lactate dehydrogenase
B. Serum procalcitonin

C. Serum C-reactive protein
D. White blood cell count

Q7. In a patient with pneumonia, which *one* of the following causative organisms could be identified by Gram stain?
A. *Legionella*
B. *Mycobacterium*
C. *Mycoplasma*
D. *Chlamydophila*
E. *H. influenzae*

Q8. In patients with pneumonia, which *one* of the following microbiological tests is considered the gold standard for diagnosing influenza virus infection?
A. Sputum polymerase chain reaction (PCR)
B. Viral culture
C. Enzyme-linked immunosorbent assay (ELISA)
D. Sputum Gram stain

Q9. Which *one* of the following is the most commonly identified infectious cause of community-acquired pneumonia?
A. *Pseudomonas*
B. Rhinovirus
C. *S. pneumoniae*
D. Respiratory syncytial virus
E. *K. pneumoniae*

ANSWERS

A1. **D.** In intravenous drug users, the common organisms causing pneumonia are *S. aureus*, *M. tuberculosis* and *S. pneumoniae*.

A2. **A.** The most common causes of pneumonia in patients exposed to birds are *Cryptococcus neoformans*, *Chlamydia psittaci* and *Histoplasma capsulatum*.

A3. **B.** *M. pneumoniae* adheres to the cell surface and impairs the ciliary activity and generates toxic substances. On the other hand, *Chlamydophila pneumoniae* adheres to specific receptors and replicates with lung cells. Influenza virus directly invades columnar epithelium cells resulting in pathological changes (vacuolisation and desquamation) of these cells.

A4. **A.** In patients with pneumonia, tachycardia and SaO_2 of less than 90% should be considered as impending respiratory distress. An increase of respiratory rate up to 25/min should also be considered as a serious sign.

A5. **B.** *Aspergillus* usually present as a growth/mass within a cavity causing a distinct appearance of 'a fungus ball' surrounded by a halo of air. On the other hand, 'patchy' pneumonia may be due to bacteria, viruses, *Mycoplasma* or *Chlamydophila*. *P. jirovecii* causes a diffuse interstitial infiltrate.

A6. **B.** Elevated serum procalcitonin level increases the likelihood of a bacterial infection, whereas a low level opposes such diagnosis. This may help in the early diagnosis of bacterial pneumonia and the commencement of antibiotics. However, in up to 25% of patients with bacterial pneumonia, the procalcitonin level is normal.

A7. **E.** *Legionella*, *Mycobacterium*, *Mycoplasma* and *Chlamydophila* do not readily accept Gram stain.

A8. **A.** PCR is the gold standard for the diagnosis of influenza pneumonia and not viral culture. ELISA can detect pneumococcal cell wall or capsular polysaccharide in the urine with pneumococcal pneumonia. *Legionella* pneumonia, *H. capsulatum* and *Cryptococcus* can also be detected by ELISA.

A9. **C.** *S. pneumoniae* is the most common organism identified in CAP. *Pseudomonas* and other Gram-negative bacteria generally cause pneumonia in patients who have pathological damage (underlying chronic respiratory disease affecting the lungs) or those on corticosteroids, or who are immunocompromised. *Klebsiella* is not a common organism in CAP. Viruses may become a common cause in epidemics.

TAKE-HOME MESSAGE

- Pneumonia is exudative inflammatory solidification of the lung parenchyma; most is managed in primary care.
- The most common symptoms are fever, expectoration, dyspnoea, pleuritic pain and haemoptysis.
- The most common clinical signs are fever, tachycardia, tachypnoea and signs of consolidation.
- In the elderly, the presentation may be different than classical presentation. For example, pneumonia may present with confusion.
- *S. pneumoniae* is the commonest pathogen in CAP even in patients with COPD.
- *H. influenzae* is the second commonest, particularly in older people.
- Other organisms include atypical organisms in younger people and *S. aureus*, *M. catarrhalis* and influenza viruses A and B in older people.
- Gram-negative bacteria and anaerobic bacteria are usually associated with aspiration.
- The pathology typically is lobar consolidation and herpetic cold sores are common.
- The severity of pneumonia can be determined by using CURB-65 score.
- Common complications in pneumonia include respiratory failure, pleural effusion, empyema (less common), lung abscess (rare), cavitation and lung fibrosis.

- Management includes appropriate antibiotic treatment for 1–2 weeks, support, monitoring for complications, treatment of complications, oxygen therapy and ventilation support when needed, patient education and prevention (e.g. vaccination).
- Vaccination by pneumococcal vaccine is recommended in the following: (i) those older than 65 years; (ii) asplenic patients; (iii) splenic dysfunction (e.g. celiac disease); (iv) chronic respiratory, heart, renal or liver conditions; (v) immunosuppressed patients; and (vi) patients with cerebrospinal fluid leak.

FURTHER READINGS

Barlow GD, Lamping DL, Davey PG, Nathwani D. Evaluation of outcomes in community-acquired pneumonia: a guide for patients, physicians, and policy-makers. *Lancet Infect Dis.* 2003;3(8):476-488. Review.

Corrales-Medina VF, Musher DM, Shachkina S, Chirinos JA. Acute pneumonia and the cardiovascular system. *Lancet.* 2013;381(9865):496-505. Review.

Cunha BA, Burillo A, Bouza E. Legionnaires' disease. *Lancet.* 2016;387(10016):376-385. Review.

File TM. Community-acquired pneumonia. *Lancet.* 2003;362(9400):1991-2001. Review.

Garau J. Treatment of drug-resistant pneumococcal pneumonia. *Lancet Infect Dis.* 2002;2(7):404-415. Review.

Musher DM, Thorner AR. Community-acquired pneumonia. *N Engl J Med.* 2014;371(17):1619-1628. Review.

Prina E, Ranzani OT, Torres A. Community-acquired pneumonia. *Lancet.* 2015;386(9998):1097-1108. Review.

van der Poll T, Opal SM. Pathogenesis, treatment, and prevention of pneumococcal pneumonia. *Lancet.* 2009;374(9700):1543-1556. Review.

CASE 2.4

'I Have Been Smoking for Over 20 Years . . . '

Ahmed Ayhan, a 68-year-old gardener, presents to the emergency department with severe shortness of breath and cough. Ahmed has a history of progressive dyspnoea for the past 2–3 years and chronic cough which is productive particularly in the morning; he usually coughs up white sputum. Ahmed has no chest pain and gives no history of palpitation or high blood pressure. He has smoked two packs of cigarettes daily for over 20 years. On examination, the pulse rate is 110/min, respiratory rate 28 breaths/min, blood pressure 130/88 mm Hg and temperature 37.0°C. He has no clubbing of fingers. His chest is barrel-shaped and he uses accessory muscles of respiration. A prolonged expiratory phase is noted. He has no cyanosis and a mild oedema of the ankles. On auscultation, the heart sounds are distant, with some wheezes all over his lungs. Pulse oximeter reading is 93%. Pulmonary function tests, in his hospital file, show a decrease of forced expiratory volume in 1 second (FEV_1) and a decrease of FEV_1/forced vital capacity (FVC) ratio. Chest X-ray shows hyperinflation of lungs, low diaphragms and increased retrosternal airspace.

CASE DISCUSSION

Q1. On the basis of Ahmed's presentation, what is your diagnosis?

Q2. What is your differential diagnosis?

Q3. What are the key clinical features of this disease? What are the scientific bases for these features?

Q4. What is the pathophysiology underlying these changes?

Q5. What are your management goals and management options?

ANSWERS

1. The presentation of this patient is suggestive of chronic obstructive pulmonary disease (COPD). The supportive evidence for the diagnosis is a history of progressive shortness of breath and productive cough in a patient older than 40 years together with a history of smoking two packs of cigarettes daily for over 20 years. On examination, the patient has a barrel-shaped chest and uses accessory muscles of respiration. He has a prolonged expiratory phase and a mild oedema of the ankles.

On auscultation, the heart sounds are distant, with some wheezes all over his lungs. Pulmonary function tests show a decrease of FEV_1 and a decrease of FEV_1/FVC ratio. These findings are supportive of the diagnosis of COPD.

2. The differential diagnosis of COPD includes the following:
   - Asthma: In asthma, patients present at an earlier age, usually have a history of atopy and not necessarily give a history of smoking. They usually show variability of symptoms over time and the obstruction of airways is reversible after using bronchodilators.
   - Bronchiectasis: These patients give a history of cough and expectoration (purulent sputum) and chest CT scans show a predominant bronchitis component. These patients have finger clubbing (no clubbing of fingers in patients with COPD).
   - Bronchiolitis obliterans: These patients have severe irreversible airway obstruction, shortness of breath, a dry cough, wheezing and tiredness. The disease may be associated with collagen vascular disease, usually seen after lung transplantation or bone marrow transplantation and also described after exposure to certain industrial inhalants. If patients are not smokers and have the symptoms of the disease, the diagnosis can be made on the basis of history. Chest X-ray is usually normal. The diagnosis is based on CT scan of the chest, pulmonary function tests or lung biopsy.

3. The following are essential for the diagnosis of COPD:
   - Symptoms: These include progressive shortness of breath, chronic cough, sputum production, wheezing, impaired exercise tolerance, history of smoking (20% of patients have no history of smoking) and history of occupational exposure to toxicants.
   - Clinical signs: There are no findings; clinical signs include a barrel-shaped chest, low diaphragm (by percussion), prolonged expiratory phase, use of accessory muscles of respiration, distant heart sounds, chest auscultation (rhonchi, wheezes, rattles), cyanosis (may be present), pedal oedema, distended jugular veins and cor pulmonale.
   - In advanced disease, cachexia (loss of muscles and subcutaneous fat) is present.
   - There is *no* clubbing. The presence of clubbing of a finger should suggest another diagnosis.
   - Laboratory findings: The key point here is that COPD is an irreversible airflow obstruction.
     (i) Spirometry:
        - It involves the measurement of post-bronchodilator FEV_1 and FVC.
        - A post-bronchodilator FEV_1/FVC ratio <0.7 is consistent with the diagnosis of airflow obstruction.
     (ii) Chest X-ray:
        - It shows gross hyperinflation, flattened hemidiaphragms, horizontal rib configuration and 'stretched' cardiac silhouette.

　　　– A chest X-ray also helps in the detection of bullae, heart failure or lung cancer.

(iii) Full blood count:
　　　– The presence of polycythaemia (secondary to decreased oxygen saturation) may require further assessment.

(iv) α_1-Antitrypsin concentration:
　　　– Should be measured in all patients who present at a young age, have a family history of COPD or have a minimal smoking history (<20 pack-years)

(v) Pulse oximeter and arterial blood gases:
　　　– Pulse oximetry may prompt referral for a domiciliary oxygen assessment if <93%.

(vi) CT chest scan:
　　　– May be required in cases that are difficult to diagnose or there is difficulty to manage the patient

(vii) Other tests:
　　　– Sputum culture
　　　– Full pulmonary function tests
　　　– Echocardiogram to assess elevated pulmonary artery pressure and right ventricular dysfunction
　　　– Health status questionnaire which provides valuable clinical information to the treating doctor

4. Pathological features:
- The underlying pathophysiology is chronic inflammation triggered by inhalation of toxic particles and gases (e.g. tobacco smoke).
- The chronic inflammation results in narrowing of small airways and release of proteases that result in two main changes:
First, damage of the airspaces distal to the terminal bronchioles and loss of the diffusing surface and exchange of gases (emphysema)
Second, dissolved elastin and loss of lung elasticity and the ability of airways to keep open during expiration (loss of the elastic recoil of the lungs)
- In COPD, several factors affect the severity of inflammation/damage of the airways and lungs including genetics, oxidative stress, endogenous antioxidants, disease exacerbation and exposure to toxins.

5. Management goals:
- Reducing frequency of exacerbation
- Slowing disease progression
- Monitoring for complications
- Patient education:
　(1) Inhalation therapy:
　　　– Maximal bronchodilation using both short- and long-acting β_2-adrenoceptor agonists and antimuscarinic agents plus anti-inflammatory (inhaled corticosteroids)

(2) Oral theophylline (slow release):
  – The serum theophylline concentration should be checked 3–5 days after the start of treatment and 1 week later and then once every 6 months.

(3) Oral mucolytic therapy:
  – Particularly in patients who have cough and sputum load

(4) Oxygen therapy:
  – Long-term oxygen therapy should be considered in a patient with arterial partial pressure of oxygen <7.3 kPa
  – It should be used for a minimum of 15 hours/day.

(5) Smoking cessation:
  – It is important to teach the patient about the role of smoking in the progression of the disease and to start a program to complete cessation of smoking.
  – Reduction of the number of cigarettes smoked each day has little effect.

(6) Pulmonary rehabilitation:
  – Exercise should be encouraged at all stages.
  – A multidisciplinary program involving physical training, patient education, nutritional counselling and vaccination should be started at earlier stages.

(7) Surgical intervention:
  – Bullectomy (removal of a bulla)
  – Lung volume reduction surgery
  – Lung transplantation in selected patients with advanced disease

BACK TO BASIC SCIENCES

Q1. What is the definition of COPD?
- COPD is a chronic, persistent, progressive and irreversible airway limitation.
- It is characterised by narrowing of the small airways, decreased elastic recoil of the lungs and decreased capacity of the airways to remain open during expiration resulting in air trapping and hyperinflation.
- It results from pathological structural changes due to chronic inflammation.
- Patients usually give a history of smoking and/or exposure to chemicals.
- COPD can be differentiated from asthma by observing a change in the post-bronchodilator FEV_1/FVC ratio. A change in the post-bronchodilator FEV_1/FVC ratio less than 70% is diagnostic for COPD and can differentiate COPD from asthma, which shows a *reversible* airway obstruction.

Q2. Briefly discuss the pathophysiology of COPD.
- The underlying pathophysiology is chronic inflammation triggered by inhalation of toxic particles and gases (e.g. tobacco smoke).
- The chronic inflammation results in narrowing of small airways and release of proteases that result in two main changes:
  First, damage of the airspaces distal to the terminal bronchioles and loss of the diffusing surface and exchange of gases (emphysema)

Second, dissolved elastin and loss of lung elasticity and the ability of airways to keep open during expiration (loss of the elastic recoil of the lungs)

- In COPD, several factors affect the severity of inflammation/damage of the airways and lungs including genetics, oxidative stress, endogenous antioxidants, disease exacerbation and exposure to toxins.

Q3. Briefly discuss the effects of loss of elasticity and the meaning of static and dynamic hyperinflation.

Progressive loss of elasticity of the lung results in the development of static and dynamic hyperinflation.

a. Static hyperinflation: It is due to loss of recoil properties of the lungs and inability to exhale fully.

b. Dynamic hyperinflation: It is due to the start of inhalation before full exhalation. Air trapping occurs because the air volume inspired exceeds the expiratory air volume resulting in increased tidal volume and increased respiratory rate.

These changes of air trapping and hyperinflation of the lungs result in reducing the effectiveness of the diaphragm and stimulate the use of accessory muscles of breathing and also cause a decrease in chest wall compliance.

Q4. What are the risk factors for COPD development?

- Smoking (however, 20% or more of COPD patients are nonsmokers; factors related to smoking include age at which the patient started to smoke, maternal smoking during pregnancy, active smoking during adolescence, total pack-years smoked and current smoking status, plus other comorbidities)
- Being a relative to a patient with COPD (possibly environmental or genetic)
- Genetics (α_1-antitrypsin deficiency)
- Childhood viral respiratory infections
- Childhood asthma
- Occupational exposure to toxicants
- Environmental pollution
- Recurrent respiratory infections

Q5. What does elastic recoil of the lung refer to?

It refers to the lung's tendency to deflate after inflation.

Q6. What are the main lung and heart pathophysiological changes in COPD?

- Loss of lung elasticity
- Increased airway resistance to airflow in small airways
- Airflow obstruction (narrow airways)
- Impaired left ventricular filling
- Decreased stroke volume
- Decreased cardiac output (*no* reduction in the ejection fraction)

Q7. How is gas exchange affected in COPD?

- Early stages of COPD: Hypoxaemia (due to ventilation–perfusion mismatch)
- Severe COPD: Hypercapnia (may be absent), wasted ventilation due to inadequate pulmonary blood flow and A–a gradient for oxygen larger than expected for the patient's age; can be clinically corrected by low concentration of oxygen

REVIEW QUESTIONS

Q1. In COPD, which *one* of the following is the single best indicator of severity?
A. First second (FEV_1)
B. Total lung capacity
C. Residual volume
D. Chest X-ray
E. Chest CT scan

Q2. Emphysema associated with α_1-antitrypsin deficiency is characterised by all of the following *except*
A. Panacinar type of emphysema.
B. Predominantly basal emphysema.
C. Predominantly apical emphysema.
D. Patients with MZ heterozygote.

Q3. Which *one* of the following is a genetic risk with a major impact on COPD development?
A. Defective DNA repair
B. α_1-Antitrypsin deficiency
C. CFTR gene
D. Deletion of part of chromosome 3

Q4. In COPD, which *one* of the following changes does not occur?
A. Enlargement of the bronchial mucous glands
B. Expansion of the epithelial goblet cell population
C. Decreased $CD8^+$ lymphocytes in cartilaginous airway
D. Mucous plugging

Q5. Which *one* of the following about α_1-antitrypsin is correct?
A. It is a protein inhibitor of neutrophil elastase.
B. It is responsible for centriacinar emphysema in humans.
C. Cigarette smoking decreases cell-derived proteinases.
D. It is largely produced in the lungs.

Q6. In patients with advanced COPD, the distal airway walls are characteristically infiltrated with
A. CD8$^+$.
B. CD4$^+$.
C. B lymphocytes.
D. Eosinophils.
E. CD8$^+$, CD4$^+$, B lymphocytes.

ANSWERS

A1. **A.** First second (FEV$_1$) is the single best indicator of the severity of COPD. None of the other items stated has such ability.

A2. **C.** Emphysema in patients with α_1-antitrypsin deficiency is of panacinar type and is predominantly basal. Patients with MZ heterozygote have α_1-antitrypsin level about half of normal and are at risk of developing emphysema.

A3. **B.** α_1-Antitrypsin deficiency is the only genetic risk factor proven to have a role in the development of COPD. The CFTR gene mutation is responsible for cystic fibrosis. A small deletion of chromosome 3 is associated with small cell lung cancer.

A4. **C.** Inflammatory response consisting of neutrophils, macrophages and CD8$^+$ T lymphocytes is seen in the cartilage airways of COPD patients. In older patients with established COPD, the inflammatory response becomes more intense. The distal airways (small airways) are mainly involved causing thicker airways and smaller lumens and airway resistance.

A5. **A.** α_1-Antitrypsin is a protein inhibitor of neutrophil elastase. Its deficiency is responsible for panacinar emphysema development. Cigarette smoking increases cell-derived proteinases, which result in degrading the lung elastic tissues and other matrix compartments including collagen, proteoglycans and fibronectin and the development of COPD. Neutrophils produce a number of serine proteinases including proteinase 3, cathepsin G and matrix metalloproteinases.

A6. **E.** In COPD, the infiltration of the distal airway walls comprises CD4$^+$, CD8$^+$ and B lymphocytes. These changes are responsible for the development of smooth muscles, increased goblet cells and stimulation of connective tissue matrix synthesis.

TAKE-HOME MESSAGE

- COPD is caused by tobacco smoking, and it is the third leading cause of death worldwide.
- Smoking cessation is an important approach for preventing and delaying the disease progression and should be considered in every patient.

- The disease is characterised by progressive shortness of breath, chronic cough, sputum production, wheezing, impaired exercise tolerance, history of smoking or exposure to chemicals.
- COPD is an irreversible airway obstruction, whereas bronchial asthma is reversible. This is important in differentiating between these two diseases.
- A post-bronchodilator FEV_1/FVC ratio of <0.7 is consistent with the diagnosis of airway obstruction.
- α_1-Antitrypsin deficiency is the only genetic risk factor proven to have a role in the development of COPD. Patients with α_1-antitrypsin deficiency usually present with COPD at a younger age and have a minimal smoking history (<20 pack-years).
- The aims of management are reducing frequency and exacerbations, slowing disease progression and minimising complications (mainly respiratory failure, right-sided heart failure and lung cancer).

FURTHER READINGS

Bateman ED, Reddel HK, van Zyl-Smit RN, Agusti A. The asthma-COPD overlap syndrome: towards a revised taxonomy of chronic airways diseases? *Lancet Respir Med.* 2015;3(9):719-728. Review.

Casaburi R, ZuWallack R. Pulmonary rehabilitation for management of chronic obstructive pulmonary disease. *N Engl J Med.* 2009;360(13):1329-1335. Review.

Niewoehner DE. Clinical practice. Outpatient management of severe COPD. *N Engl J Med.* 2010; 362(15):1407-1416. Review.

Postma DS, Bush A, van den Berge M. Risk factors and early origins of chronic obstructive pulmonary disease. *Lancet.* 2015;385(9971):899-909. Review.

Postma DS, Rabe KF. The asthma-COPD overlap syndrome. *N Engl J Med.* 2015;373(13):1241-1249. Review.

Rabe KF, Watz H. Chronic obstructive pulmonary disease. *Lancet.* 2017;389(10082):1931-1940. Review.

Rennard SI, Drummond MB. Early chronic obstructive pulmonary disease: definition, assessment, and prevention. *Lancet.* 2015;385(9979):1778-1788. Review.

Silverman EK, Sandhaus RA. Clinical practice. Alpha1-antitrypsin deficiency. *N Engl J Med.* 2009; 360(26):2749-2757. Review.

Vanfleteren LEGW, Spruit MA, Wouters EFM, Franssen FME. Management of chronic obstructive pulmonary disease beyond the lungs. *Lancet Respir Med.* 2016;4(11):911-924. Review.

Wenzel RP, Fowler AA III, Edmond MB. Antibiotic prevention of acute exacerbations of COPD. *N Engl J Med.* 2012;367(4):340-347. Review.

CASE 2.5

'Nearly Fainted in the Bathroom …'

John Michael, a 67-year-old journalist, received palliative chemotherapy for inoperable colorectal cancer. Today he is seen at the emergency department because he is suffering from sudden onset of shortness of breath. He gives a history of near fainting while in the bathroom 2 hours earlier. On admission, his pulse rate is 110 beats/min, respiratory rate 25 breaths/min, blood pressure 110/75 mm Hg, temperature 36.9°C and oxygen saturation 92%. His jugular veins are distended. On heart auscultation, S1 and S2 are heard. No murmur or added sounds are present. There are no clinical signs supportive of deep vein thrombosis. Chest X-ray shows no evidence of metastasis and both lung fields are clear.

CASE DISCUSSION

Q1. On the basis of John's presentation, what is your diagnosis?

Q2. What is your differential diagnosis?

Q3. What are the key clinical features of this disease? What are the scientific bases for these features?

Q4. What is the pathophysiology underlying these changes?

Q5. What are your management goals and management options?

ANSWERS

1. The presentation of this patient is suggestive of pulmonary embolism. As per the Wells clinical prediction rule for the likelihood of pulmonary embolism, this patient has a heart rate of >100 beats/min = 1.5 points; malignancy = 1 point; and an alternative diagnosis less likely than pulmonary embolism = 3 points. Therefore, he has a clinical probability of 5.5 (a moderate score of pulmonary embolism as per Wells criteria is 2–6 points). The next step is to order D-dimer test and if the results are positive, the patient should be evaluated to undergo computed tomography pulmonary angiography (CTPA) to confirm the diagnosis of pulmonary embolism.

2. The differential diagnosis of pulmonary embolism includes the following:
   - Heart failure
   - Pneumonia
   - Lung cancer/pulmonary metastasis
   - Asthma

- Chronic obstructive pulmonary disease
- Acute coronary syndrome
- Pericarditis
- Rib fracture

3. The following are essential for the diagnosis of pulmonary embolism:
   - Symptoms: These include dyspnoea of sudden onset, at rest or with minimal effort (the shortness of breath is progressive in severity), pleuritic chest pain may be present, haemoptysis (particularly in the presence of pulmonary infarction), risk factors for thrombotic pulmonary embolism (surgery, immobilisation, cancer), deep venous thrombosis (DVT; leg pain, swelling, tenderness along deep leg veins, dusky blue colour of the skin) and lightheadedness/syncope.
   - Clinical signs: These include tachypnoea, tachycardia, hypoxaemia, palpitations, anxiety, central and peripheral cyanosis, a gallop rhythm (heart failure); distended jugular veins if heart failure develops, a widely split second heart sound and loud pulmonic component, and right ventricular heave (massive pulmonary embolism and high pulmonary pressure).
   - Hypotension plus hypoxaemia and increased cardiac work may trigger angina or acute myocardial infarction.
   - Table 2.5.1 summarises the Revised Geneva score and Wells score for clinical prediction of the diagnosis of pulmonary embolism.

Table 2.5.1 Revised Geneva and Wells clinical predictions for calculating the probability of pulmonary embolism

Revised Geneva score		Wells score	
Variables	Scores	Variables	Scores
Age 65 years or above	1	Previous DVT or pulmonary embolism	1.5
Previous DVT or pulmonary embolism	3	Recent surgery or immobilisation	1.5
Surgery or fracture within 1 month	2	Cancer	1
Active malignancy	2	Haemoptysis	1
Unilateral lower limb pain	3	Heart rate greater than 100 beats/min	1.5
Haemoptysis	2	Clinical signs of DVT	3
Heart rate 75–94/min	3	Other diagnosis less likely than pulmonary embolism	3
Heart rate ≥95/min	5		
Pain on deep palpation of lower limb and unilateral oedema	4		
Clinical probability: • Low, 0–3 • Intermediate, 4–10 • High, >11		Clinical probability: • Low, <2 • Intermediate, 2–6 • High, >6	

DVT, deep venous thrombosis.

4. Investigations:
- The symptoms and signs of pulmonary embolism including evidence of DVT and routine tests such as hypoxaemia and hypocapnia have low sensitivity and specificity for the diagnosis of pulmonary embolism.
- ECG and chest X-ray also have low sensitivity and specificity (ECG may show sinus tachycardia, or atrial fibrillation, right-axis deviation).
- However, the combination of symptoms and predisposing factors could determine the probability of the clinical diagnosis of pulmonary embolism.
- The use of Wells score or Geneva score is recommended and they help in the process of clinical diagnosis (Table 2.5.1).

(i) D-dimer test:
  - It is recommended in patients with clinical suspicion of the diagnosis of pulmonary embolism.
  - A D-dimer level <0.5 mg/L rules out the presence of circulating fibrin and intravascular thrombosis.
  - A negative D-dimer may eliminate the need for further testing in approximately 30% of patients suspected of having pulmonary embolism.
  - However, D-dimer can be elevated in patients older than 80 years, hospitalised patients (venipuncture and venous stasis), patients with cancer and pregnant women.

(ii) Imaging of the leg veins:
  - Ultrasonographic examination of proximal and distal veins of the legs
  - Single-detector CT angiography or multidetector CT angiography
  - Identification of DVT, which may be sufficient to confirm the venous thromboembolism

(iii) CT Pulmonary Angiogram (CTPA):
  - Multidetector CTPA is the recommended imaging for nonmassive pulmonary embolism detection.
  - This technique can diagnose pulmonary embolism with 98% sensitivity.
  - In patients with a negative CTPA, even if there were a clinical possibility of pulmonary embolism, it is reasonable to exclude pulmonary embolism and consider further imaging of the leg by ultrasound or invasive angiography.

(iv) Ventilation/perfusion lung scan (V/Q scan):
  - V/Q scan is an alternative to CTPA when injection of a contrast dye is a concern.
  - Normal scan rules out the diagnosis particularly when the clinical evidence is low.
  - A high probability scan together with a high clinical evidence supports the diagnosis of pulmonary embolism.

(v) Other tools:
  - Bedside echocardiography may be valuable if CT scan is not available or if the patient is unstable.

– Magnetic resonance imaging does not have adequate sensitivity for distal pulmonary branches.

5. Management goals:
    • Prevention in patients at a higher risk of developing pulmonary embolism (aspirin or low-molecular-weight heparin [LMWH], mobility as in long travel).
    • Management of the first idiopathic pulmonary embolism with LMWH and anticoagulants (warfarin for 3–6 months)
    • Thromboembolic therapy in patients with massive pulmonary embolism
    • Management of patients with recurrent idiopathic pulmonary embolism (lifelong anticoagulants)

BACK TO BASIC SCIENCES

Q1. What are the risk factors for venous thromboembolism?

• Genetic factors such as abnormalities associated with hypercoagulability (e.g. factor V Leiden and prothrombin 20110 gene mutation)
• Obesity
• Active cancer
• Advanced age
• Previous venous thrombosis
• Limited mobility
• Surgery (e.g. total knee replacement)
• Pregnancy
• Oestrogen therapy
• Indwelling central venous catheters

Q2. What are the roles of LMWH in the management of pulmonary embolism?

• LMWH is used in nonmassive pulmonary embolism.
• It is superior to unfractionated heparin because dosing and administration are simple and monitoring is not required except in obesity, pregnancy and renal failure.
• In patients with an intermediate to high probability of pulmonary embolism, LMWH should be instituted immediately before imaging.
• In massive pulmonary embolism, unfractionated heparin should be considered or thrombolysis (first line of pulmonary embolism with shock – massive embolism).

Q3. What is the role of oral anticoagulation in the management of pulmonary embolism?

• For the pulmonary embolism occurring for the first time, oral anticoagulation is administrated for 3–6 months (the International Normalised Ratio [INR] should be in the range of 2:0–3:0).
• Prolonged treatment for 6 months may be recommended for idiopathic pulmonary embolism, whereas 3 months is recommended in the first pulmonary embolism in which the cause has been identified.

- In patients with first pulmonary embolism but persisting risk factor, anticoagulation should be lifelong.

Q4. What is the role of thrombolytic therapy in the management of pulmonary embolism?

- Thrombolytic therapy is recommended as the first line of treatment in patients with massive pulmonary embolism (shock – massive pulmonary embolism).
- Thrombolytic therapy should not be used in patients with nonmassive pulmonary embolism because the risk of bleeding is approximately 2.2%.

Q5. What are the mechanisms underlying warfarin anticoagulation?

- Warfarin inhibits the synthesis of prethrombotic factors II, VII, IX and X.
- Warfarin inhibits the production of normal anticoagulant promoter protein C and its cofactor protein S.

REVIEW QUESTIONS

Q1. Regarding patients with multiple pulmonary emboli over an extended period of time, which *one* of the following is correct?

A. Patients have more right ventricular failure than occurs with acute large pulmonary embolism.

B. Patients have increasing dyspnoea and progressive decreasing exercise tolerance.

C. Patients have a decrease in cardiac output.

D. Patients develop systemic hypotension.

Q2. Which *one* of the following pathological changes *does not occur* in patients with a large thromboembolic embolism?

A. Ventilation–perfusion mismatch

B. Increased alveolar dead space

C. Increased pulmonary vascular resistance

D. Right ventricular hypertrophy

E. Reduced cardiac output

Q3. Which *one* of the following is *not* a risk factor for DVT?

A. Factor V Leiden

B. Prothrombin 20210 gene mutation

C. Active malignancy

D. Pregnancy

E. Progesterone therapy

Q4. Regarding D-dimer, which *one* of the following statements is *not* correct?

A. It can be measured in whole blood or plasma.

B. Elevated D-dimer has 85%–98% sensitivity for pulmonary embolism diagnosis.

C. False-positive D-dimer elevation occurs in advanced age.

D. False-positive D-dimer elevation occurs in patients with cancer.

E. D-dimer test has a high specificity.

Q5. Regarding computed tomography pulmonary angiogram (CTPA) in a patient with pulmonary embolism, which *one* of the following is *not correct*?

A. It has largely replaced V/Q scanning for pulmonary embolism diagnosis.

B. It can provide alternative diagnosis in patients with no pulmonary embolism.

C. The test has a high sensitivity and specificity.

D. When combined with CT venography, there are no changes in sensitivity or specificity for diagnosing pulmonary embolism.

Q6. Regarding V/Q scanning, which *one* of the following is *not correct*?

A. The test comprises two parts, a ventilation phase and a perfusion phase.

B. By comparison of the area with abnormal perfusion because of pulmonary embolism and ventilation status, the diagnosis can be made.

C. CTPA is preferred over V/Q scanning during pregnancy.

D. The CTPA has largely replaced V/Q scanning.

ANSWERS

A1. **B.** Because the changes took place over time, there has been time for adaptation to the changes. Therefore, the patients have no hypotension and no decrease in cardiac output. Also they have less right heart failure than occurs with acute large pulmonary embolism. However, these patients usually have increasing dyspnoea particularly because these emboli affect peripheral and medium-sized pulmonary vessels.

A2. **D.** Right ventricular dilatation and right ventricular failure usually occur rather than right ventricular hypertrophy. This is because of the thin right ventricular wall and its inability to maintain output in face of increased pulmonary arterial pressure.

A3. **E.** Oestrogen therapy is a risk factor for thrombosis.

A4. **E.** The D-dimer test lacks specificity and the value of the D-dimer assay resides with its high negative predictive value and therefore a normal D-dimer can reduce the probability of pulmonary embolism sufficiently to avoid further diagnostic testing (this is particularly important in patients with a low or moderate pretest likelihood, as per Wells clinical criteria, to have pulmonary embolism).

A5. **D.** The combination of CTPA and CT venography increases the sensitivity for diagnosing pulmonary embolism from 80%–83% to 90%–92% but this combination does not affect the specificity.

A6. **C.** During pregnancy, lung scanning is favoured over CTPA because lung scanning produces less maternal–fetal radiation exposure.

TAKE-HOME MESSAGE

- High-risk population for developing pulmonary embolism and DVT include those with surgery, immobilisation and cancer.
- The presenting symptoms of pulmonary embolism may include the following: (i) Dyspnoea of sudden onset, at rest or with minimal effort (the shortness of breath is progressive in severity); (ii) pleuritic chest pain may be present; (iii) haemoptysis (particularly in the presence of pulmonary infarction); (iv) risk factors for thrombotic pulmonary embolism (surgery, immobilisation, cancer); (v) DVT (leg pain, swelling, tenderness along deep leg veins, dusky blue colour of the skin); and (vi) lightheadedness/syncope.
- The signs of pulmonary embolism may include tachypnoea, tachycardia, hypoxaemia, palpitations, anxiety, central and peripheral cyanosis, a gallop rhythm (heart failure), distended jugular veins if heart failure develops, a widely split second heart sound and loud pulmonic component, and right ventricular heave (massive pulmonary embolism and high pulmonary pressure).
- The Wells clinical prediction rule for the likelihood of the diagnosis of pulmonary embolism is of clinical help.
- D-dimer test is the first test to start with in patients with clinical susceptibility of the diagnosis of pulmonary embolism.
- CTPA is the recommended imaging technique for the diagnosis of pulmonary embolism.
- Radioisotope V/Q scan is an alternative to CTPA when injection of contrast dye is a concern.
- Other tests include imaging of the leg veins (ultrasound examination) and bedside echocardiography in massive pulmonary embolism.
- LMWH is safe and is simple to administer and should be used in patients with a high probability of pulmonary embolism.
- For the pulmonary embolism occurring for the first time, oral anticoagulation is administrated for 3–6 months (INR should be in the range of 2:0–3:0).
- Prolonged treatment for 6 months may be recommended for idiopathic pulmonary embolism, whereas 3 months is recommended in the first pulmonary embolism in which the cause has been identified.
- In patients with first pulmonary embolism but persisting risk factor, anticoagulation should be lifelong.
- Thrombolytic therapy is recommended as the first line of treatment in patients with massive pulmonary embolism (shock – massive pulmonary embolism).
- It should not be used in patients with nonmassive pulmonary embolism because of the risk of bleeding.

FURTHER READINGS

Agnelli G, Becattini C. Acute pulmonary embolism. *N Engl J Med.* 2010;363(3):266-274. Review.

Di Nisio M, van Es N, Büller HR. Deep vein thrombosis and pulmonary embolism. *Lancet.* 2016; 388(10063):3060-3073. Review.

Goldhaber SZ. Pulmonary embolism. *Lancet.* 2004;363(9417):1295-1305. Review.

Goldhaber SZ, Bounameaux H. Pulmonary embolism and deep vein thrombosis. *Lancet.* 2012;379(9828): 1835-1846. Review.

Goldhaber SZ, Visani L, De Rosa M. Acute pulmonary embolism: clinical outcomes in the International Cooperative Pulmonary Embolism Registry (ICOPER). *Lancet.* 1999;353(9162):1386-1389.

Konstantinides S. Clinical practice. Acute pulmonary embolism. *N Engl J Med.* 2008;359(26):2804-2813. Review.

Kunutsor SK, Seidu S, Khunti K. Statins and primary prevention of venous thromboembolism: a systematic review and meta-analysis. *Lancet Haematol.* 2017;4(2):e83-e93. Review.

Kyrle PA, Eichinger S. Deep vein thrombosis. *Lancet.* 2005;365(9465):1163-1174. Review.

Piazza G, Goldhaber SZ. Chronic thromboembolic pulmonary hypertension. *N Engl J Med.* 2011;364(4): 351-360. Review.

Rahim SA, Panju A, Pai M, Ginsberg J. Venous thromboembolism prophylaxis in medical inpatients: a retrospective chart review. *Thromb Res.* 2003;111(4-5):215-219.

Tapson VF. Acute pulmonary embolism. *N Engl J Med.* 2008;358(10):1037-1052. Review.

CASE 2.6

'Like a Stone on My Chest . . . '

Clark Master, a 69-year-old volunteer worker, is brought by an ambulance to the emergency department of a local hospital because he is suffering from sudden, severe, substernal, crushing chest pain for the past 3–4 hours. He says, 'I feel like a stone on my chest, I never had such severe pain.' The pain radiates to the lower jaw, both shoulders and along the left arm. It did not resolve with rest. Mr Master also has nausea and excessive sweating started with the pain. He was diagnosed to have high blood lipids about 10 years ago and high blood pressure about 8 years ago. He is not taking his medications regularly. He is conscious and oriented; his pulse rate is 115/min (regular), respiratory rate 25/min, blood pressure 145/90 mm Hg and temperature 37.0°C; on auscultation of the heart, S1 + S2 and S4 gallop are heard. Chest auscultation shows bilateral fine crackles.

CASE DISCUSSION

Q1. On the basis of Mr Master's presentation, what is your diagnosis?

Q2. What is your differential diagnosis?

Q3. What are the key clinical features of this disease? What are the scientific bases for these features?

Q4. What is the pathophysiology underlying these changes?

Q5. What are your management goals and management options?

ANSWERS

1. The presentation of this patient is suggestive of acute myocardial infarction and pulmonary oedema. The supportive evidence for the diagnosis is a history of sudden, severe, substernal pain that radiates to the jaw, both shoulders and left arm. The pain is described by the patient as 'like a stone on the chest, and he never had such severe pain'. Also the pain did not improve on rest. These characteristics of the pain together with symptoms/signs triggered by sympathetic overactivity (sweating, tachycardia, increased respiratory rate, nausea and breathlessness), S4 gallop on auscultation and the presence of risk factors such as high blood lipids, high blood pressure and poor compliance suggest the diagnosis of acute myocardial infarction. The increased respiratory rate and the presence of bilateral basal crackles support pulmonary oedema.
2. The differential diagnosis of acute myocardial infarction includes the following:
   - Gastro-oesophageal reflux

- Musculoskeletal pain
- Anxiety/panic attacks
- Pleurisy
- Pulmonary embolism
- Acute aortic dissection
- Acute pericarditis
- Acute myocarditis

3. The following are essential for the diagnosis of acute myocardial infarction:
- Symptoms: Chest pain/discomfort – sudden, severe, described by the patient as pressing, crushing, squeezing, pressure-like, band-like and constricting. It is not a stabbing pain.
- The pain is typically retrosternal, substernal or felt in the precordium, and may radiate to the neck, the epigastrium, the lower jaw, teeth, the left shoulder or both shoulders and the left arm or both arms.
- The chest discomfort continues for 20 minutes or up to several hours (this differentiates the pain of myocardial infarction from the brief pain of angina).
- The chest pain is usually associated with shortness of breath, nausea, vomiting and sweating (indicating sympathetic overactivity).
- Approximately 20%–25% of patients have no pain (atypical or silent infarction). This is typically noted in elderly patients, especially diabetics and women.
- Other presenting symptoms include light-headedness, sudden syncope, loss of consciousness, new murmur and unexplained drop of blood pressure.
- Clinical signs: S4 gallop is present on auscultation; blood pressure may be raised initially (sympathetic stimulation) and then becomes normal or low. Signs of sympathetic overactivity (sweating, tachycardia, hypertension, increased respiratory rate) are present.
- Patients with inferior myocardial infarction may show signs of parasympathetic overactivity (low blood pressure and bradycardia).
- Watch for signs of heart failure (search for the cause: hypovolaemia, right-sided failure, left-sided failure), poor peripheral perfusion, changes in the heart rhythm, appearance of a new murmur and mechanical complications (new murmurs).
- ECG and laboratory findings:
  (a) ECG changes:
    - ST-segment elevation in V1–V2 indicates myocardial injury and impending infarction.
    - Presence of Q waves indicates progression to infarction.
    - ST segments and/or T-wave inversion indicates ischaemic changes.
    - Posterior infarction shows a depression in V1–V4.
    - Anteroseptal infarction may show changes extended to V3 and V4 (Fig. 2.6.1).
    - Anterior infarction changes are present in V2 and V5.
  (b) Cardiac troponin (cTn):
    - Isoforms I and T are the preferred diagnostic biomarkers.
    - They are highly sensitive and specific for myocardial infarction within 2–3 hours and peak within 24–48 hours (Fig. 2.6.2).

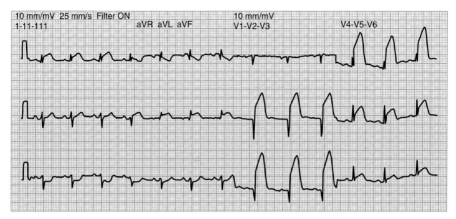

Figure 2.6.1 Changes in ECG in a patient with acute anterolateral myocardial infarction. *(Source: Andreoli TE, Benjamin IJ, Griggs RC, Wing EJ. Andreoli and Carpenter's Cecil Essentials of Medicine. 8th ed. Philadelphia, PA: Elsevier; 2010.)*

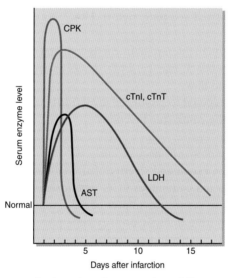

Figure 2.6.2 Typical time course for detection of enzyme released after myocardial infarction. *(Source: Andreoli TE, Benjamin IJ, Griggs RC, Wing EJ. Andreoli and Carpenter's Cecil Essentials of Medicine. 8th ed. Philadelphia, PA: Elsevier; 2010.)*

- The cTn blood level continues to be elevated for 7–10 days and up to 14 days or longer in patients with renal failure, making it difficult to detect new infarctions.
- High-sensitivity cardiac troponin T (hs-cTnT) has led to a further increase of 20% in the diagnosis.
- The use of the ECG criteria together with hs-cTnT results is critical in making the diagnosis.
- The limitation is the high levels in blood up to 10 days.

      (c) Creatine kinase myocardial band (CK-MB):
- Follows similar kinetics of cTn
- Is specific to myocardial injury
- Limitation: Not sensitive to small infarctions
- Can be used to detect the recurrence of myocardial infarction

4. Pathological features:
   - The spectrum of myocardial injury varies depending on several factors including the intensity of impairment, duration and the level of metabolic demand at the time of onset.
   - The injury results in coagulation necrosis of the myocardium → later the formation of myocardial scarring → myocardial fibrosis → changes in the contractile functions of the myocardium.
   - Reperfusion injury develops as a result of restoration of blood flow to the damaged myocardium. The underlying mechanism is related to oxygen free radicals and intracellular calcium → acceleration of myocardial damage.
   - Reperfusion injury of the myocardium is protected by nitric oxide (released from endothelium–derived releasing factor). How? Nitric oxide inactivates oxygen free radicals.
   - Stunned myocardium refers to transient dysfunction of the left ventricle following myocardial ischaemia. It may persist for hours or days following re-establishment of coronary blood flow.
   - However, areas exposed to prolonged myocardial ischaemia may have permanent impairment of the contractile functions.

5. Management goals:
   - Control of symptoms and adequate analgesia
   - Assessment of the extent and severity of arterial disease
   - Bed rest, oxygen and continuous ECG monitoring
   - Drug treatment to reduce the impact of the thrombus and maintenance of the cardiac functions (thrombolysis, primary angioplasty)
   - Management of complications (cardiac arrest, bradycardia, tachyarrhythmias, right ventricular failure, pericarditis, mitral regurgitation, systemic embolism)
   - Identification and control of risk factors (smoking, hypertension, dyslipidaemia, obesity)
   - Improving life expectancy in higher risk groups

   Key points in emergency management:
- On the way to hospital (ambulance officers):
   (i) Aspirin 300 mg chewed
   (ii) Nitroglycerin sublingual
   (iii) Analgesia – morphine 5–10 mg IV + metoclopramide 10 mg IV
- On arrival:
   (i) Primary angioplasty or thrombolysis
   (ii) Beta-blocker (atenolol 5 mg IV)

   (iii) Angiotensin-converting enzyme (ACE) inhibitor (lisinopril 2.5 mg)
   (iv) Clopidogrel 300 mg loading followed by 75 mg/day for 30 days
- Subsequent management:
  - **(i)** Bed rest and continuous ECG monitoring
  - **(ii)** Daily examination to detect any complications
  - **(iii)** Prophylaxis against thromboembolism
  - **(iv)** Aspirin 75 mg (to decrease vascular events)
  - **(v)** Long-term beta-blockers
  - **(vi)** Continuing ACE inhibitors in all patients
  - **(vii)** Starting statins
  - **(viii)** Discussing and encouraging exercise, and controlling diabetes, hypertension and dyslipidaemia
  - **(ix)** Introducing the patient to cessation smoking program
  - **(x)** Exercise ECG
  - **(xi)** Patient education
  - **(xii)** Review at 5 weeks post–myocardial infarction
  - **(xiii)** Review at 3 months and checking fasting blood lipids

BACK TO BASIC SCIENCES

Q1. What is the definition of atherosclerosis?
- Atherosclerosis is a chronic inflammatory change in response to the accumulation of lipids in the arterial walls.
- It is characterised by the presence of intimal plaques that develop gradually in the walls of arteries. Fissuring of the plaques stimulates thrombus formation and acute ischaemic changes.
- Atherosclerosis is the major cause of myocardial infarction, ischaemic strokes, peripheral artery disease, chronic heart failure and vascular dementia.

Q2. Discuss risk factors for the development of atherosclerosis.
- An elevation of low-density lipoprotein (LDL) cholesterol
- Cigarette smoking
- Type 2 diabetes mellitus
- Hypertension
- Family history of premature stroke or ischaemic heart disease
- A low high-density lipoprotein cholesterol
- Abdominal obesity
- Hypertriglyceridemia
- Physical inactivity
- High level of lipoprotein(a)
- Elevated C-reactive protein (reflects the presence of inflammation)

Other risk factors:
- Depression
- Stress (financial, family, work-related)
- Elevated uric acid
- Elevated total homocysteine
- Renal impairment
- Systemic inflammatory conditions (e.g. SLE, rheumatoid arthritis)

Q3. Discuss the pathogenesis of atherosclerosis development.
- One or more cardiovascular risk factors are present (see Q2).
- Initial step is entrapment of LDL in the intima of arteries (apolipoprotein B, accumulation of LDL, lipoprotein lipase role, extracellular matrix, proteoglycans, sphingomyelins).
- Activation of endothelial cells and macrophages results in the production of cytokines and leukocyte adhesion molecules, T-cell influx to the intima and development of monocytes to macrophages.
- Macrophages take up the oxidised LDL by scavenger receptors resulting in the formation of cholesterol-laden foam cells and the production of proinflammatory mediators: TNF-alpha, IL-1, radical oxygen and nitrogen species and prothrombotic factors.
- T-cells in the intima, particularly TH_1 type, secrete interferon-gamma, TNF and lymphotoxin, which contribute to the pathological changes in the walls of arteries and stimulate macrophages.
- Other cells involved in the pathogenesis of atherosclerosis are dendritic cells and mast cells. Dendritic cells take up the presenting antigens and mast cells secrete enzymes and bioactive mediators.
- Triglyceride-rich lipoproteins are added into the subendothelial space and contribute to the pathological changes in the arterial wall.

Q4. What are the main differences between warfarin and heparin?
The main differences are summarised in Table 2.6.1.

Table 2.6.1 Main differences between warfarin and heparin

Parameter	Warfarin	Heparin
Uses/group	Oral anticoagulant Acts only in vivo	A family of sulphated glycosaminoglycans (mucopolysaccharides) Doses are presented in units of activity Given by subcutaneous routes (intramuscular injections cause bleeding and haematoma formation) Acts both in vivo and in vitro
Mechanism(s) of action	It interferes with the post-translational γ-carboxylation of glutamic acid residues in clotting factors II, VII, IX and X	Heparin acts as anti–thrombin III and accelerates the rate of action of anti–thrombin III

Continued

Table 2.6.1 Main differences between warfarin and heparin—cont'd

Parameter	Warfarin	Heparin
Clinical effect	Its effect is not immediate. This depends on the half-lives of clotting factors II, VII, IX and X	Acts immediately after intravenous injections
Factors potentiating its effect	Liver disease Cimetidine and amiodarone Cephalosporins Broad-spectrum antibiotics Nonsteroidal anti-inflammatory drugs Aspirin	Liver disease
Factors decreasing its effect	Hypothyroidism Vitamin K Barbiturates Rifampicin	Anti–thrombin III deficiency (rare) Platelets, plasma proteins and fibrin may interfere with its action
Side effects	Haemorrhage from the brain and bowel	Heparin-induced thrombocytopenia and thrombosis, osteoporosis (on long-term treatment), and hypersensitivity LMWH less likely to cause thrombo-cytopenia

Modified from Azer SA. Basic Biomedical Sciences, Core Clinical Cases. Hodder Arnold, UK, 2006.

Q5. Briefly discuss the cardiac biomarkers of necrosis.

- Cardiac-derived cTn I and cTn T are proteins of the sarcomere of the cardiac muscle cells and are sensitive assays of cardiac muscle damage.
- They are first detectable 2–4 hours after the onset of acute myocardial infarction; levels peak at 10–24 hours and persist for 5–14 days.
- Therefore, the measurement of cTn I and cTn T may replace other markers for the diagnosis of myocardial infarction in patients who present late (1 or 2 days) after the start of symptoms.
- However, the levels of cTn I and cTn T remain high for 5–14 days, making these tests less useful in diagnosing reinfarction. Because CK-MB level returns to normal after 72 hours, it should be recommended for such situations.
- The sensitivity and specificity of cTn I and cTn T make these the gold standard biomarkers in diagnosing myocardial infarction.
- However, cTn T and cTn I may show false positive (high levels) in the following situations/conditions: renal failure, sepsis, pregnancy, pericarditis and severe systemic illness.

REVIEW QUESTIONS

Q1. The mechanisms by which cholesterol-lowering statins reduce atherosclerosis lesions include all of the following *except*

A. Statins prevent nitrogen-induced endothelial dysfunction.

B. Statins inhibit immune activity and inflammation.

C. Statins inhibit the progression of atherosclerotic lesion.

D. Statins inhibit platelet aggregation.

Q2. Current secondary prevention of coronary artery disease includes all of the following *except*

A. Smoking cessation.

B. Dietary and pharmacological reduction of LDL cholesterol.

C. Management of high blood pressure.

D. Control of hyperglycaemia.

E. Beta-adrenergic receptor agonist therapy.

ANSWERS

A1. **D.** There is no evidence that statins cause inhibition of platelet aggregation.

A2. **E.** Drugs such as statins, aspirin, beta-adrenergic receptor blockers, ACE inhibitors together with control of hyperglycaemia are essential in the secondary prevention of coronary artery disease.

TAKE-HOME MESSAGE

- Atherosclerosis is a chronic inflammatory change in response to the accumulation of lipids in the arterial walls.
- It is characterised by the presence of intimal plaques that develop gradually in the walls of arteries. Fissuring of the plaques stimulates thrombus formation and acute ischaemic changes.
- Atherosclerosis is the major cause of myocardial infarction, ischaemic strokes, peripheral artery disease, chronic heart failure and vascular dementia.
- Symptoms suggestive of acute myocardial infarction are chest pain/discomfort – sudden, severe, described by the patient as pressing, crushing, squeezing, pressure-like, band-like and constricting. It is not a stabbing pain.
- The pain is typically retrosternal, substernal or felt in the precordium, and may radiate to the neck, the epigastrium, the lower jaw, teeth, the left shoulder or both shoulders and the left arm or both arms.
- The chest discomfort continues for 20 minutes or up to several hours (this differentiates the pain of myocardial infarction from the brief pain of angina).
- The chest pain is usually associated with shortness of breath, nausea, vomiting and sweating (indicating sympathetic overactivity).
- Approximately 20%–25% of patients have no pain (atypical or silent infarction). This is typically noted in elderly patients, especially diabetics and women.
- Other presenting symptoms are light-headedness, sudden syncope, loss of consciousness, new murmur and unexplained drop of blood pressure.

- Clinical signs of myocardial infarction include the following: S4 may be heard on auscultation; blood pressure may be raised initially (sympathetic stimulation) and then becomes normal or low. Signs of sympathetic overactivity (sweating, tachycardia, hypertension, increased respiratory rate) are present.
- ECG changes and cTn or hs-cTnT results are used in assessing the patient and making the diagnosis.
- The aims of management are (i) control of symptoms and adequate analgesia; (ii) assessment of the extent and severity of arterial disease; (iii) bed rest, oxygen and continuous ECG monitoring; (iv) drug treatment to reduce the impact of the thrombus and maintenance of the cardiac functions (thrombolysis, primary angioplasty); (v) management of complications (cardiac arrest, bradycardia, tachyarrhythmias, right ventricular failure, pericarditis, mitral regurgitation, systemic embolism); (vi) identification and control of risk factors (smoking, hypertension, dyslipidaemia, obesity); and (vii) improving life expectancy in higher risk groups.

FURTHER READINGS

Azer SA. Basic Biomedical Science. Core Clinical Cases. United Kingdom: Hodder-Arnold; 2006.

Anderson JL, Morrow DA. Acute myocardial infarction. *N Engl J Med.* 2017;376(21):2053-2064. Review.

Hansson GK. Inflammation, atherosclerosis, and coronary artery disease. *N Engl J Med.* 2005;352(16): 1685-1695. Review.

Patrono C, García Rodríguez LA, Landolfi R, Baigent C. Low-dose aspirin for the prevention of atherothrombosis. *N Engl J Med.* 2005;353(22):2373-2383. Review.

Reed GW, Rossi JE, Cannon CP. Acute myocardial infarction. *Lancet.* 2017;389(10065):197-210. Review.

Wang K, Asinger RW, Marriott HJ. ST-segment elevation in conditions other than acute myocardial infarction. *N Engl J Med.* 2003;349(22):2128-2135. Review.

White HD, Chew DP. Acute myocardial infarction. *Lancet.* 2008;372(9638):570-584. Review.

Windecker S, Bax JJ, Myat A, Stone GW, Marber MS. Future treatment strategies in ST-segment elevation myocardial infarction. *Lancet.* 2013;382(9892):644-657. Review.

Yellon DM, Hausenloy DJ. Myocardial reperfusion injury. *N Engl J Med.* 2007;357(11):1121-1135. Review.

CASE 2.7

'Not Feeling Well ...'

Fatma Ahmed, a 55-year-old housewife, comes in to see a general practitioner because she is suffering from progressive shortness of breath; she always feels tired and has progressive decline in her exercise tolerance. She says, 'I am not feeling well'. She is unable to lie in bed and has to use three pillows to prop up herself. She gives a history of hospital admission because of rheumatic fever when she was 7 years old. On examination, her pulse rate is 115/min (irregularly irregular pulse, a pattern suggestive of atrial fibrillation), respiration rate 25/min, blood pressure 125/85 mm Hg and temperature 36.8°C. Her jugular venous pressure is raised. On cardiac auscultation, S1 (loud) + S2 and S3 gallop, a mid-diastolic rumble murmur and an opening snap are heard. On chest auscultation, bilateral crackles are heard over both the lungs and pitting oedema of lower extremities is present.

CASE DISCUSSION

Q1. On the basis of Fatma's presentation, what is your diagnosis?

Q2. What is your differential diagnosis?

Q3. What are the key clinical features of this disease? What are the scientific bases for these features?

Q4. What is the pathophysiology underlying these changes?

Q5. What are your management goals and management options?

ANSWERS

1. The presentation of this patient is suggestive of heart failure secondary to mitral valve stenosis. The supportive evidence for the diagnosis is a history of progressive shortness of breath, orthopnoea (dyspnoea in recumbent position), feeling tired and not good and progressive decline in her exercise tolerance. She gives a history of hospital admission because of rheumatic fever (this provides a clue about the murmur heard on auscultating the heart and the cause of her heart failure). The clinical findings including raised jugular venous pressure, loud S1, diastolic rumble murmur, opening snap, chest crackles and pitting oedema of the lower extremities are suggestive of right-sided heart failure and mitral valve stenosis.

   Mitral stenosis is prevalent in developing countries because of its association with rheumatic fever (prevalent in these communities). However, it can be seen in developed countries.

2. The differential diagnosis of heart failure includes the following:
   * Bronchial asthma
   * Chronic obstructive pulmonary disease
   * Pneumonia
   * Liver cirrhosis
   * Peripheral venous insufficiency
   * Nephrotic syndrome

3. The following are essential for the diagnosis of heart failure secondary to mitral stenosis:
   (i) Shortness of breath (dyspnoea); the underlying mechanisms are as follows:
      - Pulmonary congestion
      - Increased interstitial or intra-alveolar fluid
      - Decreased lung compliance
      - Increased work of breathing.
   (ii) Orthopnoea (dyspnoea when the patient is trying to lie flat); the underlying mechanisms are as follows:
      - Increased venous return from extremities and splanchnic circulation
      - Increased pulmonary venous congestion and pulmonary capillary hydrostatic pressure
   (iii) Bendopnoea (severe dyspnoea while bending over); the underlying mechanisms are as follows:
      - Gravity effect
      - Limitation of chest expansion
      - Pressure made by the viscera, limiting diaphragmatic movement
   (iv) Paroxysmal nocturnal dyspnoea (acute severe shortness of breath, waking the patient from sleep); the underlying mechanisms are as follows:
      - Increased venous return
      - Mobilisation of interstitial fluids
      - Alveolar oedema
   (v) Fatigue: Due to hypoxaemia
   (vi) Chest pain due to myocardial ischaemia, and mismatch between oxygen supply and oxygen demand
   (vii) Cognitive dysfunction; the underlying mechanisms are as follows:
      - Hypoperfusion of the brain
      - Memory impairment and poor concentration
      - Depression
      - Sleep disturbances
      - Drugs' side effects
   (viii) Sleep disorders; the underlying mechanisms are as follows:
      - Obstructive sleep apnoea
      - Central sleep apnoea/Cheyne–Stokes respiration
      - Gasping during sleep
      - Recurrent awakenings

4. Clinical signs:
   - Pale
   - Diaphoretic
   - Unable to speak or complete a sentence
   - Unable to lie recumbent in bed (because of dyspnoea)
   - Increased heart rate >100 minutes
   - Arrhythmias such as atrial fibrillation and pulsus alternans, which are common
   - Blood pressure normal or high (can be low due to decreased output in heart failure)
   - A narrow pulse pressure <30 mmHg (in severe failure)
   - Weight (helps in assessing the severity of heart failure and cardiac cachexia)
   - Increased respiratory rate
   - Increased jugular venous pressure
   - Examination of the lungs: Rales and crackles because of fluid accumulation (acute pulmonary oedema and fluid accumulation in the pleural space [pleural effusion] may be present)
   - Cardiac examination: (i) a right ventricular heave, (ii) apex beat displaced in case of left ventricular failure, (iii) increased intensity of the second heart sound (pulmonary hypertension), (iv) S3 gallop in severe left ventricular dysfunction and (v) S4 gallop in ischaemic heart disease or hypertension (diabetic dysfunction)
   - Abdominal examination: Enlarged tender pulsatile liver in right ventricular failure + ascites (usually there is elevated right heart pressure and tricuspid regurgitation)
   - Examination of extremities: Peripheral oedema. The underlying mechanisms include (i) sodium retention, (ii) decreased cardiac output, (iii) decreased renal perfusion, (iv) increased right-sided filling pressure and (v) increased hydrostatic pressure (Fig. 2.7.1). The cool extremities suggest low cardiac output and/or concomitant peripheral arterial disease.

5. Radiological and laboratory investigations:
   (i) Chest radiography:
      - There may be no changes or mild changes depending on the degree of stenosis.
      - Typical changes in severe cases:
        - A large left atrium causing elevation of the left mainstem bronchus
        - A large left atrium causing double density in the posterior–anterior view
        - Prominent pulmonary artery causing 'mitralisation of the left border of the heart'
        - Mitral valve calcification (may be present [lateral views])
        - 'Kerley B lines' (may be present in severe cases)
        - Pulmonary congestion of the upper lobes
        - Pulmonary oedema in left ventricular failure
   (ii) Electrocardiography:
      - It may be normal.
      - It may show atrial fibrillation.

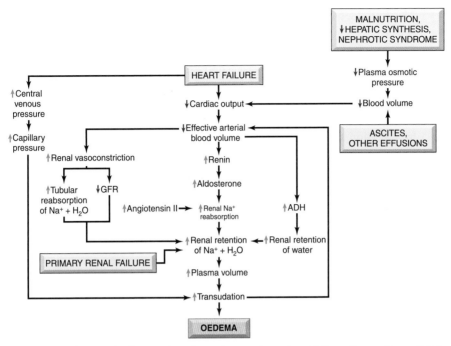

Figure 2.7.1 Pathogenesis of systemic oedema due to primary heart failure. *(Source: Kumar V, Abbas AK, Fausto N, Mitchell R. Robbins Basic Pathology. 8th ed. London, UK: Elsevier; 2007.)*

  - In sinus rhythm, there may be broad M-shaped configuration of the P-wave in lead II (P mitral).
  - There may be biphasic P-wave in lead V1 (P negative V1) suggesting increased left atrial pressure.
(iii) Cardiac echocardiogram (2D):
  - Confirms the diagnosis of mitral stenosis
  - Enables the assessment of mitral valve motion, left ventricular function, left atrial size and left atrial clots
(iv) Cardiac catheterisation:
  - Not generally needed for the diagnosis
  - Recommended if the diagnosis not certain
6. Pathological features:
   • The normal valve area is 4–6 cm^2.
   • Symptoms appear when the valve area is <1.5 cm^2.
   • The shortness of breath correlates with an increase in the mean of left atrial pressure (in mitral stenosis, the left atrial pressure increases).
   • In developing countries, mitral stenosis is related to the prevalence of rheumatic fever. The disease is accelerated in cases with a recurrent rheumatic fever, compressing the natural history of the disease by 5–10 years.

- The pathological changes are summarised in Q2 in the section 'Back to Basic Sciences'.
- The appearance of atrial fibrillation (usually complicates mitral stenosis) → irregular RR intervals, lack of atrial contractions, increase of dyspnoea and development of atrial blood clots.
- The main complications of mitral stenosis are (i) atrial fibrillation, (ii) pulmonary congestion, (iii) pulmonary oedema and left-sided heart failure, (iv) pulmonary hypertension and (v) congestive heart failure.

7. Management goals:
   - Control the patient's symptoms.
   - Slow the heart rate to increase the diastolic filling time.
   - Decrease the vascular volume.
   - Manage new-onset atrial fibrillation.
   - Educate the patient.

   Options:
   - Drug treatment
   - Percutaneous balloon valvuloplasty
   - Surgical mitral commissurotomy
   - Patient education

   The benefit of balloon valvuloplasty to mortality in mitral stenosis might be similar to that of surgery but needs further study (Chandrashekhar, Westaby, 2009).

BACK TO BASIC SCIENCES

Q1. What are the causes of mitral stenosis?
(1) Rheumatic fever: It is common in developing countries. Not every patient will remember or know that he/she had a rheumatic fever. It is estimated that only 50% of patients who had rheumatic fever will report this in history.
(2) Degenerative causes: It is common in developed countries.
(3) Other rare causes include congenital deformities (usually present in infancy or childhood).

Q2. Briefly summarise the pathology of mitral stenosis.
- Leaflets thickened
- Show nodularity
- Commissural fusion
- Narrowing of the valve (takes the shape of a fish mouth)
- Gradual narrowing of the valve area by 0.1–0.3 cm^2/year
- Calcification
- Chordal fusion and shortening
- Continuous inflammation
- Possibility that left ventricular function may not be reduced or reduced later

- Systolic dysfunction (one-third of patients)
- Reduced preload
- Reflex increase in the afterload

Q3. Define heart failure.
- Heart failure results from structural and functional abnormalities of the myocardium that impair cardiac output or decrease filling of the ventricles.
- Common presentations of patients with heart failure include dyspnoea, fatigue, fluid retention (ascites, pleural effusion, oedema) and impaired exercise tolerance.

Q4. What are the common causes of heart failure?
- Coronary artery disease
- Hypertension
- Diseases of cardiac muscles (dilated cardiomyopathy, hypertrophic cardiomyopathy, muscle dystrophy)
- Valvular disease (valvular stenosis, valvular regurgitation)
- Chemotherapy causing cardiac toxicity (e.g. anthracyclines)
- Chest radiation therapy
- Toxins such as excessive drinking of alcohol and use of cocaine
- Persistent tachycardia and abnormal cardiac rhythms
- Pulmonary heart disease (e.g. cor pulmonale)
- Infections (e.g. viral infection, Chagas disease)
- Constrictive pericarditis
- Nutritional disorders (beriberi)
- High-output states such as chronic anaemia and thyrotoxicosis

Q5. What are the common causes of heart failure in developing countries?
Rheumatic valvular disease is a common cause of heart failure in developing countries. However, it may be a common cause in certain communities in Western countries.

Q6. What are the factors that contribute to the pathological development and/or precipitate acute heart failure?
- Myocardial infarction
- Arrhythmias
- Hypertension
- Discontinuation of medications
- Alcohol consumption
- Fever and infection
- Anaemia
- Thyroid problems
- High altitude
- Pregnancy

- Worsening valvular diseases
- Fluid overload/transfusion

REVIEW QUESTIONS

Q1. In mitral stenosis, which *one* of the following combinations is *not correct*?
A. Dysphagia – the enlarged left atrium impinges the oesophagus
B. Hoarseness – the enlarged left atrium impinges on the left recurrent laryngeal nerve
C. Haemoptysis – high left atrial pressure rupture of the anastomosis of small bronchial veins occurs
D. S1 becomes soft – the transmitral gradient holds the mitral valve open through diastole

Q2. Which *one* of the following is *not* a clinical sign observed in mitral stenosis?
A. A loud S1
B. Soft pulmonary component of S2 if pulmonary hypertension develops
C. S4 gallop sound
D. An opening snap
E. A low-pitched diastolic rumbling murmur

Q3. Which *one* of the following is *not found* on a chest X-ray of a patient with mitral stenosis?
A. Straightening of the left border of the heart
B. Kerley B lines
C. A double density at the right heart border
D. Decreased lung vascularity

Q4. Patients with concomitant mitral stenosis and atrial fibrillation should
A. Undergo anticoagulation with warfarin.
B. Take the prescribed diuretics.
C. Undergo valve replacement.
D. Be appropriately treated for beta-haemolytic streptococcal infection.

Q5. The commonest arrhythmia in patients with mitral stenosis is
A. Heart block.
B. Atrial fibrillation.
C. Ventricular tachycardia.
D. Supraventricular tachycardia.

ANSWERS

A1. **D.** In mitral stenosis, S1 is typically loud and is an important sign in mitral stenosis. However, as the disease becomes advanced and mitral valve is damaged, S1 becomes soft (mitral valve neither opens nor closes well).

A2. **B.** Pulmonary hypertension results in a loud pulmonary component of S2.

A3. **D.** Usually there is increased lung vascularity because of pulmonary venous hypertension.

A4. **A.** The patients are at a higher risk for systemic embolism. They should undergo anticoagulation with warfarin (INR target 2.5–3.5).

A5. **B.** Stretching and enlargement of the left atrium contribute to the pathogenesis of atrial fibrillation in patients with mitral stenosis.

TAKE-HOME MESSAGE

- The normal mitral valve area is 4–6 cm^2. Symptoms appear when the valve area is <1.5 cm^2.
- The causes of mitral stenosis are (i) rheumatic fever, which is common in developing countries (not every patient will remember or know that he/she had a rheumatic fever; it is estimated that only 50% of patients who had rheumatic fever will report this in history); (ii) degenerative causes, which is common in developed countries; and (iii) other rare causes such as congenital deformities (usually present in infancy or childhood).
- Not all patients with mitral stenosis will give a history of rheumatic fever.
- Patients with mitral stenosis present with shortness of breath on exercise, tiredness, fatigue, palpitation, orthopnoea and oedema of the lower limbs.
- Heart failure results from structural and functional abnormalities of the myocardium that impair cardiac output or decrease filling of the ventricles.
- Common presentations of patients with heart failure include dyspnoea, fatigue, fluid retention (ascites, pleural effusion, oedema) and impaired exercise tolerance.
- The main complications of mitral stenosis are (i) atrial fibrillation, (ii) pulmonary congestion, (iii) pulmonary oedema and left-sided heart failure, (iv) pulmonary hypertension and (v) congestive heart failure.
- The management of mitral stenosis includes (i) drug treatment, (ii) percutaneous balloon valvuloplasty, (iii) surgical mitral commissurotomy and (iv) patient education.

FURTHER READINGS

Chandrashekhar Y, Westaby S, Narula J. Mitral stenosis. *Lancet.* 2009;374(9697):1271-1283. Review.

Conrad N, Judge A, Tran J, et al. Temporal trends and patterns in heart failure incidence: a population-based study of 4 million individuals. *Lancet.* 2018;391(10120):572-580.

Nishimura RA, Otto CM, Bonow RO, et al. 2014 AHA/ACC guideline for the management of patients with valvular heart disease: a report of the American College of Cardiology/American Heart Association Task Force on Practice Guidelines. *J Am Coll Cardiol.* 2014;63(22):e57.

Nishimura RA, Vahanian A, Eleid MF, Mack MJ. Mitral valve disease—current management and future challenges. *Lancet.* 2016;387(10025):1324-1334. Review.

Shah AM, Mann DL. In search of new therapeutic targets and strategies for heart failure: recent advances in basic science. *Lancet.* 2011; 378(9792):704-712.

CASE 2.8

'In the Backyard . . . '

George Clark, a 74-year-old, is brought by an ambulance to a local hospital because of a brief loss of consciousness. His son who lives with him accompanies him to the emergency department, and says, 'Dad was doing gardening in the backyard and it was too hot. Suddenly he lost consciousness. This is not the first time, two weeks ago dad was attending the funeral of a relative and again lost consciousness.' Mr Clark, who regained his consciousness, says, 'I sometimes have substernal chest pain, shortness of breath on exertion and an awareness of my heartbeats.' On examination, the pulse rate is 90/min (low volume), blood pressure 100/85 mm Hg, respiratory rate 18/min, temperature 36.8°C and oxygen saturation 98%. The carotid pulse is weak and delayed. Cardiac examination shows that the apex beat is not displaced but enlarged, and an ejection murmur is heard in the aortic area and it radiates to the neck. S4 gallop is also heard. Lungs are clear to auscultation. ECG shows left ventricular hypertrophy.

CASE DISCUSSION

Q1. On the basis of Mr Clark's presentation, what is your diagnosis?

Q2. What is your differential diagnosis?

Q3. What are the key clinical features of this disease? What are the scientific bases for these features?

Q4. What is the pathophysiology underlying these changes?

Q5. What are your management goals and management options?

ANSWERS

1. The presentation of this patient is suggestive of aortic stenosis. The supportive evidence for the diagnosis is a history of recurrent syncope, shortness of breath on exertion, angina and awareness of his heartbeats (palpitations). On examination, his pulse is of low volume and the pulse pressure is reduced (normally about 35–40 mm Hg). The carotid pulse is weak and delayed. The apex beat is not displaced but enlarged; an ejection murmur is heard in the aortic area and it radiates to the neck. S4 gallop is also heard. Lungs are clear to auscultation and an ECG shows left ventricular hypertrophy. These findings are consistent with the diagnosis of aortic valve stenosis.
2. The differential diagnosis of aortic valve stenosis includes the following:
   - Acute coronary syndrome
   - Myocardial infarction

- Hypovolemic shock
- Mitral valve prolapse
- Mitral regurgitation
- Mitral stenosis

Table 2.8.1 summarises key differences between chronic acquired valvular heart diseases regarding physical findings, echocardiogram, and radiological changes.

Table 2.8.1 Key differences between chronic acquired valvular heart diseases

	Physical findings[a]	Electrocardiogram	Radiograph
Aortic stenosis	Pulsus parvus et tardus (may be absent in older patients or in patients with associated aortic regurgitation); carotid *shudder* (coarse thrill) Ejection murmur radiates to base of neck; peaks late in systole if stenosis is severe Sustained but not significantly displaced LV impulse A_2 decreased, S_2 single or paradoxically split S_4 gallop, often palpable	LV hypertrophy Left bundle branch block is also common Rare heart block from calcific involvement of conduction system	LV prominence without dilation Post-stenotic aortic root dilation Aortic valve calcification
Aortic regurgitation	Increased pulse pressure Bifid carotid pulses Rapid pulse upstroke and collapse LV impulse hyperdynamic and displaced laterally Diastolic decrescendo murmur; duration related to severity Systolic flow murmur S_{3G} common	LV hypertrophy, often with narrow, deep Q waves	LV and aortic dilation
Mitral stenosis	Loud S_1 OS S_2–OS interval inversely related to stenosis severity S_1 not loud, and OS absent if valve heavily calcified Signs of pulmonary arterial hypertension	Left atrial abnormality Atrial fibrillation common RV hypertrophy pattern may develop if associated pulmonary arterial hypertension is present	Large LA: Double-density, posterior displacement of oesophagus, elevation of left mainstem bronchus Straightening of left heart border as a result of enlarged left appendage Small or normal-sized LV Large pulmonary artery Pulmonary venous congestion

Continued

Table 2.8.1 Key differences between chronic acquired valvular heart diseases—cont'd

	Physical findings[a]	Electrocardiogram	Radiograph
Mitral regurgitation	Hyperdynamic LV impulse S_3 Mitral regurgitation Widely split S_2 may occur Holosystolic apical murmur radiating to axilla (murmur may be atypical with acute mitral regurgitation, papillary muscle dysfunction or mitral valve prolapse)	LA abnormality LV hypertrophy Atrial fibrillation	Enlarged LA and LV Pulmonary venous congestion
Mitral valve prolapse	One or more systolic clicks, often mid-systolic, followed by late systolic murmur Auscultatory findings dynamic Symptoms may include tall, thin habitus, pectus excavatum, straight back syndrome	Often normal Occasionally ST-segment depression and/or T-wave changes in inferior leads	Depends on degree of valve regurgitation and presence or absence of those abnormalities
Tricuspid stenosis	Jugular venous distention with prominent α wave if sinus rhythm Tricuspid OS and diastolic rumble at left sternal border; may be overshadowed by concomitant mitral stenosis Tricuspid OS and rumble increased during inspiration	Right atrial abnormality Atrial fibrillation common	Large RA
Tricuspid regurgitation	Jugular venous distention with large regurgitant (systolic) wave Systolic murmur at left sternal border, increased with inspiration Diastolic flow rumble RV S_3 increased with inspiration Hepatomegaly with systolic pulsation	RA abnormality; findings are often related to cause of the tricuspid regurgitation	RA and RV are enlarged; findings are often related to cause of the tricuspid regurgitation

LA, left atrium; LV, left ventricle; OS, opening snap; RA, right atrium; RV, right ventricle.
[a]Findings are influenced by the severity and chronicity of the valve disorder.
Source: Andreoli TE, Benjamin IJ, Griggs RC, Wing EJ. Andreoli and Carpenter's Cecil Essentials of Medicine. 8th ed. Philadelphia, PA: Elsevier; 2010.

3. The following are essential for the diagnosis of aortic valve stenosis:
   - Symptoms: These include shortness of breath, angina, syncope, palpitations and heart failure.
   - Angina: Due to myocardial ischaemia, demands exceed supply (e.g. exercising, sweating in hot environment).

- Syncope: It occurs due to inadequate cerebral perfusion particularly during exercise (decreased systemic blood pressure and decreased cerebral perfusion are the main factors responsible).
- Heart failure: Both systolic failure and diastolic failure may occur.
- Clinical signs: Classic ejection murmur is heard during examination. The murmur is loudest in the aortic area and radiates to the neck. The intensity of the murmur increases with cycle length. In mild stenosis, the murmur peaks in early systole and mid-systole, and in severe stenosis, the murmur peaks later in late systole.
- Delay in carotid pulse compared to apex beat timing is the most helpful sign in assessing severe aortic stenosis.
- Left apical impulse is not displaced but is enlarged and forceful.
- S1 is normal. In calcified disease, S2 may be single and soft (aortic component is lost – neither opens nor closes well).
- An S4 gallop is common.
- Diagnosis: ECG shows left ventricular hypertrophy (may be absent). Chest X-ray is nondiagnostic; cardiac silhouette is enlarged (a boot-shaped configuration); and pulmonary congestion, aortic valve calcification and cardiomegaly are present.
- Echocardiography: It is done for the assessment of the extent of left ventricular hypertrophy, systolic ejection performance and severity of stenosis.
- Stress testing is *contraindicated* in symptomatic patients because of a high risk of complications.
- Brain natriuretic peptide (BNP) levels may be higher in patients who will become symptomatic. Levels >550 pg/mL may indicate a poor prognosis.
- Cardiac catheterisation: It is done for coronary angiography, and is undertaken before surgery.

4. Pathology:
   - The normal aortic valve is 3–4 cm^2. There are no significant haemodynamic changes expected to occur with a reduction of the aortic valve orifice to one-third of normal.
   - Normally the left ventricle and aortic pressure are equal during systole.
   - However, with the development of stenosis, a gradient pressure develops at the valve area because of increased pressure in the left ventricle of approximately 10–15 mm Hg at a valve area of 1.3–1.5 cm^2.
   - The gradient increases to 70 mm Hg at the valve area of 0.6 cm^2.
   - The increase in left ventricle pressure results in two main pathological changes (i) left ventricular hypertrophy (concentric hypertrophy) and (ii) preservation of ejection fraction and cardiac output; however, in long-standing cases, heart failure will gradually occur.
   - During exercise, this preservation of ejection fraction is affected and the patient may have syncope, palpitation and angina.

5. Management goals:
   - The appearance of symptoms suggests a worsening progress and an indication for surgery (e.g. exertional syncope is an indication for valve replacement).

- The onset of symptoms such as angina, syncope or heart failure is associated with a poor survival rate and is an indication for preparing the patient for surgery.
- Patients who are unable to have valve surgery are treated with diuretics and perhexiline maleate.
- Aortic valvuloplasty is not useful in adults because of early restenosis (within 6–9 months) and is rarely performed.
- Aortic valve replacement is not contraindicated in advanced age up to the age of 85, and in extreme old age (>85 years) or the presence of comorbidities, surgery may not be the proper approach for treatment.
- The following investigations are usually needed for patients prepared for valve replacement: (i) cardiac catheterisation (calculate the valve area, cardiac output, valve gradient, systolic ejection time) and (ii) echo measurements.

BACK TO BASIC SCIENCES

Q1. What are the causes of aortic stenosis?
- Bicuspid and other anomalies of aortic valve: Approximately 1% of the population is born with a bicuspid aortic valve. Stenosis usually develops at 40–60 years of age.
- Tricuspid aortic valve stenosis: Valves become thickened due to an inflammatory process similar to coronary heart disease. Stenosis in these patients is diagnosed at 60–80 years of age.
- Rheumatic aortic valve disease: It may be seen in developing countries.

Q2. Briefly discuss the pathophysiology of aortic stenosis.
- Pressure overload on the left ventricle (the left ventricle and aortic pressures are normally nearly equal during systole). The high pressure is compensated by left ventricular hypertrophy (concentric hypertrophy).
- The progression of the disease results in reduced coronary blood flow reserve causing angina, and reduced cerebral blood flow due to reduced blood pressure particularly during exercising.
- Left ventricular hypertrophy and afterload excess contribute to left ventricular dysfunction and heart failure.

REVIEW QUESTIONS

Q1. Which *one* of the following about the normal aortic valve area is correct?
A. 0.5–1.0 cm^2
B. 1.5–2.0 cm^2
C. 2.5–3.0 cm^2
D. 3.0–4.0 cm^2

Q2. Which *one* of the following best describes the pathophysiological process of stenosis of the tricuspid aortic valve?

A. An inflammatory process similar to that of coronary heart disease

B. Calcification secondary to excessive vitamin D receptor stimulation

C. Plaque formation secondary to increased blood phosphate

D. Imbalance between calcium and phosphate ratio

Q3. In patients with asymptomatic aortic stenosis, which *one* of the following is a recommended management option?

A. Commencing patients on statins

B. Close follow-up, no treatment

C. Diuretics

D. Nitrates

Q4. In patients with symptomatic aortic stenosis, which *one* of the following is *not* recommended?

A. Diuretics

B. Aortic valve replacement

C. Angiotensin-converting enzyme (ACE) inhibitors

D. Balloon aortic valvotomy

ANSWERS

A1. **D.** The normal aortic valve area is 3.0–4.0 cm^2.

A2. **A.** Stenosis in the aortic valve arises as an active inflammatory process similar to that of coronary artery disease. The risk factors such as hypertension, hyperlipidaemia, and increased lipoprotein(a) may play a role.

A3. **B.** No treatment is shown to be useful in asymptomatic aortic stenosis patients. Close follow-up is recommended.

A4. **C.** Although ACE inhibitors are a cornerstone of therapy for heart failure, in aortic stenosis they produce vasodilation and reduce pressure distal to the obstruction against fixed valvular obstruction causing syncope.

TAKE-HOME MESSAGE

- The main causes of aortic stenosis are (i) bicuspid and other anomalies of the aortic valve, (ii) tricuspid aortic valve stenosis and (iii) rheumatic aortic valve disease.
- The symptoms of aortic stenosis include shortness of breath, angina, syncope, palpitations and heart failure.
- The pressure overload on the left ventricle is compensated by left ventricle hypertrophy (concentric hypertrophy).

- The progression of the disease results in reduced coronary blood flow (angina) and reduced cerebral blood flow (syncope).
- Left ventricular hypertrophy and afterload excess contribute to right ventricular dysfunction and heart failure.
- The clinical signs of aortic stenosis include (i) delay in the carotid pulse and (ii) S1 is normal + S2 may be single or soft + S4 gallop.
- Classic ejection murmur (peak in early systole, mid-systole) is present.
- Low pulse volume is present.
- The pulse pressure is narrow, <30 mm Hg.
- ECG: Left ventricular hypertrophy may be present.
- Echocardiography: It shows left ventricular hypertrophy, systolic ejection performance and severity of stenosis.
- Stress testing is contraindicated in symptomatic patients.
- Coronary catheterisation is needed before the surgery.
- The appearance of symptoms suggests the worsening progress of the condition and the need for surgery.
- Aortic valve replacement is not contraindicated in advanced age (up to 85 years old).
- In patients with extreme old age or when surgery is contraindicated because of comorbidities, patients are treated with diuretics and perhexiline maleate.

FURTHER READINGS

Carabello BA. Clinical practice. Aortic stenosis. *N Engl J Med.* 2002;346(9):677–682. Review.

Carabello BA, Crawford Jr FA. Valvular heart disease. *N Engl J Med.* 1997;337(1):32–41. Review.

Carabello BA, Paulus WJ. Aortic stenosis. *Lancet.* 2009;373(9667):956–966. Review.

Manning WJ. Asymptomatic aortic stenosis in the elderly: a clinical review. *JAMA.* 2013;310(14):1490–1497. Review.

Otto CM, Prendergast B. Aortic-valve stenosis—from patients at risk to severe valve obstruction. *N Engl J Med.* 2014;371(8):744–756. Review.

Zakkar M, Bryan AJ, Angelini GD. Aortic stenosis: diagnosis and management. *BMJ.* 2016;355:i5425. Review.

CASE 2.9

'While at the University Campus . . .'

Alfred Michael, a 22-year-old university student, is brought by an ambulance to the emergency department because of a history of a syncope episode while at the university campus. Alfred gives a history to the paramedic officer of dizziness for 1 hour and palpitations prior to the syncope attack. He has a history of similar symptoms twice about 6–8 months ago but did not seek medical advice. He has no chest pain, nausea, vomiting, fever or diarrhoea. On examination, he looks unwell, but is alert and oriented. The electrocardiogram (ECG) shows tachycardia, pre-excitation and a delta wave in the QRS complexes.

CASE DISCUSSION

Q1. On the basis of Alfred's presentation, what is your diagnosis?

Q2. What is your differential diagnosis?

Q3. What are the key clinical features of this disease? What are the scientific bases for these features?

Q4. What is the pathophysiology underlying these changes?

Q5. What are your management goals and management options?

ANSWERS

1. The findings of dizziness, palpitations and syncope episodes together with the ECG changes of tachycardia, pre-excitation and a delta wave in the QRS complexes are suggestive of the diagnosis of Wolff–Parkinson–White (WPW) syndrome.
2. The differential diagnosis of loss of consciousness may include the following:
    *   Acute myocardial infarction
    *   Acute coronary syndromes
    *   Pulmonary embolism
    *   Bleeding and hypovolaemia
    *   Dissection of the aorta
    *   Orthostatic hypotension
    *   Cardiac arrhythmias
    *   Structural anomalies in the cardiovascular system

- Hypoglycaemia
- Intoxication
- Seizure
- Vertebrobasilar migraine
- Transient ischaemic attacks
- Vasovagal attack
- Panic attack

The differential diagnosis for cardiac causes of syncope:

(A) Tachyarrhythmias:
  - WPW syndrome
  - Idiopathic ventricular tachycardia/fibrillation
  - Long QT syndrome
  - Brugada syndrome

(B) Bradyarrhythmias:
  - Heart block

(C) Coronary artery syndromes

(D) Vascular/cardiac defects:
  - Pulmonary hypertension
  - Pulmonary embolism
  - Atrial septal defect
  - Tetralogy of Fallot

(E) Outflow obstruction:
  - Mitral valve prolapse
  - Hypertrophic obstructive cardiomyopathy
  - Left atrial myxoma
  - Pulmonary stenosis

3. Clinical picture:

Symptoms and signs: An eyewitness is usually needed for a number of reasons:
- Approximately one-third of patients with syncope may have a retrograde amnesia for the event and cannot recall what happened.
- An eyewitness helps in differentiating a syncope from seizures.

Common symptoms encountered in syncope and tachycardia are as follows:
- Light-headedness is present.
- Palpitations occur.
- There is shortness of breath.
- Chest pain may be present.
- The patient goes 'white'.
- Loss of consciousness is brief.

The assessment in syncope includes the following:
- History (eyewitness report is important)
- Physical examination, particularly the heart and nervous system
- Measurement of blood pressure (lying and standing)

- A 12-lead ECG
- The presence of structured heart disease is always an indicator of a cardiac cause of syncope, and further assessment of the cardiovascular functions will help in detecting the exact cause

4. Laboratory findings:
   - Echocardiography
   - Stress test
   - ECG monitoring
   - Electrophysiological studies
   - Complete blood count
   - Thyroid function tests
   - Blood urea/creatinine and electrolytes
   - Drug screening

5. Pathology and pathophysiology:
   - Accessory AV pathway (known as Kent bundle) is responsible for the connection between the atrium and the ventricle in the WPW syndrome.
   - Conduction in the WPW syndrome via the Kent bundle can be antegrade or retrograde (from the ventricle to the atrium).
   - The presence of a bystander accessory pathway together with the natural AV node and His–Purkinje tract is responsible for the reentrant tachycardia circuits (pre-excited tachycardia).
   - These different pathways have different conduction properties and are responsible for the differences in the PR interval and the QRS width.

6. Management goals:
   - Termination of an acute episode
   - Blocking or slowing the accessory pathway, or blocking the AV node
   - Managing the triggers
   - Patient education
   - Termination of an acute episode: Vagal manoeuvres, IV adenosine or IV verapamil
   - Radiofrequency ablation of the accessory pathway
   - Slowing the accessory pathway by antiarrhythmic drugs
   - Blocking the AV node in adults in some types of arrhythmias
   - Managing the triggers, e.g. coronary artery disease, ischaemic cardiomyopathy, pericarditis, anaemia and thyroid dysfunctions

BACK TO BASIC SCIENCES

Q1. What are the causes of syncope?

1. Cardiac and vascular causes:
   - Heart valve disease, e.g. aortic stenosis and mitral stenosis
   - Hypertrophic cardiomyopathy

- Obstruction of major blood vessels, e.g. pulmonary embolism
- Cardiac arrhythmias, e.g. sinus bradycardia, heart block, ventricular tachycardia, ventricular fibrillation, AV block, long QT interval, WPW syndrome and paroxysmal supraventricular tachycardia
- Orthostatic hypotension
- Vasovagal (cardioneurogenic)
- Carotid sinus hypersensitivity (patients older than 50 years)

2. Noncardiac causes:
   - Transient ischaemic attacks
   - Normal-pressure hydrocephalus
   - Subclavian steel syndrome
   - Seizure
   - Panic attack

3. Metabolic causes
   - Hypoglycaemia
   - Hyperventilation

Q2. Which groups of people are likely to experience syncope?

- Military recruits
- Elderly people
- Medical students
- Pregnant women

Q3. How would you evaluate a patient with syncope?

- History is the basis for the diagnosis. An eyewitness whenever possible will be of help to differentiate syncope from a seizure.
- Physical examination helps to identify the potential cause for the syncope (particular focus on the cardiovascular and neurological examinations).
- Measure the blood pressure (standing and lying).
- Perform a 12-lead ECG.
- Search for any structured heart disease (mitral stenosis, mitral valve prolapse, aortic stenosis and hypertrophic cardiomyopathy). Perform appropriate tests to confirm these disorders.
- In the elderly, search for causes such as vasovagal, orthostatic syncope, autonomic dysfunction, postprandial hypotension, carotid sinus hypersensitivity (rare) and arrhythmias.
- Other areas to check are family history of sudden cardiac death, history of myocardial infarction, history of seizure, history of heart problems, investigations and hospital admissions.
- Cardiac evaluation for patients with unexplained syncope: (i) echocardiography, (ii) stress test, (iii) ECG monitoring and (iv) electrophysiological studies.

Q4. How would you manage a patient with syncope?

- Identify the cause.
- Patients with structural heart disease should be admitted and referred to a cardiologist.
- All patients who develop syncope during exercise and have a cardiac cause should be admitted for cardiac/vascular evaluation.
- Patients with noncardiac causes could be evaluated as outpatients.
- Assess whether the patient is fit to drive or not.

Q5. What are the characteristics of the WPW syndrome on ECG?

- A shortened PR interval
- A slow rise of the initial upstroke of the QRS complex (delta wave)
- A widened QRS complex (>0.12 second)
- ST segment–T wave directed opposite the major delta wave and QRS complex

REVIEW QUESTIONS

Q1. Which *one* of the following is consistent with syncope rather than with seizure?
A. Presence of aura
B. Cyanosis
C. Patient going 'white'
D. Rigidity occurring with loss of consciousness
E. Faecal incontinence

Q2. Which *one* of the following is *not* correct regarding the management of syncope?
A. Monitor patients with no structural heart disease for 24 hours
B. History and physical examinations are the basis for the diagnosis
C. Measure the blood pressure (lying and standing)
D. CT scan of the brain is of no value in assessment

Q3. Which *one* of the following is *not* a tachyarrhythmia associated with syncope?
A. WPW syndrome
B. Idiopathic ventricular tachycardia
C. Brugada syndrome
D. Long QT syndrome
E. Atrial fibrillation

ANSWERS

A1. **C.** In syncope, the patient is usually in the upright position, there may be predisposing factors, loss of consciousness is usually brief, patients usually recover if allowed to lie flat and the patient's colour goes 'white' as he/she loses consciousness. Cyanosis and incontinence are more with seizures.

A2. **A.** It is not productive and unnecessary to do 24-hour monitoring in a patient with no structured heart disease. CT scan of the brain is of no use in assessing syncope.

A3. **E.** Atrial fibrillation is not usually associated with syncope.

TAKE-HOME MESSAGE

- Tachyarrhythmias may include (i) WPW syndrome, (ii) idiopathic ventricular tachycardia/fibrillation, (iii) long QT syndrome and (iv) Brugada syndrome.
- Accessory AV pathway (known as Kent bundle) is responsible for the connection between the atrium and the ventricle in the WPW syndrome.
- Conduction in the WPW syndrome via the Kent bundle can be antegrade or retrograde (from the ventricle to the atrium).
- The presence of a bystander accessory pathway together with the natural AV node and His–Purkinje tract is responsible for the reentrant tachycardia circuits (pre-excited tachycardia).
- These different pathways have different conduction properties and are responsible for the differences in the PR interval and the QRS width.
- The goals of management are (i) termination of an acute episode; (ii) blocking or slowing the accessory pathway or blocking the AV node; (iii) managing the triggers; and (iv) patient education.

FURTHER READINGS

Delacrétaz E. Clinical practice. Supraventricular tachycardia. *N Engl J Med*. 2006;354(10):1039-1051. Review.

Link MS. Clinical practice. Evaluation and initial treatment of supraventricular tachycardia. *N Engl J Med*. 2012;367(15):1438-1448. Review.

Page RL. Clinical practice. Newly diagnosed atrial fibrillation. *N Engl J Med*. 2004;351(23):2408-2416. Review.

Roden DM. Drug-induced prolongation of the QT interval. *N Engl J Med*. 2004;350(10):1013-1022. Review.

Roden DM. Clinical practice. Long-QT syndrome. *N Engl J Med*. 2008;358(2):169-176. Review.

Zimetbaum P. Amiodarone for atrial fibrillation. *N Engl J Med*. 2007;356(9):935-941. Review.

CASE 2.10

'I Am Coughing Up Blood . . .'

Andrew Morgan, a 65-year-old personal coach, comes in to see his general practitioner because he is suffering from a cough for the past 2–3 months, progressive shortness of breath and loss of 3 kg of body weight. Early in his illness, he was seen by another doctor, who prescribed him a broad-spectrum antibiotic and Andrew feels that his cough has increased. Chest X-ray reveals a mass of 3.5 × 4.0 cm at the right hilum. Mr Morgan is referred for bronchoscopy, which confirms the presence of a tumour mass in the right lower lobe. A biopsy of the mass and histopathological examination reveals squamous cell carcinoma of moderate differentiation. A CT scan of the chest shows the tumour mass at the apex of the right lower lobe and the presence of two subcarinal nodes and three lymph nodes in the mediastinum. Mr Morgan is referred to a cardiothoracic surgeon for further assessment and management.

CASE DISCUSSION

Q1. On the basis of Andrew's presentation, what is your diagnosis?

Q2. What is your differential diagnosis?

Q3. What are the key clinical features of this disease? What are the scientific bases for these features?

Q4. What is the pathophysiology underlying these changes?

Q5. What are your management goals and management options?

ANSWERS

1. The findings of persistent cough, progressive shortness of breath, weight loss and a mass at the right hilum on chest X-ray together with confirmation of mass in the right lower lobe that turned out to be squamous cell carcinoma of moderate differentiation of histopathological examination and the chest CT scan findings are consistent with the diagnosis of squamous cell lung carcinoma.
2. The differential diagnosis includes the following:
   * Pulmonary tuberculosis
   * Bacterial pneumonia
   * Viral pneumonia
   * Bronchitis

- Pleural effusion
- Mycoplasma pneumonia
- Lung abscess
- Hamartoma
- Granuloma
- Carcinoid lung tumours
- Benign lung tumours
- Metastatic cancer
- Mediastinal lymphomas

3. Clinical signs:

Symptoms: The clinical picture of lung cancer is reflected in local and metastatic effects and some tumours such as small cell lung cancer have paraneoplastic effects.

1. Cough: It may be dry or productive (secondary infection).
2. Haemoptysis: It occurs particularly in central bronchial tumours or if the tumour invades a large vessel (massive haemoptysis).
3. Breathlessness: It occurs due to collapse, pneumonia or large pleural effusion. In some cases, a large tumour presses on the phrenic nerve causing diaphragmatic paralysis.
4. Chest pain: Compression of intercostal nerve causes dermatomal chest pain.
5. Pleural pain: Invasion of the pleura causes pleural pain.
6. Horner syndrome: This occurs in carcinoma of the apex of the lung → involvement of sympathetic chain → ipsilateral partial ptosis, enophthalmos, miosis and hypohidrosis (or anhidrosis) of the face.
7. Pancoast syndrome → apical tumour invading the T1 and C8 roots of the bronchial plexus → shoulder pain, pain in the inner aspect of the arm and wasting in the hand.
8. Dysphagia: It occurs due to mediastinal spread and involvement of the oesophagus.
9. Pericarditis and pericardial effusion: They spread to the mediastinum → involvement of the pericardium and development of pericardial effusion. Arrhythmias may occur secondary to pericardial involvement.
10. Superior vena cava obstruction → pressure on the superior vena cava by enlarged lymph nodes → cough, dyspnoea, swelling of the face and neck, facial cyanosis, conjunctival oedema, dilated veins on the chest wall, papilloedema and headache.
11. Voice changes: Involvement of the left recurrent laryngeal nerve by the tumour → vocal cord paralysis and voice changes. Also the cough becomes not explosive in character.
12. Metastasis to the nervous system → seizures, personality changes, focal neurological deficit and spinal cord metastasis.
13. Bone pain → metastasis to the bones.

14. Clubbing of fingers: It may be associated with hypertrophic pulmonary osteo-arthropathy of the distal tibia, fibula, radius and ulna (X-ray shows subperiosteal new bone formation).
15. Enlargement of the supraclavicular lymph nodes occurs.
16. Syndrome of inappropriate antidiuretic hormone secretion (SIADH) and adrenocorticotrophic hormone (ACTH) secretion (Cushing syndrome) occur in patients with small cell lung cancer.
17. Hypercalcaemia occurs in patients with squamous cell carcinoma.
18. Other paraneoplastic syndromes that may occur in addition to SIADH (ectopic production of ACTH) and hypercalcaemia are as follows:
    – Clubbing: All types of lung cancers
    – Eaton–Lambert syndrome: Small cell carcinoma
    – Trousseau syndrome: Adenocarcinoma

4. Laboratory investigations:
   • Plain chest X-ray: It may show central tumour, hilar glandular enlargement, peripheral well-circumscribed opacity, lobar or segmental collapse, plural effusion, mediastinal changes, elevation of a hemidiaphragm and invasion.
   • Flexible bronchoscopy for central masses: It involves visualisation and taking biopsies from the lesion for cytological studies, and assessment of operability.
   • Percutaneous needle biopsy under chest CT or ultrasound guidance: It is performed for peripheral lesions that cannot be examined via flexible bronchoscopy – get histological diagnosis.
   • Sputum examination: Three samples of sputum are calculated for cytological studies. This may be used in patients with chronic obstructive lung diseases and difficulties in assessing them using percutaneous needle biopsy.
   • Pleural aspiration: In patients with pleural effusion, pleural aspiration and biopsy could offer great help in the investigation.
   • Thoracoscopy: It can be used in specialised centres.
   • Staging: This includes the following:
     (a) Computed tomography scan of the lower neck, chest and upper abdomen
     (b) Positron emission tomography (PET) – malignant lung neoplasms have higher metabolic activities than benign tumours
     (c) Brain magnetic resonance imaging
     (d) Complete blood count and differential
     (e) Blood biochemistry studies – blood urea, creatinine, electrolytes and liver function tests
     (f) Pulmonary function tests
     (g) Mediastinoscopy – review the TNM staging for lung cancer (Table 2.10.1)

5. Pathological features:
   • Lung carcinoma can be classified into two main groups: (i) non-small cell lung cancer (85% of all types) and (ii) small cell lung cancer forming remaining 15%.

Table 2.10.1 TNM staging system for lung cancer

Primary tumour (T)

T1: Tumour ≤3 cm diameter without invasion more proximal than lobar bronchus

T2: Tumour >3 cm diameter *or* tumour of any size with any of the following characteristics:
    Invasion of visceral pleura
    Atelectasis of less than entire lung
    Proximal extent at least 2 cm from carina

T3: Tumour of any size with any of the following characteristics:
    Invasion of chest wall
    Involvement of diaphragm, mediastinal pleura or pericardium
    Atelectasis involving entire lung
    Proximal extent within 2 cm of carina

T4: Tumour of any size with any of the following:
    Invasion of mediastinum
    Invasion of heart or great vessels
    Invasion of trachea or oesophagus
    Invasion of vertebral body or carina
    Presence of malignant pleural or pericardial effusion
    Satellite tumour nodule(s) within same lobe as primary tumour

Nodal involvement (N)

N0: No regional node involvement

N1: Metastasis to ipsilateral hilar and/or ipsilateral peribronchial nodes

N2: Metastasis to ipsilateral mediastinal and/or subcarinal nodes

N3: Metastasis to contralateral mediastinal or hilar nodes *or* ipsilateral or contralateral scalene
    or supraclavicular nodes

Metastasis (M)

M0: Distant metastasis absent

M1: Distant metastasis present (includes metastatic tumour nodules in a different lobe from the
    primary tumour)

Stage groupings of TNM subsets

Stage IA	T1 N0 M0	Stage IIIA	T3 N1 M0
Stage IB	T2 N0 M0		T1–3 N2 M0
Stage IIA	T1 N1 M0	Stage IIIB	Any T N3 M0
Stage IIB	T2 N1 M0		T4 Any N M0
	T3 N0 M0	Stage IV	Any T Any N M1

Adapted from Greene FL, Page DL, Fleming ID. AJCC Cancer Staging Manual, 6th ed. New York, Springer, 2002.
Source: Andreoli TE, Benjamin IJ, Griggs RC, Wing EJ. Andreoli and Carpenter's Cecil Essentials of Medicine. 8th ed. Philadelphia, PA: Elsevier; 2010.

- Non-small cell lung cancer comprises (i) squamous cell carcinoma, (ii) adenocarcinoma, (iii) bronchoalveolar carcinoma, (iv) large cell cancer, (v) carcinoid and (vi) others.
- The commonest forms are adenocarcinoma, squamous cell cancer and large cell lung cancer.
- Approximately 85%–90% of lung cancers occur in cigarette smokers. Smokers are at risk of both non-small cell lung cancer and small cell lung cancer.
- Nonsmokers who develop lung cancer usually have adenocarcinoma.

6. Management goals:

The goals and options depend on the type:

1. Non-small cell lung cancer:
   - Surgery: For stages I–II, surgery is the best chance of cure (anatomical lobectomy or pneumonectomy).
   - Adjuvant therapy: Adjuvant postoperative chemotherapy is indicated for patients with recurrence.
   - Radiotherapy: External beam radiotherapy is done for patients not fit for surgery.
   - Stage IIIA: Surgery and adjuvant chemotherapy are performed after complete surgical resection + radiotherapy.
   - Stage IIIB: Palliative therapy or palliative radiation is performed.
   - Stage IV: It involves palliative treatment (symptomatic).

2. Squamous cell lung cancer:
   - Platinum chemotherapy doublets are the first line of treatment.
   - Immunotherapy is now considered the second line of therapy.

3. Small cell lung cancer:
   - Limited stage – surgical resection but usually benefit from chemotherapy and radiotherapy within 30 days of the start of chemotherapy
   - Extensive disease – palliative chemotherapy
   - Prophylactic cranial irradiation – because the brain is a common site of relapse in small lung cancer

BACK TO BASIC SCIENCES

Q1. What are the major forms of lung cancer?

1. Non-small cell lung cancer (about 85% of all lung cancers). It includes the following histological subtypes:
   - Squamous cell carcinoma
   - Adenocarcinoma
   - Large cell lung cancer
   - Bronchioloalveolar carcinoma
2. Small cell lung cancer (about 15% of all cases of lung cancer)

Q2. Which types of lung cancers are caused by smoking?

- All types of lung cancers are caused by smoking. However, small cell lung cancer and squamous cell carcinoma are strongly linked with smoking.
- Adenocarcinoma is the most common lung cancer that is found in nonsmokers.

Q3. Briefly discuss the pathology of small cell carcinoma.

Small cell carcinoma is a highly malignant epithelial tumour of the lung. It is closely linked to smoking. The tumour metastasises rapidly and over 70% of patients are first seen at advanced stages of the disease.

The carcinoma is characterised by neuroendocrine features, which are responsible for paraneoplastic syndromes:
- Inappropriate secretion of antidiuretic hormone.
- Ectopic ACTH secretion (Cushing syndrome)
- Eaton–Lambert syndrome

The lesion is usually in the periphery and there is always extensive lymph node metastasis. Cut sections are soft, white in colour with areas of haemorrhages and necrosis. This cancer is sensitive to chemotherapy and this is the mainstay of management.

Q4. Discuss the clinical application of the epidermal growth factor receptor (EGFR) mutation in the management of lung cancer.

EGFR mutations are more common in adenocarcinomas. These mutations are more commonly observed in women with adenocarcinomas who do not smoke and also in Asians. They are more likely to respond to the EGFR tyrosine kinase inhibitors such as gefitinib and erlotinib.

Q5. Discuss 'Pancoast tumour' and its clinical significance.

Lung tumours affecting the apex of the lung (usually squamous lung cancer) are called Pancoast tumours. These tumours are capable of involving the eighth cervical and first and second thoracic nerves resulting in shoulder pain and pain along the medial aspect of the arm (ulnar nerve distribution).

This tumour can also involve the cervical sympathetic chain resulting in Horner syndrome on the same side: (i) enophthalmos, (ii) ptosis of the upper eyelid, (iii) construction of the pupil (miosis) and (iv) loss of sweating (anhidrosis).

Q6. Discuss paraneoplastic syndromes in lung cancer.

1. A number of disorders are associated with lung cancer such as acanthosis nigricans, dermatomyositis, polymyositis, myasthenia (Eaton–Lambert syndrome) and clubbing
2. Endocrine syndromes such as inappropriate secretion of antidiuretic hormone, Cushing syndrome (in small cell carcinoma) and hypercalcaemia (in squamous cell carcinoma)

REVIEW QUESTIONS

Q1. Which type of lung cancer is usually present in people who never smoked and develop lung cancer?

A. Squamous cell carcinoma

B. Small cell carcinoma

C. Adenocarcinoma

D. Lymphoma

E. Large cell carcinoma

Q2. Which *one* of the following statements about lung cancer is *not* correct?
A. It was regarded as a rare tumour in the year 1940.
B. Over 80% of lung carcinomas are non-small cell lung cancer.
C. K-ras mutation confers poor prognosis in patients with adenocarcinoma.
D. It is particularly dominant in males.

Q3. Regarding molecular pathogenesis of lung cancer, which *one* of the following is *not* correct?
A. Mutations in *p53* are identical in more than 80% of small cell carcinoma.
B. Mutations in *retinoblastoma (Rb)* gene occur in more than 80% of small cell carcinoma.
C. Overexpression of *Myc* oncogene occurs in all lung cancers but not in small cell carcinoma.
D. Deletion of the short arm of chromosome 3 (3p) occurs in all lung cancers.

Q4. Which *one* of the following is *not* correct about squamous cell carcinoma?
A. Mostly arises in the central portion of the lung
B. Arises in scars left from old tuberculosis
C. Central cavitation frequent
D. Microscopically has 'keratin pearls' surrounded by concentric 'onion skin' layers

Q5. Which *one* of the following is *not* correct about adenocarcinoma?
A. Demonstration of mucin using periodic acid–Schiff (PAS) stain excludes its diagnosis.
B. It is the most common type in women.
C. It arises in the periphery in the subpleural region.
D. Cut section is glistening greyish white in appearance.
E. The most common histologic type of adenocarcinoma is the acinar pattern.

Q6. Which *one* of the following is *not* correct about bronchoalveolar carcinoma?
A. It is a subtype of adenocarcinoma.
B. It is strongly linked to smoking.
C. Copious mucin in the sputum is seen in 10% of patients.
D. Two-thirds of this carcinoma is nonmucinous.

ANSWERS

A1. **C.** Nonsmokers who develop lung carcinoma usually have an adenocarcinoma.

A2. **D.** The distribution of lung cancer shows a rising trend in women, particularly with the increased smoking among women.

A3. **C.** Overexpression of *Myc* oncogene occurs in approximately 40% of small cell lung carcinoma. It is rare in other types.

A4. **B.** Adenocarcinoma was thought to arise from scars of old tuberculosis. Now we know that most of these scars in adenocarcinoma represent a desmoplastic response to the tumour.

A5. **A.** The demonstration of mucin using mucicarmine or PAS stains helps in differentiating adenocarcinoma (produces mucin) from large cell carcinomas.

A6. **B.** Like adenocarcinoma, bronchoalveolar carcinoma is not linked to smoking. Two-thirds of bronchoalveolar carcinoma is nonmucinous and only one-third is mucinous.

The production of large amounts of mucin in the sputum is characteristic but only occurs in 10% of patients.

TAKE-HOME MESSAGE

- Lung carcinoma can be classified into two main groups: (i) non-small cell lung cancer (85% of all types) and (ii) small cell lung cancer forming remaining 15%.
- Non-small cell lung cancer comprises (i) squamous cell carcinoma, (ii) adenocarcinoma, (iii) bronchoalveolar carcinoma, (iv) large cell cancer, (v) carcinoid and (vi) others.
- The commonest forms are adenocarcinoma, squamous cell cancer and large cell lung cancer.
- Approximately 85%–90% of lung cancers occur in cigarette smokers. Smokers are at risk of both non-small cell lung cancer and small cell lung cancer.
- Nonsmokers who develop lung cancer usually have adenocarcinoma.
- Symptoms of lung cancer may include cough, haemoptysis, shortness of breath, chest pain, Horner syndrome, Pancoast syndrome, dysphagia, superior vena cava obstruction, vocal changes, bone pains, symptoms related to metastasis and paraneoplastic syndrome.
- Investigations include (i) plain chest X-ray; (ii) flexible bronchoscopy for central masses; (iii) percutaneous needle biopsy under chest CT or ultrasound guidance – performed for peripheral lesions; (iv) sputum examination – three samples of sputum are calculated for cytological studies; (v) pleural aspiration – in patients with pleural effusion, pleural aspiration and biopsy could offer great help in the investigation; and (vi) thoracoscopy in specialised centres.
- The management depends on the type and stage of cancer.

FURTHER READINGS

Hirsch FR, Scagliotti GV, Mulshine JL, et al. Lung cancer: current therapies and new targeted treatments. *Lancet.* 2017;389(10066):299-311. Review.

Hirsch FR, Suda K, Wiens J, Bunn Jr PA. New and emerging targeted treatments in advanced non-small-cell lung cancer. *Lancet.* 2016;388(10048):1012-1024. Review.

Oudkerk M, Devaraj A, Vliegenthart R, et al. European position statement on lung cancer screening. *Lancet Oncol.* 2017;18(12):e754-e766. Review.

Perrot M, Wu L, Wu M, Cho BCJ. Radiotherapy for the treatment of malignant pleural mesothelioma. *Lancet Oncol.* 2017;18(9):e532-e542. Review.

Titulaer MJ, Lang B, Verschuuren JJ. Lambert-Eaton myasthenic syndrome: from clinical characteristics to therapeutic strategies. *Lancet Neurol.* 2011;10(12):1098-1107. Review.

SECTION 3

Nervous System

CASE 3.1

Tremor in Hands

Ahmad Murad, a 65-year-old pensioner, comes in with his wife to see a local general practitioner. Ahmad has difficulty with his gait for the past 8–10 months. He has no pains but he walks slowly and remembers occasional falls particularly when changing his direction. He also noted difficulty in turning himself in bed. His wife noted tremor in his hands. On examination, he has an expressionless face, and there is saliva drooling from his mouth; he has a resting tremor in his hands that disappears with intentional movement. He walks slowly with his body leaning forward.

CASE DISCUSSION

Q1. On the basis of Ahmad's presentation, what is your diagnosis?

Q2. What is your differential diagnosis?

Q3. What are the key clinical features of this disease? What are the scientific bases for these features?

Q4. What is the pathophysiology underlying these changes?

Q5. What are your management goals and management options?

ANSWERS

1. The findings of rest tremor, expressionless face, rigidity, bradykinesia, gait impairment and falling tendency on changing directions are consistent with the diagnosis of Parkinson disease. The mean age of the disease is about 60 years but it can be seen in patients in their 20s.
2. The differential diagnosis:
   - Parkinson disease: Genetic and sporadic (about 80%–90% of cases)
   - Atypical parkinsonism: Multiple system atrophy, cerebellar type, Parkinson type and progressive supranuclear palsy
   - Secondary parkinsonism: Drug-induced (reserpine, metoclopramide, antipsychotic agents), infection, vascular, trauma, normal-pressure hydrocephalus, liver failure and toxins
   - Other neurodegenerative disorders: Wilson disease, Huntington disease, Creutzfeldt–Jakob disease and Alzheimer disease with parkinsonism
   - Essential tremor

The following are essential for the diagnosis of Parkinson disease:
- Rest tremor, rigidity, bradykinesia and gait impairment are cardinal for the diagnosis. A sustained response to therapy with levodopa is also important.
- Other features are postural instability, speech difficulty, autonomic disorders, mood disorders, sleep disturbance, cognitive disturbance and dementia.

3. Symptoms and signs:
   - Cardinal symptoms: (i) Tremor (at rest, enhanced by stress), (ii) rigidity (causes flexed posture), (iii) bradykinesia (slow voluntary movements, reduction in swinging of the arms while walking), (iv) postural instability and (v) mild decline in intellectual functions
   - Tremor: Important in the diagnosis, may be absent in some patients, 2–6 cycles/s, observed in resting hands, become less noticed during voluntary movement, enhanced by stress, usually limited to one limb for months or years, and may be present around the mouth and lips
   - Immobility of facial muscles: Infrequent blinks, fixed facial expression and seborrhoea of the face
   - Positive Myerson sign: A sustained blinking on repetitive tapping over the bridge of the nose
   - Other clinical findings: Drooling of saliva from the mouth, dysphagia, micrographia, slowness of voluntary movements and voice change
   - No changes in muscle tone or muscle weakness, and no changes in tendon reflexes or plantar responses
   - Gait: Moving forward, unsteady on turning, small shuffling steps and loss of arm swinging while walking

4. Pathological features:
   - Degeneration of dopaminergic neurons in the substantia nigra
   - Reduced striatal dopamine
   - Intracytoplasmic proteinaceous inclusions known as Lewy bodies

   Recent studies showed that norepinephrine neurons of the locus coeruleus and serotonin neurons in the raphe nuclei in the brainstem and neurons of the olfactory system are affected earlier in the disease together with cerebral hemisphere, spinal cord and peripheral autonomic neurons system. The nondopaminergic pathological changes occur earlier in the disease and are responsible for a number of symptoms such as constipation, anosmia, rapid eye movement, sleep disturbance and autonomic disturbances. These changes usually precede the classic motor features of the disease.

5. Management goals:
   - Improve the clinical symptoms of parkinsonism.
   - Ameliorate dyskinesia and replace the deficiency of dopamine in the striatum of Parkinson disease patients.
      - **A.** Pharmacological treatment: Levodopa, nonergot dopamine agonists and monoamine oxidase B inhibitors are used for the initial therapy. Details of medications are summarised in Table 3.1.1.

Table 3.1.1 Drugs used to treat patients with Parkinson disease

Group	Examples	Mechanisms of action	Advantages	Side effects
Carbidopa/levodopa	Immediate and sustained release	Levodopa, the metabolic precursor of dopamine, crosses the blood–brain barrier and is converted to dopamine in the brain	Most effective, improves disability, improves patient's daily activities	Dyskinesia, dystonia, confusion, psychosis, sedation
Dopamine agonists	Ergot – bromocriptine Nonergot – pramipexole	Bromocriptine stimulates centrally located dopaminergic receptors The postsynaptic D2 stimulation is the primary action responsible for the parkinsonian effect	Can be used as monotherapy in early disease Or added to levodopa Less risk of developing motor complications	Ergot – pulmonary fibrosis, cardiac valve fibrosis, erythromelalgia All: (i) dopaminergic adverse effects (nausea, vomiting, orthostatic hypotension), (ii) neuropsychiatric side effects (hallucinations, psychosis, impulse control disorders)
Monoamine oxidase B inhibitors	Selegiline Rasagiline	Unknown One possible mechanism is related to its MAO–B inhibitory activity → increased extracellular levels of dopamine in the striatum → increased dopaminergic activity	Can be used as monotherapy in early disease Once daily Well tolerated	Amphetamine and methamphetamine metabolites may cause side effects Serotonin syndrome
Catechol O-methyltransferase inhibitors	Entacapone Tolcapone	Inhibit COMT in peripheral tissues → changing the plasma pharmacokinetics of levodopa	Can treat motor complications Decreased 'off time'[a] No titration Mild improvement in daily activities	Dopaminergic adverse effects (nausea, vomiting, orthostatic hypotension) Discolouration of urine Tolcapone > severe diarrhoea and liver toxicity

Continued

Table 3.1.1 Drugs used to treat patients with Parkinson disease—cont'd

Group	Examples	Mechanisms of action	Advantages	Side effects
Anticholinergics	Benztropine	Benztropine is selectively M1 muscarinic acetylcholine It also partially blocks cholinergic activity in the CNS which is responsible for symptoms in Parkinson disease	Useful in treating tremor in patients younger than 60 years without cognitive impairment	Anticholinergic side effects
N-methyl-o-aspartate receptor inhibitor	Amantadine	Mechanism not fully known It is possibly related to the release of dopamine from nerve endings in the brain cells together with the stimulation of the norepinephrine response	Can treat dyskinesias in late disease	Cognitive effects, livedo reticularis, oedema, development of tolerance, potential for withdrawal
Injectable dopamine agonists	Apomorphine	Unknown Stimulation of postsynaptic D2-type receptors within the brain	Reduces 'off time[a]' in late disease	Require initiation in hospital, subcutaneous injections

[a]Severe debilitating symptoms with periods of decreased motor and nonmotor functions.

B. Surgery: Most patients will eventually develop disabling symptoms despite optimum medications and become candidates for deep brain stimulation, which targets either the subthalamic nucleus or the globus pallidus (GP) interna.

BACK TO BASIC SCIENCES

Q1. What are the major neuropathic findings in Parkinson disease?
The major neuropathic findings in Parkinson disease are loss of pigmented dopaminergic neurons of the substantia nigra pars compacta and the presence of Lewy bodies and Lewy neuritis.

Q2. What are the anatomical structures forming the basal ganglia?
Basal ganglia are a group of nuclei situated deep at the base of the forebrain. They are connected with the cerebral cortex, forebrain, midbrain and thalamus as well as other areas of the brain. They include the caudate nucleus, putamen, nucleus accumbens, amygdala and the globus pallidus (GP).

The caudate and putamen have similar functions and are called neostriatum or striatum.

Medial to the putamen is the GP. The GP has two parts: GP (external) and GP (internal). The putamen and GP are shaped like a lens and hence called 'lenticular nucleus'.

Q3. What are the functions of the basal ganglia?
   (i) The basal ganglia play a role in controlling movement and facilitate desired movements and inhibit unwanted movements.
  (ii) They are involved in neuronal pathways having emotional, motivational, associative and cognitive functions.
 (iii) They are involved in involuntary and stereotyped movements or paucity of movements.

Q4. What are the cells producing dopamine in the substantia nigra?
These include cells in the pars compacta of the substantia nigra.

Q5. What are the subtypes of dopamine receptors?
There are five subtypes of the dopamine receptors: D1, D2, D3, D4 and D5. They are encoded in humans by genes *DRD1*, *DRD2*, *DRD3*, *DRD4* and *DRD5*, respectively.

The receptors are classified as D1-class receptors (D1 and D5) and D2-class receptors (D2, D3 and D4).

Q6. Give examples of physiological functions mediated by dopamine.
Examples include voluntary movement, reward, sleep regulation, feeding, affect, attention, cognitive function, olfaction, vision, hormonal regulation, sympathetic regulation

and penile erection. The dopamine receptors also influence the immune system and the cardiovascular, renal and gastrointestinal functions.

Q7. Briefly discuss the direct and indirect pathways in the basal ganglia that regulate movement.
Direct pathway: The striatal cells project directly to GP (internal) → increased excitatory drive from the thalamus to the cortex (mediated by glutamate) → excite striatal neurons (inhibiting transmitter GABA) → inhibit GP (internal) cells → less inhibition of the motor thalamus and turning up the motor cortex.
Indirect pathway: The striatal neurons of this pathway project to GP (external) → GP (external) neurons project to the subthalamic nucleus → project to GP (internal) → project to the thalamus → decreased excitatory drive from the thalamus to the cortex → turn down the motor cortex → thus turning down the motor activity.

Q8. Discuss dopaminergic modulation of direct and indirect pathways in the basal ganglia.
Dopamine via D1 receptors has an *excitatory* effect on cells in the striatum (direct pathway).
　　Dopamine via D2 receptors has an *inhibitory* effect on striatal cells (indirect pathway).

REVIEW QUESTIONS

Q1. Which *one* of the following is not a component of the basal ganglia?
A. Thalamus
B. Putamen
C. Caudate nucleus
D. GP
E. Amygdala

Q2. Regarding basal ganglia circuits (pathways), which *one* of the following statements is correct?
A. They affect movements of the contralateral body.
B. They affect movements of the ipsilateral body.
C. They affect movement of both sides of the body.
D. Regardless of the pathway, they finally turn up the motor cortex.

Q3. Which *one* of the following is not a neurotransmitter?
A. Dopamine
B. Acetylcholine
C. Noradrenaline
D. Adrenaline
E. Cyclic AMP

Q4. Which *one* of the following drugs may cause parkinsonism?
A. Apomorphine
B. Metoclopramide
C. Dopamine
D. Benzhexol

Q5. Which *one* of the drugs used in treating Parkinson disease may reduce the 'off-time' effect?
A. Carbidopa/levodopa
B. Bromocriptine
C. Selegiline
D. Catechol O-methyltransferase inhibitors
E. Amantadine

ANSWERS

A1. **A.** The components of the basal ganglia include the caudate nucleus, putamen, nucleus accumbens, amygdala and GP.

A2. **A.** The output neurons of the basal ganglia circuits project to the ipsilateral motor thalamus via the ansa lenticularis. However, they affect the movements of the contralateral side of the body.

A3. **E.** Cyclic AMP is not a neurotransmitter. It is a second messenger important in biological processes.

A4. **B.** Drugs that may cause parkinsonism include reserpine, metoclopramide and anti-psychotic agents. Benzhexol is used in treating drug-induced parkinsonism.

A5. **D.** Catechol O-methyltransferase inhibitors such as entacapone and tolcapone can decrease the 'off-time' effect. Also, apomorphine can reduce the 'off time' in late disease.

TAKE-HOME MESSAGE

- Parkinson disease is a progressive neurodegenerative disorder that mainly affects the substantia nigra and the development of Lewy bodies in the residual dopaminergic neurons.
- The cardinal clinical features of the disease are resting tremor, rigidity, bradykinesia and postural instability. The symptoms respond to levodopa, the primary treatment for Parkinson disease.
- The disease may be detected many years before the appearance of the motor symptoms – nondopaminergic pathological changes responsible for a number of symptoms such as constipation, anosmia, rapid eye movement, sleep disturbance and autonomic disturbances.

- There are several conditions that mimic the disease, making it difficult to diagnose in the early stages.
- The diagnosis of Parkinson disease is based on clinical assessment and the response of symptoms to levodopa.
- Levodopa, nonergot dopamine agonists and monoamine oxidase B inhibitors are used for the initial therapy. Dopamine agonists are inferior to levodopa in controlling motor symptoms. However, the long use of levodopa is limited by the development of drug-induced dyskinesia.
- In advanced disease, surgical approach such as deep brain stimulation of the subthalamic nucleus is used to ameliorate the symptoms.

FURTHER READINGS

Beaulieu JM, Espinoza S, Gainetdinov RR. Dopamine receptors - IUPHAR Review 13. *Br J Pharmacol.* 2015;172(1):1-23. Review.

Gazewood JD, Richards DR, Clebak K. Parkinson disease: an update. *Am Fam Physician.* 2013;87(4): 267-273.

Lewitt PA. Levodopa for the treatment of Parkinson's disease. *N Engl J Med.* 2008;359(23):2468-2476. Review.

Muzerengi S, Clarke CE. Initial drug treatment in Parkinson's disease. *BMJ.* 2015;351:h4669. Review.

Nutt JG, Wooten GF. Clinical practice. Diagnosis and initial management of Parkinson's disease. *N Engl J Med.* 2005;353(10):1021-1027. Review.

Rao SS, Hofmann LA, Shakil A. Parkinson's disease: diagnosis and treatment. *Am Fam Physician.* 2006; 74(12):2046-2054.

Scottish Intercollegiate Guidelines Network. *Diagnosis and pharmacological management of Parkinson's disease. A national clinical guideline. No 113. NHS.* January 2010. (A summary of guidelines appeared in BMJ 2010; 340. https://doi.org/10.1136/bmj.b5614)

CASE 3.2

Not Moving

Lilian Andrew, a 67-year-old widow, is brought by an ambulance to the emergency department because she is suffering from acute-onset inability to move her right arm and leg for the past 1 hour. She is also unable to speak since about the same time. Her daughter who comes with her says, 'About 1–2 months and on two occasions mum had brief visual disturbances, inability to talk and numbness of extremities, which were recovered in about 10–20 minutes. She cannot remember which side was affected.' Mrs Andrew has had high blood pressure and diabetes mellitus for nearly 10 years, but she lacks adherence to treatment and does not see her GP regularly. She ceased smoking about 4 years after the death of her husband. On examination, she is conscious, unable to move her right side and unable to speak but appears to understand. Her pulse is 95/min (regular), blood pressure 160/95 mm Hg, respiratory rate 24/min and temperature 36.8°C. Neurological examination shows right-sided weakness and loss of sensations. Deep tendon reflexes on the right side (triceps, biceps, brachioradialis, knee and ankle) are exaggerated and Babinski reflex is positive. There is no weakness on the left side and corresponding reflexes on the left side are all normal. A noncontrast computed tomography (CT) of the head showed no intracranial bleeding or subarachnoid haemorrhage (SAH) but was not informative about stroke. Magnetic resonance imaging (MRI) scan of the head confirmed stroke.

CASE DISCUSSION

Q1. On the basis of Mrs Andrew's presentation, what is your diagnosis?

Q2. What is your differential diagnosis?

Q3. What are the key clinical features of this disease? What are the scientific bases for these features?

Q4. What is the pathophysiology underlying these changes?

Q5. What are your management goals and management options?

ANSWERS

1. The findings of acute onset, aphasia and right-sided hemiplegia within 1–2 hours of onset of symptoms together with a history of transient ischaemic attacks on two occasions and risk factors (diabetes mellitus, hypertension, smoking and poor compliance) in an elderly patient are consistent with the diagnosis of stroke involving the left middle cerebral artery territory.

2. The differential diagnosis:
   - Transient ischaemic attack
   - Subdural or epidural haemorrhage
   - Hypoglycaemia
   - Ischaemic stroke
   - Subarachnoid haemorrhage (SAH)
   - Focal seizure

3. Symptoms and signs:

   The clinical signs and symptoms in patients with ischaemic vascular disease are dependent on the arterial supply involved. The clinical presentation can be summarised as follows (for further reading, check Leung et al., 2010):
   - Anterior cerebral artery: (i) Contralateral leg involvement more than (>) arm paresis; and (ii) contralateral leg involvement > arm sensory deficit/loss
   - Middle cerebral artery: (i) Contralateral hemiparesis (face, arm > leg), (ii) contralateral sensory deficit (face, arm > leg), (iii) contralateral visual field deficit, (iv) aphasia (depending on the dominant hemisphere) and (v) contralateral hemisphere neglect
   - Posterior cerebral artery: (i) Contralateral homonymous hemianopia and (ii) contralateral sensory deficit/loss (thalamic involvement)
   - Posterior inferior cerebellar artery: (i) Ipsilateral sensory loss over the face, (ii) dysphasia, (iii) ipsilateral Horner syndrome and (iv) ataxia
   - Internal carotid artery: (i) Ipsilateral visual loss and (ii) ipsilateral middle cerebral artery syndrome
   - Lacunar syndromes: (i) Pure motor stroke, (ii) pure sensory stroke, (iii) ataxic hemiparesis and (iv) clumsy hand-dysarthria (Fig. 3.2.1 shows the extracranial and intracranial arterial supply of the brain)

   The principal types of aphasia associated with middle cerebral artery ischaemia are summarised in Table 3.2.1.

4. Investigations:
   - Laboratory investigations:
     - Complete blood count (look for polycythaemia, raised white blood cells may indicate infection such as bacterial endocarditis)
     - Platelet count (thrombocytopenia can lead to platelet thrombi)
     - ESR (raised may indicate inflammation or systemic infection)
     - Prothrombin time/INR
     - Activated partial thromboplastin time
     - Blood glucose level
     - Renal function tests
     - Liver function tests
     - Pregnancy test in young women
     - Toxicology tests and blood screen for drugs and alcohol
     - A thrombin time
     - Troponin test
     - Oxygen saturation

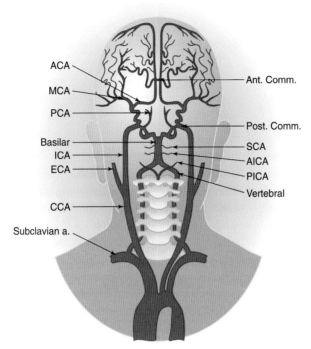

Figure 3.2.1 Extracranial and intracranial arterial supply of the brain. *(Source: Andreoli TE, Benjamin IJ, Griggs RC, Wing EJ. Andreoli and Carpenter's Cecil Essentials of Medicine. 8th ed. Philadelphia, PA: Elsevier; 2010.)*

Table 3.2.1 Principal types of aphasia

Type	Lesion site	Fluency	Comprehension	Repetition	Naming	Other signs
Broca	Inferior frontal lobe	↓	Good	↓	↓	Contralateral weakness
Wernicke	Posterior superior temporal lobe	Good	↓	↓	↓	Homonymous hemianopia
Conduction	Supramarginal gyrus	Good	Good	↓	↓	None
Global	Frontal lobe (large)	↓	↓	↓	↓	Hemiplegia

Source: Andreoli TE, Benjamin IJ, Griggs RC, Wing EJ. Andreoli and Carpenter's Cecil Essentials of Medicine. 8th ed. Philadelphia, PA: Elsevier; 2010.

- Electrocardiogram (ECG): It may show myocardial infarction, ST-segment changes, atrial fibrillation and other types of arrhythmias.
- Imaging: CT brain scan or MRI brain scan:
  - Usually we start with CT scan and it can help us in (i) locating the area of damage, (ii) distinguishing a brain haemorrhage from an ischaemic stroke, (iii) identifying localised mass/tumour and (iv) identifying subdural haematoma (Fig. 3.2.2).

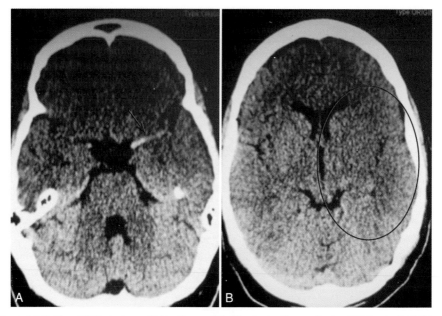

Figure 3.2.2 (A and B) Early signs of infarction on CT of the brain. *(Source: Andreoli TE, Benjamin IJ, Griggs RC, Wing EJ. Andreoli and Carpenter's Cecil Essentials of Medicine. 8th ed. Philadelphia, PA: Elsevier; 2010.)*

- An MRI scan is needed if the CT scan cannot show the lesion. In acute phase, the CT scan is often normal and MRI is more sensitive for detecting ischaemic changes (Fig. 3.2.3).
- MRI brain scan is also needed if the lesion involves the posterior cerebral region, brainstem and cerebellum. Usually CT scan cannot visualise these areas.
- However, MRI scans cannot be used in patients with metal implants or cardiac pacemakers. CT scans should be used.
- Other investigations include (i) carotid duplex ultrasonography (examination of carotid arteries for stenosis, usually not done during the acute stage) and (ii) CT or MR angiography to provide more details.

5. Pathology
- The common risk factors for stroke are (i) cigarette smoking, (ii) physical inactivity, (iii) alcohol consumption, (iv) sleep-disordered breathing, (v) hypertension, (vi) diabetes mellitus, (vii) atrial fibrillation and (viii) carotid stenosis (Poorthuis et al., 2017).
- Although stroke can lead to the development of sleep-disordered breathing, the current evidence shows that sleep-disordered breathing may function as a risk factor for stroke (Yaggi, Mohsenin, 2004).
- Causes of acute ischaemic stroke are (i) vasculitis, (ii) sickle cell disease, (iii) atrial myxoma, (iv) coagulation disorders, (v) hyperviscosity (polycythaemia, multiple myeloma), (vi) cerebral artery dissection and (vii) Fabry disease.

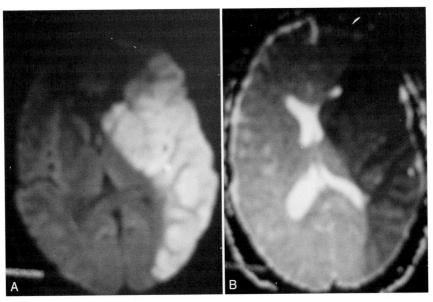

Figure 3.2.3 (A and B) MRI scan of the brain of the same patient shown in Fig. 3.2.2. *(Source: Andreoli TE, Benjamin IJ, Griggs RC, Wing EJ. Andreoli and Carpenter's Cecil Essentials of Medicine. 8th ed. Philadelphia, PA: Elsevier; 2010.)*

6. Management goals:
   - Prevention
   - Patient education
   - Management of transient ischaemic attacks
   - Management of cases presenting with acute ischaemic stroke
   - Rehabilitation
     A. Prevention: (i) A healthy lifestyle, (ii) stopping smoking, (iii) a diet low in sodium and rich in fruits, (iv) 30 minutes of physical activities/exercise on a daily basis, (v) keeping BMI at <25 kg/m^2 and (vi) reducing alcohol to <1 drink daily for women or 1–2 drinks daily for men (Davis and Donnan, 2012)
     B. For patients with risk factors: (i) Controlling blood pressure <140/90 mm Hg; (ii) regular monitoring of blood pressure; (iii) controlling diabetes (HbA$_{1c}$ <7%); (iv) starting patients, especially diabetics, on statins (Chou et al., 2016); (v) treating patients with atrial fibrillation with warfarin or novel oral anti-coagulants; and (vi) in case of carotid stenosis, no evidence that patients with asymptomatic carotid stenosis will benefit from carotid endarterectomy
     C. Patient education
     D. Managing transient ischaemic attacks (Leung et al., 2010, 2014)
     E. Managing patients presenting with acute ischaemic stroke and assessing within 1 hour of arrival in the emergency department for IV thrombolytic therapy (for further reading, check Wechsler, 2011.)
     F. Rehabilitation (for further reading, check Dobkin, 2004.)

BACK TO BASIC SCIENCES

Q1. Briefly discuss autoregulation of cerebral blood flow.

Autoregulation can be represented by the following equation:

$$\text{Cerebral blood flow} = \text{Cerebrovascular resistance}/\text{Mean arterial pressure}$$

- If the mean arterial pressure is decreased (e.g. in haemorrhage) → there is compensatory decrease in resistance → dilatation of the cerebral arterioles to maintain cerebral blood flow.
- If the mean arterial pressure is raised (e.g. in high blood pressure) → there is compensatory increase in resistance → constriction of the cerebral arterioles to maintain cerebral blood flow.
- However, there are limitations to these physiological mechanisms.

Q2. Discuss the metabolic factors that can affect cerebral blood flow.

- Hypercapnia → cerebral vasodilatation → increased cerebral blood flow
- Hypocapnia → cerebral vasoconstriction → decreased cerebral blood flow
- Acute hypoxia → cerebral vasodilatation → increased cerebral blood flow
- Increased nitric acid locally → cerebral vasodilatation → increased cerebral blood flow
- Increased adenosine production locally → cerebral vasodilatation → increased cerebral blood flow

Q3. What is the blood–brain barrier?

- The blood–brain barrier is critical for maintaining the environment necessary for normal neuronal functions.
- The blood–brain barrier comprises (i) the capillary endothelial cells, (ii) a basement membrane with pericytes and (iii) astrocytic perivascular footplates.
- The brain's vascular endothelial cells lack the transport channels found in other organs. This means that hydrophilic and large particles cannot enter the brain.
- On the other hand, oxygen and carbon dioxide rapidly cross the blood–brain barrier.

REVIEW QUESTIONS

Q1. Which *one* of the following is an initial investigation in a patient with stroke?
A. A noncontrast CT scan of the head
B. A contrast CT scan of the head
C. MRI scan of the head
D. A lumbar puncture

Q2. Which *one* of the following best describes the use of MRI of the head in a patient with stroke?
A. An initial evaluation of a patient with stroke
B. When the initial CT scan was not informative

C. The presence of mononuclear visual loss

D. In cardioembolic stroke

Q3. Which *one* of the following statements about transient ischaemic attack (TIA) is correct?

A. Transient ischaemic attack is not a neurological emergency.

B. Patients are at a higher risk of ischaemic stroke 6 months later.

C. Patients with ABCD score of 3 or greater are less likely to develop stroke.

D. Patients should undergo neuroimaging with noncontrast CT or MRI within 24 hours.

Q4. Which *one* of the following is not correct about cardioembolic stroke?

A. Most common cause is atrial fibrillation.

B. Transthoracic echocardiography is indicated.

C. Neuroimaging may show more than one infarct involving the territories of both internal carotids.

D. It is associated with a carotid bruit.

Q5. Regarding lacunar infarcts (small subcortical infarcts), which *one* of the following is not correct?

A. Visual field loss and aphasia are lacking.

B. The main risk factor is hypertension.

C. They typically present with motor and sensory findings.

D. Vascular imaging is required.

Q6. Regarding SAH, which *one* of the following is *not* correct?

A. Patients present with severe headache.

B. A common clinical sign is impairment of consciousness.

C. Subhyaloid haemorrhage on fundoscopy is present.

D. The fourth cranial nerve palsy and pupillary constriction are common.

Q7. Which *one* of the following about the blood–brain supply is *not* correct?

A. Common carotid arteries bifurcate at the level of the thyroid cartilage.

B. The internal carotid enters the skull through the foramen lacerum.

C. The ophthalmic artery can originate from the internal carotid artery in carotid siphon.

D. The internal carotid gives the superficial temporal arteries.

ANSWERS

A1. **A.** A noncontrast CT scan of the head will identify intracranial cerebral haemorrhage and SAH and is the initial radiological investigation of patients with stroke. Patients with suspected SAH in whom head CT scan is normal should have a lumbar puncture for evidence of blood or xanthochromia. MRI is of greater cost and is less widely available, and therefore cannot be used as the initial investigation.

A2. **B.** Because MRI scan is expensive and less readily available, the use of MRI scan is recommended when the initial noncontrast CT scan was not informative. Echocardiogram is needed to confirm cardioembolic stroke, and vessel imaging is recommended when there is clinical evidence of extracranial large artery atherosclerosis and monocular blindness.

A3. **D.** Transient ischaemic attack is a neurological emergency, needs hospital admission and patients who have ABCD scores of 3 or more must be admitted to a hospital and should undergo neuroimaging with noncontrast CT within 24 hours. These patients are at a higher risk of developing ischaemic stroke within 48 hours and 90 days. The ABCD system comprises A, age >60 years; B, blood pressure >140/90 mm Hg; C, clinical picture showing focal weakness and speech impairment; and D, duration of TIA and diabetes mellitus.

A4. **D.** The commonest cause of cardioembolic stroke is atrial fibrillation. Other causes include calcific mitral stenosis, ventricular thrombus, apical aneurysm and congenital anomalies. Transthoracic echocardiography is among the investigations needed for assessing the cause of cardioembolic stroke. Carotid bruit is usually present in cases caused by large artery atherosclerosis.

A5. **C.** In lacunar infarcts, hypertension is the main risk factor. Vascular imaging is needed. The lesion is characterised by motor *or* sensory findings, not both of them. Visual field defects and aphasia are lacking.

A6. **D.** Usually oculomotor nerve palsies with pupillary dilatation are noted in SAH.

A7. **D.** The external carotid arteries give extracranial branches such as superficial temporal arteries.

TAKE-HOME MESSAGE

- The common risk factors for stroke are (i) cigarette smoking, (ii) physical inactivity, (iii) alcohol consumption, (iv) sleep-disordered breathing, (v) hypertension, (vi) diabetes mellitus, (vii) atrial fibrillation and (viii) carotid stenosis.
- Although stroke can lead to the development of sleep-disordered breathing, the current evidence shows that sleep-disordered breathing may function as a risk factor for stroke.
- Causes of acute ischaemic stroke are (i) vasculitis, (ii) sickle cell disease, (iii) atrial myxoma, (iv) coagulation disorders, (v) hyperviscosity (polycythaemia, multiple myeloma), (vi) cerebral artery dissection and (vii) Fabry disease.
- The clinical presentation will depend on the blood artery involved.
- The differential diagnosis may include transient ischaemic attack, subdural or epidural haemorrhage, hypoglycaemia, subdural haemorrhage or epidural haemorrhage and focal seizure.
- The goals of management are (i) prevention, (ii) patient education and (iii) management of cases presenting with acute ischaemic stroke.

FURTHER READINGS

Chou R, Dana T, Blazina I, Daeges M, Jeanne TL. Statins for prevention of cardiovascular disease in adults: evidence report and systematic review for the US Preventive Services Task Force. *JAMA*. 2016;316(19):2008-2024. Review.

Davis SM, Donnan GA. Clinical practice. Secondary prevention after ischemic stroke or transient ischemic attack. *N Engl J Med*. 2012;366(20):1914-1922. Review.

Dobkin BH. Strategies for stroke rehabilitation. *Lancet Neurol*. 2004;3(9):528-536.

Grotta JC. Clinical practice. Carotid stenosis. *N Engl J Med*. 2013;369(12):1143-1150. Review.

Hackshaw A, Morris JK, Boniface S, Tang JL, Milenkovic D. Low cigarette consumption and risk of coronary heart disease and stroke: meta-analysis of 141 cohort studies in 55 study reports. *BMJ*. 2018;360:j5855.

Jolliffe L, Lannin NA, Cadilhac DA, Hoffmann T. Systematic review of clinical practice guidelines to identify recommendations for rehabilitation after stroke and other acquired brain injuries. *BMJ Open*. 2018;8(2):e018791.

Leung ES, Hamilton-Bruce MA, Koblar SA. Transient ischaemic attacks - assessment and management. *Aust Fam Physician*. 2010;39(11):820-824. Review.

Leung ES, Price C, Hamilton-Bruce MA, Stocks N, Koblar SA. Stroke. *Aust Fam Physician*. 2014;43(11):750-751.

Poorthuis MH, Algra AM, Algra A, Kappelle LJ, Klijn CJ. Female- and male-specific risk factors for stroke: a systematic review and meta-analysis. *JAMA Neurol*. 2017;74(1):75-81. Review.

Saver JL. Clinical Practice. Cryptogenic Stroke. *N Engl J Med*. 2016;374(21):2065-2074. Review.

Wechsler LR. Intravenous thrombolytic therapy for acute ischemic stroke. *N Engl J Med*. 2011;364(22):2138-2146. Review.

Yaggi H, Mohsenin V. Obstructive sleep apnoea and stroke. *Lancet Neurol*. 2004;3(6):333-342.

CASE 3.3

Is It Because of My Back Pain?

Othman Ibrahim, a 45-year-old factory worker, comes in to see a general practitioner because he is suffering from back pain in the lower part of his back for about a week. The pain is a dull ache and is precipitated by sudden movements of the trunk and by coughing or sneezing. The pain radiates to the right buttocks, back of the calf muscles, outer aspect of the right knee joint and the outer toes. He has no changes in urination or defecation. He took paracetamol tablets three to four times but there were no changes to the pain. On examination, he looks unwell and in pain. He leans to the left and places his weight on the left leg. Pulse rate is 85/min, blood pressure 120/80 mm Hg, temperature 36.5°C and respiratory rate 16/min. Straight leg raising is restricted to only 30° on the right side. The left side is normal. Reflexes are normal except the right ankle reflex is lost. Chest X-ray and CT scan of the lower back are normal. An MRI scan of the back shows mild bulging of the intervertebral disc at L5/S1. There are no bony abnormalities. There is no metastasis or tumour.

CASE DISCUSSION

Q1. On the basis of Mr Ibrahim's presentation, what is your diagnosis?

Q2. What is your differential diagnosis?

Q3. What are the key clinical features of this disease? What are the scientific bases for these features?

Q4. What is the pathophysiology underlying these changes?

Q5. What are your management goals and management options?

ANSWERS

1 The findings of lower back pain, the pain being precipitated by movements of the trunk, by coughing or sneezing, radiation of the pain to the right buttocks, back of the calf muscles, the outer aspect of right knee and the outer toes, and the pain not being relieved by simple analgesics, together with findings from examination – the straight leg raising is restricted on the right side, the right ankle reflex is lost and the MRI scan of the back shows bulging of the intervertebral disc at L5/S1 – are all suggestive of the diagnosis of disc prolapse at the level of L5/S1 resulting in compression on the nerve on the right side.

2 The differential diagnosis of back pain may include the following:
- Age-related degeneration of discs
- Facet dysfunction
- Ligament-related injury
- Muscle-related injury
- Nerve root syndrome, e.g. in herniated disc
- Spinal stenosis
- Cauda equina syndrome
- Fibromyalgia
- Osteomyelitis
- Spinal abscess
- Sacroiliitis
- Malignancy

Other conditions to be considered in the differential diagnosis:
- Appendicitis
- Nephrolithiasis
- Perirectal abscess
- Prostatitis

In females, consider the following:
- Ectopic pregnancy
- Cystitis
- Ovarian cyst
- Pelvic inflammatory disease

3. Clinical picture:

Symptoms and signs:
- There is a history of lifting a heavy object or twisting the trunk while carrying a heavy object.
- There is prolonged sitting such as taxi drivers.
- There is a history of falls.
- Assess the patient's pain in regard to the following aspects:
  - Intensity, location, character of pain, rating the pain on a scale of 0–10, what makes the pain better, what makes the pain worse
  - Impact of the pain on daily functions, activities and sleep
  - Emotional component of the pain, how the pain is perceived, fears, etc.
- There is a history of surgery, medications, hospital admission, other illnesses and psychological illnesses (depression, heavy alcohol consumption, poor job satisfaction, problems at home).
- Ask the patient, 'What do you think is the cause of your pain?'
- History should aim at differentiating serious causes of back pain from simple back pain, radicular pain and inflammatory pain.
- Inflammatory pain is likely to occur in patients with a history of inflammatory bowel disease, uveitis or psoriasis.

- Serious causes of back pain include (i) spinal fracture, (ii) primary or metastasis of a malignant tumour, (iii) infection such as tuberculosis and epidural abscess, (iv) cauda equina compression and (v) multiple myeloma.
- History points that may highlight serious causes of back pain:
  - Systemic symptoms
  - Fever
  - Weight loss
  - Night sweats
  - Night wakening with pain
  - Rapid onset of neurological changes, e.g. saddle anaesthesia and bladder/bowel abnormalities suggestive of cauda equina compression (these patients need urgent reference to a neurosurgeon, urgent MRI scan and urgent decompression)
  - Patients with breast cancer, prostate cancer, multiple myeloma or other causes of metastases to bones
  - Patients with a history of trauma/falls
  - Patients with a history of osteoporosis
  - Infections – history of immunosuppression and HIV infection
- Clinical examination: Table 3.3.1 summarises the changes associated with disc lesions, common root syndromes and localisation of the level of lesion (root affected).

4. Investigations:
   - Most patients do not require investigations.
   - Patients with a history suggestive of a serious cause of back pain will require investigations:
     i. Full blood count
     ii. Blood film
     iii. Erythrocyte sedimentation rate

Table 3.3.1 Common root syndromes of intervertebral disc disease

Disc space	Root affected	Muscles affected	Distribution of pain	Distribution of sensory symptoms	Reflex affected
C4–5	C5	Deltoid, biceps	Medial scapula, shoulder	Shoulder	Bicep
C5–6	C6	Wrist extensors	Lateral forearm	Thumb, index finger	Triceps
C6–7	C7	Triceps	Medial scapula	Middle finger	Brachioradialis
C7–T1	C8	Hand intrinsics	Medial forearm	Fourth and fifth fingers	Finger flexion
L3–4	L4	Quadriceps	Anterior thigh	Across knee joint	Knee jerk
L4–5	L5	Peronei	Great toe, dorsum of foot	Great toe	
L5–S1	S1	Gastrocnemius, glutei	Calf	Lateral sole of foot	Ankle jerk

Source: Andreoli TE, Benjamin IJ, Griggs RC, Wing EJ. Andreoli and Carpenter's Cecil Essentials of Medicine. 8th ed. Philadelphia, PA: Elsevier; 2010.

    iv. Serum C-reactive protein

    v. Liver function tests

    vi. Blood urea

    vii. Serum creatinine

    viii. Electrolytes

    ix. Myeloma screen

    x. Prostate-specific antigen

    xi. Plain X-ray

    xii. MRI scan with and without contrast

    xiii. Biopsy

5. Pathological features: The pathology of back pain can be divided into four main groups: (i) mechanical pain – simple back pain is seen in over 90% of cases, usually responding to nonsteroidal anti-inflammatory drugs (NSAIDs); (ii) inflammatory pain – seen in patients with inflammatory conditions such as inflammatory bowel disease and seronegative spondyloarthropathy; (iii) radicular pain – unilateral, with signs and symptoms suggestive of radicular nerve entrapment; and (iv) serious back pain such as vertebral wedge fracture, malignancy, metastasis and infection.

6. Management goals:
   - Relieve pain.
   - Identify cases with serious back pain early and manage according to the cause.
   - Improve function.
   - Reduce time away from work or normal activities.
   - Optimise treatment and physiotherapy.
   - Develop coping strategies.
   - Educate the patient.

BACK TO BASIC SCIENCES

Q1. Discuss red flags in the medical history that may give a clue of a serious cause of back pain. What would you look for in clinical examination?

Table 3.3.2 summarises red flags in the medical history that may give a clue of a serious cause of back pain.

Table 3.3.2 Red flags in the medical history that may give a clue of a serious cause of back pain

Red flags in the medical history	Possible causes	What to look for in the medical examination?
1. History of cancer or bone metastasis, unexplained weight loss	Cancer/ metastasis	Vertebral tenderness Neurological signs Plain X-ray, MRI/CT scan
2. Severe pain, history of lumbar spine surgery, immune suppression, history of IV drug use, and possibly has a fever	Infection	Temperature (sometimes afebrile), sweating, vertebral tenderness, urinary tract infection

Continued

Table 3.3.2 Red flags in the medical history that may give a clue of a serious cause of back pain—cont'd

Red flags in the medical history	Possible causes	What to look for in the medical examination?
3. History of trauma, falls, accident, history of osteoporosis, old age	Vertebral fracture	Vertebral tenderness, pain, loss of function, limitation of movement Plain X-ray, MRI/CT scan
4. Bladder incontinence, bowel incontinence, urine retention, progressive sensory loss	Cauda equina syndrome	Saddle anaesthesia, loss of anal tone, sensory loss, motor weakness, history of fall or motor accident

Q2. Discuss the categories of back pain and state examples of causes for each category.

1. Mechanical pain: This is the commonest type and represents over 90% of all causes of back pain. Under this category come the idiopathic causes. Examples of causes are problems or dissatisfaction at work, problems at home, claim for compensation, overprotective family, poor support, fears, anxiety and spasm of muscles of the back. Usually these patients do not need investigation of the cause of back pain.

2. Inflammatory category: The patients in this group may have a history of chronic inflammatory conditions such as inflammatory bowel disease, psoriasis, uveitis or family history of seronegative spondyloarthropathy. MRI scan may be indicated.

3. Radicular pain category: The patients in this group present with acute back pain and unilateral leg pain; the pain may radiate to back of the leg, foot or toes; numbness and paraesthesia follow the dermatomal distribution and can help together with the neurological examination in the localisation of the level of the lesion.

4. Serious causes of back pain: These include cancer, metastasis, myeloma, fractures, infection or cauda equina syndrome. These patients should be referred immediately for urgent management.

Q3. What is the value of erythrocyte sedimentation rate and serum C-reactive protein in a patient with back pain?

These two tests may be useful in patients suspected to have spinal infection or bone marrow neoplasm. They are most sensitive in a patient with infection because fever is usually lacking in these patients and the full blood count may be normal (for further reading, check Acosta et al., 2006).

Q4. What is the first line of treatment of back pain?

Medications including NSAIDs and muscle relaxants are usually used as the first line of treatment of back pain.

Although opioids are commonly prescribed, there is no evidence that the use of opioids makes a difference compared to that of NSAIDs or acetaminophen in regard to pain relief or time to return to work.

Q5. What is the use of epidural steroid injection in back pain management?

Usually, the use of epidural steroid injections is not beneficial and not routinely used in the treatment of back pain.

It may be used if the radicular pain is severe and did not respond to noninvasive management for 2 or 6 weeks. Transforaminal injections appear to have a more lasting effect compared to traditional interlaminar injections (for further reading, check Roberts et al., 2009).

Q6. How would you investigate a patient with back pain due to a serious cause?

The following investigations may be needed:
- Full blood count
- Blood film
- Erythrocyte sedimentation rate
- Serum C-reactive protein
- Blood urea
- Serum creatinine
- Electrolytes
- Serum vitamin D3
- Plasma parathyroid hormone
- Serum testosterone in men
- Myeloma screen
- Prostate-specific antigen
- Plain X-ray
- MRI scan with and without contrast (to detect metastasis or malignancy)
- Isotope bone scan (to detect metastasis)
- Bone densitometry (not required in patients aged 80 or above)

Q7. What are the drugs commonly used in the management of patients with back pain? State the mechanism of actions, advantages and side effects.

Table 3.3.3 summarises drugs used in back pain.

Table 3.3.3 Drugs used in back pain

Group	Examples	Mechanisms of action	Advantages	Side effects
Nonsteroidal anti-inflammatory drugs (NSAIDs)	Ibuprofen Naproxen	They have nonselective inhibition effects on cyclooxygenase, an enzyme that takes part in prostaglandin synthesis via the arachidonic acid pathway. The pharmacological mechanisms are related to inhibition of cyclooxygenase-2 (COX-2), resulting in decreased synthesis of prostaglandins (involved in mediating inflammatory changes). Also these medications have antipyretic effects through their actions on the hypothalamus. Inhibition of COX-1 may be responsible for some of the side effects of ibuprofen including gastrointestinal ulceration.	Able to reduce moderately severe pain with minimal side effects.	Fluid retention, peripheral oedema, heartburn, nausea, vomiting, anorexia, abdominal pain, dizziness, headache, acute renal failure and acute tubular necrosis may occur. Overdose may result in abdominal pain, nausea, vomiting, lethargy, vertigo, dizziness, insomnia, headache, tinnitus and acute renal failure.
Muscle relaxants	Carisoprodol (Soma) Cyclobenzaprine (Flexeril)	Cyclobenzaprine does not directly act on the neuromuscular junction or the muscle but relieves muscle spasms through a central action, possibly at the brainstem level. It binds to the serotonin receptor and is considered a 5-HT2 receptor antagonist that reduces muscle tone by decreasing the activity of descending serotonergic neurons.	The use of a muscle relaxant together with an analgesic will provide a better control of pain in patients with back pain.	Overdose may cause poor concentration, agitation, confusion, coma, drowsiness, convulsions, overactive reflexes, dilated pupils, tachycardia and irregular heart rhythm.

Table 3.3.3 Drugs used in back pain—cont'd

Group	Examples	Mechanisms of action	Advantages	Side effects
Analgesics	Acetamino-phen (paracetamol, Tylenol)	Acetaminophen acts by in-hibiting isoforms of cyclo-oxygenase, COX-1, COX-2 and COX-3 enzymes in-volved in prostaglandin (PG) synthesis. Unlike NSAIDs, acetaminophen does not inhibit cyclooxy-genase in peripheral tissues. Acetaminophen is effective in the central nervous sys-tem and in endothelial cells but not in platelets and immune cells. Studies also report that acetaminophen selectively blocks a variant of the COX enzyme. This enzyme is now referred to as COX-3. Its antipyretic properties are related to direct effects on the heat-regulating centres of the hypothalamus.	Effective in relieving mild pain.	Metabolised mainly in the liver via CYP2E1 resulting in toxic metabolites, mainly N-acetyl-p-benzoquinone imine (NAPQI). The toxic effects of acetamino-phen are mainly related to NAPQI and in an overdose liver failure occurs (a dose as low as 6 g/day has been reported to cause liver failure).
	Hydrocodone bitartrate	Hydrocodone acts as a weak agonist at OP1, OP2 and OP3 opiate receptors within the central nervous system. It primarily affects OP3 receptors. This mech-anism involves coupling with G-protein receptors. Such binding stimulates the exchange of GTP for GDP on the G-protein complex. Also it inhibits the release of vasopressin, somatostatin, insulin and glucagon. Opi-oids close N-type voltage-operated calcium channels and open calcium-depen-dent inwardly rectifying potassium channels (OP3 and OP1 receptor agonists). This results in hyperpolari-sation and reduced neuro-nal excitability.	Enables con-trol of severe pain.	Overdose causes respiratory de-pression, somno-lence, dizziness, confusion, coma, bradycardia, hy-potension, circu-latory collapse and death.

Continued

Table 3.3.3 Drugs used in back pain—cont'd

Group	Examples	Mechanisms of action	Advantages	Side effects
	Tramadol Duloxetine (Cymbalta)	Tramadol and its metabolite are selective, weak OP3 receptor agonists. Opiate receptors are coupled with G-protein receptors and function in a similar mechanism described for hydrocodone. The molecular changes result in an inhibition of the release of substance P, GABA, dopamine, acetylcholine and noradrenaline. The analgesic properties of tramadol can be attributed to norepinephrine and serotonin reuptake blockade in the CNS, which inhibits pain transmission in the spinal cord.	Enable the control of severe pain.	Overdose causes respiratory depression, somnolence, confusion, coma, hypotension, arrhythmias, circulatory collapse and death.

REVIEW QUESTIONS

Q1. Which *one* of the following is the first line of treatment of lower back pain?
A. Acetaminophen
B. Acupuncture
C. Oral steroids
D. Spinal manipulation
E. Exercise

Q2. A patient with a low back pain comes in to see his general practitioner. On examination, there is sensory loss on the posterior aspect of his left leg and lateral aspect of the left foot. Motor examination shows weakness/loss of plantar flexion, loss of ankle reflex plantar flexion and loss of ankle reflex. Which neurological level do you think matches with his clinical presentation?
A. L2–L3
B. L3–L4
C. L4–L5
D. L5–S1

Q3. Which *one* of the following is *not* among the clinical picture of cauda equina syndrome?
A. Progressive neurological deficit
B. Hyperreflexia of the knee jerk
C. Bladder or bowel dysfunction

D. Bilateral sciatica

E. Numbness of a saddle distribution

Q4. What do we mean when we say that the patient has 'a history of sciatica'?

A. The pain is localised to the lumbar region.

B. The pain radiates to both buttocks.

C. The pain radiates beyond the knee.

D. The pain does not radiate beyond the knee.

ANSWERS

A1. **A.** NSAIDs or acetaminophen is considered the first line of management of low back pain. There is no evidence to support the usefulness of acupuncture, oral steroids, spinal manipulation or exercise in the management.

A2. **D.** The neurological defect (e.g. disc herniation) is at the level of L5–S1 as shown from the loss of sensory sensation on the posterior aspect of his left leg and lateral aspect of the left foot and loss of the ankle reflex (S1).

A3. **B.** Hyperreflexia of the knee jerk is not found in cauda equina syndrome.

A4. **C.** Sciatica means that the pain radiates beyond the knee.

TAKE-HOME MESSAGE

- History should aim at differentiating serious causes of back pain from simple back pain, radicular pain and inflammatory pain.
- Inflammatory pain is likely to occur in patients with a history of inflammatory bowel disease, uveitis or psoriasis.
- The differential diagnosis of back pain may include age-related degeneration of discs, facet dysfunction, ligament-related injury, muscle-related injury, nerve root syndrome (e.g. in herniated disc), spinal stenosis, cauda equina syndrome, fibromyalgia, osteomyelitis, spinal abscess, sacroiliitis and malignancy (e.g. metastasis from prostate cancer or breast cancer).
- Serious causes of back pain include (i) spinal fracture, (ii) primary or metastasis of a malignant tumour, (iii) infection such as tuberculosis and epidural abscess, (iv) cauda equina compression and (v) multiple myeloma.
- Mechanical pain: This is the commonest type and represents over 90% of all causes of back pain.
- Inflammatory category: The patients in this group may have a history of chronic inflammatory conditions such as inflammatory bowel disease, psoriasis or uveitis.
- Radicular pain category: The patients in this group present with acute back pain and unilateral leg pain; the pain may radiate to the back of the leg, foot or toes, and there may be numbness and paraesthesia (assess for dermatomal distribution).

- Medications including NSAIDs and muscle relaxants are usually used as the first line of treatment of back pain.
- Although opioids are commonly prescribed, there is no evidence that the use of opioids makes a difference compared to that of NSAIDs or acetaminophen in regard to pain relief or time to return to work.
- Usually, the use of epidural steroid injections is not beneficial and not routinely used in the treatment of back pain.

FURTHER READINGS

Acosta Jr FL, Galvez LF, Aryan HE, Ames CP. Recent advances: infections of the spine. *Curr Infect Dis Rep.* 2006;8(5):390-393.

Carragee EJ. Clinical practice. Persistent low back pain. *N Engl J Med.* 2005;352(18):1891-1898. Review.

Cohen SP, Hooten WM. Advances in the diagnosis and management of neck pain. *BMJ.* 2017;358:j3221. Review.

Deyo RA, Mirza SK. Clinical Practice. Herniated Lumbar Intervertebral Disk. *N Engl J Med.* 2016;374(18):1763-1772. Review.

Deyo RA, Weinstein JN. Low back pain. *N Engl J Med.* 2001;344(5):363-370. Review.

Enthoven WTM, Roelofs PD, Koes BW. NSAIDs for chronic low back pain. *JAMA.* 2017;317(22): 2327-2328. Review.

John M. Eisenberg Center for Clinical Decisions and Communications Science. Early Imaging for Back Pain and Clinical Outcomes in Older Adults: A Brief Summary of Findings and Key Points for Clinician-Patient Discussions. Comparative Effectiveness Review Summary Guides for Clinicians [Internet]. Rockville, MD: Agency for Healthcare Research and Quality (US); 2007.

Paige NM, Miake-Lye IM, Booth MS, et al. Association of spinal manipulative therapy with clinical benefit and harm for acute low back pain: systematic review and meta-analysis. *JAMA.* 2017;317(14):1451-1460. Review.

Roberts ST, Willick SE, Rho ME, Rittenberg JD. Efficacy of lumbosacral transforaminal epidural steroid injections: a systematic review. *PM R.* 2009;1(7):657-668. Review.

Willick SE, Kendall RW, Roberts ST, Morton K. An emerging imaging technology to assist in the localization of axial spine pain. *PM R.* 2009;1(1):89-92.

CASE 3.4

I Have Severe Headache

Hala Demardash, a 15-year-old student, is brought by her parents to the emergency department because she is suffering from severe headache, fever and vomiting for the past 5–6 hours. She has lethargy, anorexia and muscle aches for nearly the same time. On examination, she looks ill and slightly confused. Her temperature is 39.3°C, pulse rate 125/min (regular), blood pressure 110/80 mm Hg and respiratory rate 24/min. Cranial nerve examination is normal, and there is no localisation or sensory loss. Hala has neck stiffness and both Kernig and Brudzinski signs are positive. Ophthalmoscopic examination is normal. A lumbar puncture shows elevation of opening pressure. Cerebrospinal pressure analysis shows increased protein, low glucose and intracellular Gram-negative diplococci on Gram-stained smears.

CASE DISCUSSION

Q1. On the basis of Hala's presentation, what is your diagnosis?

Q2. What is your differential diagnosis?

Q3. What are the key clinical features of this disease? What are the scientific bases for these features?

Q4. What is the pathophysiology underlying these changes?

Q5. What are your management goals and management options?

ANSWERS

1. The findings of severe headaches, fever, repeated vomiting, lethargy, anorexia, muscle aches, a rise of body temperature to 39.3°C, neck stiffness and positive Kernig and Brudzinski signs in a 15-year-old female student, Hala, together with a lumbar puncture suggestive of raised opening pressure and CSF changes showing raised protein, and intracellular Gram-negative diplococci are suggestive of the diagnosis of bacterial meningitis caused by Gram-negative organisms requiring immediate intravenous administration of broad-spectrum antibiotics covering Gram-negative bacteria, hospital admission, continuous monitoring and a follow-up of the culture results and other laboratory results.
2. The differential diagnosis includes the following:
    *   Medication-induced meningeal inflammation
    *   Encephalitis

- Brain abscess
- Brain neoplasm
- Subarachnoid haemorrhage
- Leptospirosis

3. Clinical picture:

Symptoms:

- Headache
- Drowsiness
- Fever
- Altered mental state
- Neck stiffness
- Photophobia (30%–50% of patients)
- Nausea
- Vomiting
- Purpura
- Petechiae
- The triad of fever, neck stiffness and altered mental state, which is more likely to occur in pneumococcal meningitis
- Purpura and petechiae, which may be present in meningococcal septicaemia (about 70% of cases) (however, these changes may be present without the presence of septic shock)

Signs:

- Drowsiness
- Lethargy
- Deterioration of conscious state
- Fever
- Probability of septicaemia and circulatory collapse
- Purpura and petechiae in meningococcal septicaemia
- Cranial nerve palsies (II, IV and VII) and maybe focal neurological signs
- Pneumonia, which may occur in pneumococcal meningitis especially in the elderly
- Papilloedema, which may be present as part of increased intracranial pressure
- Kernig sign present in 5% of cases
- Brudzinski sign present in 5% of cases

4. Pathological features:

- The commonest cause of bacterial meningitis in Western Europe is *Streptococcus pneumoniae*, whereas in the United States the commonest cause is *Haemophilus influenzae*.

- Other countries have both *S. pneumoniae* and *H. influenzae* as the commonest causes.
- Transmission is via droplet infection. Organisms invade the epithelium and enter the bloodstream (adhere to the mucous membrane and overcome the primary immune defence mechanisms).
- Infection may be secondary to infection causing sinusitis, middle ear or mastoid or other organ infections.
- The mechanisms used to overcome the primary immune defence mechanisms by the bacteria include the following:
  1. *S. pneumoniae* → secretes neuraminidase A → decreased viscosity of mucus and decreased mucus trapping
  2. *S. pneumoniae* → secretes pneumolysin → reduces ciliary function and reduces mucus clearance
  3. *Neisseria meningitidis* and *H. influenzae* → secrete IgA1 proteinases → prevent effective opsonisation
- Meningeal invasion → invasion of the blood–brain barrier (disturbance of intercellular tight junctions causing endothelial damage).
- Inflammation response → inflammation of the pia mater and arachnoid membrane as a result of bacterial invasion and stimulation of an immune response → inflammatory changes and increased immune cells.
- The bacteria that succeed in invading the blood–brain barrier multiply to very high titers. This is because opsonin, immunoglobulins and complement are excluded by the blood–brain barrier.
- Inflammatory response and the activation of proinflammatory pathways including TNF-alpha and IL-1b → trigger the release of other mediators including interferon-gamma, platelet-activating factor, chemokines and prostaglandins → more progression of the inflammatory response.
- The inflammatory response is accompanied by the production of thin layers of pus → adhesions → may cause obstruction of the CSF circulation → hydrocephalus (in children) and damage of cranial nerves and rise in the CSF pressure.

5. Management goals and options:
   - Immediate treatment with IV antibiotics is initiated while the patient is in the emergency room (benzylpenicillin, cefotaxime or vancomycin).
   - Corticosteroid therapy may be a useful adjunctive therapy.
   - Patients presenting in septicaemia shock have a poor prognosis and should be treated in the intensive care facility (endotracheal intubation, mechanical ventilation and prevention of acute aspiration distress syndrome).
   - Table 3.4.1 summarises the important causative agents of nonviral meningitis, their treatment and prevention.

Table 3.4.1 Causative agents, treatment and prevention of nonviral meningitis

Pathogen	Treatment[a]	Prevention
Neisseria meningitidis	Penicillin (or chloramphenicol)	Rifampicin prophylaxis for close contacts; polysaccharide vaccine (poor protection against group B)
Haemophilus influenzae	Ampicillin,[b] ceftriaxone or cefotaxime (or chloramphenicol)	Polysaccharide vaccine against type b (Hib)
Streptococcus pneumoniae	Penicillin[c] (or ceftriaxone or chloramphenicol)	Prompt treatment of otitis media and respiratory infections; poly-valent (23 serotypes) polysaccharide vaccine
Escherichia coli (and other coliforms), group B streptococci	Gentamicin + cefotaxime or ceftriaxone (or chloramphenicol)[b]	No vaccines available
Listeria monocytogenes	Penicillin or ampicillin + gentamicin	No vaccines available
Mycobacterium tuberculosis	Isoniazid and rifampin and pyrazinamide ± streptomycin	BCG vaccination; isoniazid pro-phylaxis for contacts recom-mended in the United States
Cryptococcus neoformans	Amphotericin B and flucytosine	No vaccines available

BCG, bacille Calmette–Guérin.
[a]Treatment should be initiated immediately and the susceptibility of the infecting isolate confirmed in the laboratory.
[b]If isolate is shown to be susceptible (10%–20% of isolates are resistant because they produce a plasmid-coded beta-lactamase).
[c]In areas of a high prevalence of penicillin-resistant pneumococci, initial treatment with ceftriaxone may be advised until susceptibility of isolate is known.

BACK TO BASIC SCIENCES

Q1. Why is *Escherichia coli* the most common cause of bacterial meningitis in neonates?

This is because Gram-negative bacteria including *E. coli* require IgM for neutralisation. IgM does not cross the placenta. Therefore, the lack of IgM to protect newborns makes them at a higher risk of Gram-negative meningitis including *E. coli*.

Q2. How do you explain the decrease in the incidence of *H. influenzae* meningitis in early childhood in recent years?

H. influenzae used to be a common cause of meningitis in early childhood, 3 months to 3 years. The widespread vaccination against *H. influenzae* has resulted in a decrease of meningitis in early childhood.

Q3. Which groups of people are at a higher risk of developing *S. pneumoniae* meningitis?

- Adults with a history of basilar skull fracture and CSF leak

- Alcoholics
- Patients who are asplenic
- People with splenic dysfunction as in sickle cell anaemia
- People with middle ear infection and inner ear fistulas

Q4. Which groups of people are at a higher risk of developing meningococcal meningitis?

- People in crowded places such as schools
- People living in countries with no vaccination programs against *N. meningitides*
- Individuals with defects in the pathways of complement activation, defects in properdin system and mannose-binding protein

Q5. Which groups of people are at a higher risk of developing *Listeria monocytogenes* meningitis?

- All ages are at a risk of developing such infection and it comprises 10% of all cases of bacterial meningitis
- People with T-lymphocyte defects
- People with acquired immunodeficiency syndrome
- People with malignancies

Q6. In bacterial meningitis, what are the clinical and laboratory predictors of a poor prognosis?

- Reduced consciousness or coma
- Onset of seizures
- Duration of illness before admission (delay in diagnosis)
- Low peripheral white cell count
- Thrombocytopenia
- Absence of CSF pleocytosis
- Very low CSF glucose
- High CSF protein

Q7. What are the scientific bases for giving corticosteroids with antibiotics in treating bacterial meningitis?

- Mitigating the inflammatory response
- Reduction of incidence of sensorineural hearing loss
- Usually given as intravenous dexamethasone before the first dose of antibiotic therapy

Q8. Discuss the changes in CSF in bacterial, viral, fungal and tuberculous meningitis compared to a normal CSF.

Table 3.4.2 summarises the characteristics of CSF analysis in bacterial, viral, fungal and tuberculous meningitis.

Table 3.4.2 Characteristics of CSF analysis in bacterial, viral, fungal and tuberculous meningitis

CSF	Leukocytes	Protein	Glucose	Other changes
Normal/ control	<3 cells/mm^3	0.15– 0.45 g/L	2/3 of plasma glucose	Normal pressure = 5–20 cm H$_2$O
Bacterial meningitis	>1000 polymorphonuclear/ mm^3 (lymphocytes are increased in *Listeria*)	>1.0 g/L	Low (<40% of plasma glucose)	Gram stain and culture and Polymerase Chain Reaction (PCR) reveal the bacterial cause
Viral meningitis	Mostly lymphocytes <200 cells/mm^3	Normal or elevated	Normal	Viral PCR
Fungal meningitis	Lymphocytes <50 cells/mm^2	Normal or elevated	Normal	Indian ink stain/ cryptococcal antigen
Tuberculous meningitis	Moderate lymphocytosis	++++ Increased >1.0 g/L	Low <40% of plasma glucose	Elevated opening pressure AFB positive TB culture PCR

REVIEW QUESTIONS

Q1. In patients treated with corticosteroids and appropriate antibiotics for bacterial meningitis compared to patients treated with antibiotics only, which *one* of the following complications is reduced?
A. Brain abscess
B. Subdural empyema
C. Venous thrombosis
D. Sensorineural hearing loss

Q2. Which *one* of the following empirical antibiotics is recommended in a 28-year-old presenting in the emergency room with a clinical diagnosis of bacterial meningitis?
A. Aminoglycoside
B. Benzylpenicillin
C. Third-generation cephalosporin
D. Ampicillin

Q3. Which one of the following is *not* a contraindication to lumbar puncture?
A. Bradycardia, hypertension and abnormal breathing
B. Positive Kernig sign
C. Coagulopathy
D. Continuous seizure activity
E. Cardiovascular compromise

ANSWERS

A1. **D.** A Cochrane review has shown that treatment with corticosteroids together with antibiotics in bacterial meningitis reduces the incidence of deafness.

A2. **C.** Third-generation cephalosporin ± vancomycin are the best empirical antibiotics for adults with a higher index of bacterial meningitis diagnosis.

A3. **B.** Positive Kernig sign is found in 5% of patients. When positive, it confirms the clinical diagnosis. Conducting this test is not a contraindication for lumbar puncture.

TAKE-HOME MESSAGE

- The commonest cause of bacterial meningitis in Western Europe is *S. pneumoniae*, whereas in the United States the commonest cause is *H. influenzae*.
- Other countries have both *S. pneumoniae* and *H. influenzae* as the commonest causes.
- Transmission is via droplet infection. Organisms invade the epithelium and enter the bloodstream (adhere to the mucous membrane and overcome the primary immune defence mechanisms).
- Infection may be secondary to infection causing sinusitis, middle ear or mastoid or other organ infections.
- Presenting symptoms include headache, drowsiness, fever, altered mental state, neck stiffness, photophobia (30%–50% of patients), nausea, vomiting, purpura and petechiae.
- The triad of fever, neck stiffness and altered mental state is more likely to occur in pneumococcal meningitis.
- The purpura and petechiae may be present in meningococcal septicaemia (about 70% of cases). However, these changes may be present without the presence of septic shock.
- Immediate administration of intravenous coverage of antibiotics should be initiated in the emergency department, once the diagnosis of bacterial meningitis has been established from medical history, clinical examination and the lumbar puncture preliminary results.
- Positive Kernig sign is found in 5% of patients. When positive, it confirms the clinical diagnosis. Conducting this test is not a contraindication for lumbar puncture.
- Third-generation cephalosporin ± vancomycin are the best empirical antibiotics for adults with a higher index of bacterial meningitis diagnosis.
- A Cochrane review has shown that treatment with corticosteroids together with antibiotics in bacterial meningitis reduces the incidence of deafness.

FURTHER READINGS

Chiang SS, Khan FA, Milstein MB, et al. Treatment outcomes of childhood tuberculous meningitis: a systematic review and meta-analysis. *Lancet Infect Dis*. 2014;14(10):947-957. Review.

Critchley JA, Young F, Orton L, Garner P. Corticosteroids for prevention of mortality in people with tuberculosis: a systematic review and meta-analysis. *Lancet Infect Dis*. 2013;13(3):223-237. Review.

Logan SA, MacMahon E. Viral meningitis. *BMJ*. 2008;336(7634):36-40. Review.

Loyse A, Thangaraj H, Easterbrook P, et al. Cryptococcal meningitis: improving access to essential antifungal medicines in resource-poor countries. *Lancet Infect Dis.* 2013;13(7):629-637. Review.

McGill F, Heyderman RS, Panagiotou S, Tunkel AR, Solomon T. Acute bacterial meningitis in adults. *Lancet.* 2016;388(10063):3036-3047. Review.

Morís G, Garcia-Monco JC. The challenge of drug-induced aseptic meningitis revisited. *JAMA Intern Med.* 2014;174(9):1511-1512. Review.

Rosenstein NE, Perkins BA, Stephens DS, Popovic T, Hughes JM. Meningococcal disease. *N Engl J Med.* 2001;344(18):1378-1388. Review.

Thwaites GE, van Toorn R, Schoeman J. Tuberculous meningitis: more questions, still too few answers. *Lancet Neurol.* 2013;12(10):999-1010. Review.

van de Beek D, de Gans J, Tunkel AR, Wijdicks EF. Community-acquired bacterial meningitis in adults. *N Engl J Med.* 2006;354(1):44-53. Review.

van de Beek D, Drake JM, Tunkel AR. Nosocomial bacterial meningitis. *N Engl J Med.* 2010;362(2):146-154. Review.

CASE 3.5

Because of Double Vision

Naomi Lee, a 36-year-old library assistant, comes in to see her general practitioner because she is suffering from a double vision and drooping of her right eyelid, which is worsened on the afternoons. Part of her duties is to place the books back on the book-shelves. She has been doing this job for nearly 8 years with no problems but recently she noticed that she cannot continue placing the books on the bookshelves and she has to take rest for a few minutes to continue doing this job. She does not smoke and has no significant family history. On examination, pulse rate is 88/min, blood pressure 120/85 mm Hg, temperature 36.5°C and respiratory rate 18/min. Ptosis of the right eye, which is temporary, improved on applying an ice pack to the affected eyelid for 5 minutes (ice test). The drooping of the right eyelid increases when Naomi is asked to upgaze (lid fatigability test). Eye movement is normal. There is no skeletal muscle atrophy or hypertrophy. But there is proximal muscle weakness (shoulder girdle and pelvic girdle). Reflexes are normal on both sides. Serum anti–acetylcholine receptor (AChR) antibody test is positive. Electromyogram (EMG) shows a decremental response and the Tensilon test is positive.

CASE DISCUSSION

Q1. On the basis of Naomi's presentation, what is your diagnosis?

Q2. What is your differential diagnosis?

Q3. What are the key clinical features of this disease? What are the scientific bases for these features?

Q4. What is the pathophysiology underlying these changes?

Q5. What are your management goals and management options?

ANSWERS

1. The findings of double vision, drooping right eyelid which increases in the after-noon and inability to continue placing the books on the bookshelves and having to take rest for a few minutes to keep doing the job together with the clinical examina-tion findings, mainly ptosis, positive ice test and lid fatigability test, proximal muscle weakness, positive serum anti–AChR antibody test and Tensilon test, and a decre-mental response shown on EMG (an abnormal smaller and smaller muscle response to each repetitive stimulus) are all suggestive of the diagnosis of myasthenia gravis.

2. The differential diagnosis includes the following:
   - Brainstem gliomas
   - Multiple sclerosis
   - Polymyositis
   - Drug-induced myasthenia-like syndrome
   - Eaton–Lambert syndrome
   - Basilar artery thrombosis
   - Neurosarcoidosis
   - Tolosa–Hunt syndrome
   - Chronic myelogenous leukemia
   - Amyotrophic lateral sclerosis
   - Chronic progressive external ophthalmoplegia (a mitochondrial disorder can mimic ocular symptoms of myasthenia)

3. Clinical picture:
   Symptoms and signs:
   - Weakness of ocular muscles – ptosis and diplopia (ocular myasthenia)
   - Proximal muscle weakness (weakness of the elbow and finger extension is common; patients usually find it difficult to comb their hair [females], doing jobs such as placing books on shelves in the library or climbing stairs)
   - Facial changes – difficulty with eye closure and weakness of jaw closure (difficulty in chewing)
   - Bulbar symptoms – nasal speech, nasal regurgitation and dysphagia
   - Respiratory muscle involvement causing life-threatening respiratory difficulties on lying flat
   - Trunk involvement
   - Weakness of neck muscles → head drooping
   - Muscles of upper and lower limbs – no muscle wasting; reflexes normal but may be increased or brisker
   - Slow ventilator recovery from general anaesthesia (curare-like muscle relaxants)
   - Associated autoimmune diseases including the following:
     - Thyrotoxicosis
     - Systemic lupus erythematosus
     - Rheumatoid arthritis
     - Myocarditis
   - Patients at a higher risk of developing cancer, lymphoma and diseases associated with a thymoma (blood cytopenias, hypogammaglobulinaemia, polymyositis and the POEMS syndrome)

4. Laboratory investigations:
   - Anti-AChR antibodies: These antibodies are detectable in most patients. A few have muscle-specific kinase (MuSK) antibodies. Negative results do not exclude myasthenia gravis which is common in the group of patients with pure eye form.
   - EMG shows decremental response (decreasing) action potentials with repetitive stimulation.

- The Tensilon test: Intravenous injection of edrophonium $\rightarrow$ immediate, short-acting improvement. A control (placebo) should be used and the test needs to be double blinded. The side effects include eye twitching and abdominal pain. These side effects can be prevented by the administration of atropine 0.6 mg.
- Serum skeletal muscle antibodies are common in patients with thymoma.
- Chest CT or MR scans are performed to assess thymic pathology.

5. Pathological features:
   - In myasthenia gravis, the AChRs located at the postsynaptic membrane interact with antibodies against AChRs, as well as antibodies against MuSK and lipoprotein receptor-related peptide 4 (LRP4), resulting in the development of myasthenia gravis.
   - Normally acetylcholine is degraded by local acetylcholinesterase. In myasthenia gravis, acetylcholinesterase inhibitors can lead to sympathetic improvement. This forms the basis of management.
   - Also, there are antibodies against the intramuscular proteins (titin) and (ryanodine) receptors are currently used as relevant biomarkers in identifying subgroups of myasthenia gravis.

6. Management goals:
   - Symptomatic management – acetylcholinesterase inhibition leading to symptomatic improvement
   - Immunoactive therapy to limit the progression of the disease
   - Support to help the patient accommodate to these changes
   - Providing patient education
   - Management of myasthenia gravis crisis
   - Monitoring the progression of the disease and any complications

BACK TO BASIC SCIENCES

Q1. Briefly describe the muscle weakness in myasthenia gravis.

The muscle weakness in myasthenia gravis results from the binding of antibodies to the AChRs in the postsynaptic membrane at the neuromuscular junctions. The disease is an autoimmune disorder. The weakness involves mainly skeletal muscles. The weakness is symmetrical generalised or partial and is proximal more than distal. There is no muscle atrophy or changes in the muscle reflexes (may be slightly increased). The weakness typically increases on exercising and repetitive muscle use causes fatigue. The muscle weakness varies from day to day. The muscles are usually at full strength in the morning (nearly normal), but the patient observes the weakness in the afternoon (3–5 p.m.).

Q2. Briefly discuss the diagnosis of myasthenia gravis.

The diagnosis of myasthenia gravis is based on a combination of presenting symptoms and clinical signs as well as laboratory investigations including the following:
- A positive test for antibodies against AChRs
- A positive test for antibodies against MuSK and LRP4

- Neurophysiological tests particularly in patients with antibody–negative results
- Ice pack test (placing an ice pack on the affected eyelid for 5 minutes reverses ptosis; this test supports the diagnosis of myasthenia gravis)
- Mediastinal imaging (MRI scans may help in detecting a thymoma; however, this test is not sensitive or specific)
- The Tensilon test – not currently used in all centres

Q3. What are the key differences between early-onset and late-onset myasthenia gravis?

Table 3.5.1 summarises key differences between early-onset and late-onset myasthenia gravis.

Table 3.5.1 Differences between early-onset and late-onset myasthenia gravis

Item	Early onset	Late onset
Age	<50 years Juvenile onset occurs before the age of 15 years	>50 years
Sex	More in females	More in males
Thymus	Thymus hyperplasia	Thymus atrophy
Antibodies	Acetylcholine receptor antibodies	Acetylcholine receptor antibodies Titin antibodies may be present (their presence indicates severe disease) Ryanodine receptor antibodies present in 14% of late-onset patients (also a marker of severe disease)
HLA system	HLA-DR3, HLA-B8 and non-HLA genes	HLA-DR2, HLA-B7, HLA-DRB1
Associated autoimmune disorders	More common	Less common

Q4. Briefly list the coexisting disorders that may occur in patients with myasthenia gravis.

- A second autoimmune disorder in 15% of patients
- Thyroiditis
- Systemic lupus erythematosus
- Rheumatoid arthritis
- Thymoma and disorders associated with a thymoma (blood cytopenias, hypogammaglobulinaemia, polymyositis and the POEMS syndrome, autoimmune neuropathy) The POEMS syndrome includes the following:
- Polyneuropathy
- Organomegaly (liver, spleen or lymph nodes)
- Endocrinopathy (hypothyroidism, diabetes mellitus, fatigue, sexual problems)

- Monoclonal plasmaproliferative disorder (abnormal bone marrow, abnormal plasma cells)
- Skin changes

Q5. What are the side effects of pyridostigmine?
- Diarrhoea
- Abdominal pain
- Abdominal cramps
- Increased flatus
- Nausea
- Increased sweating

Q6. Why is immunosuppressive drug therapy needed in patients with myasthenia gravis?
- Meet the treatment goals.
- Prevent/delay the generation of the disease.
- Manage ocular myasthenia gravis.
- Reduce antibodies against MuSK, titin, ryanodine receptor or Kv1–4 antibodies.

Q7. Which medications are used in immunosuppression in patients with myasthenia gravis?
- Prednisolone or prednisone
- Azathioprine
- Mycophenolate mofetil
- Methotrexate
- Cyclosporine
- Tacrolimus
- Rituximab (monoclonal antibody)

REVIEW QUESTIONS

Q1. Which *one* of the following medications may cause myasthenia gravis?
A. Prednisolone
B. Penicillamine
C. Azathioprine
D. Cyclosporine

Q2. Which *one* of the following is correct about skeletal muscle weakness in myasthenia gravis?
A. Weakness is distal.
B. Weakness is asymmetrical.
C. Muscle wasting is common.
D. Reflexes are usually normal.

Q3. Which *one* of the following about laboratory investigations of myasthenia gravis is correct?
A. Negative anti–acetylcholine receptor antibodies excludes the diagnosis.
B. Tensilon test should be conducted in patients with positive anti–acetylcholine receptor antibodies.
C. Thyroid function tests are usually abnormal.
D. Serum skeletal muscle antibodies are mostly common in patients with thymoma.

Q4. Which *one* of the following is *not* a side effect of pyridostigmine?
A. Abdominal pain
B. Nausea
C. Increased sweating
D. Increased flatus
E. Constipation

ANSWERS

A1. **B.** Penicillamine is used in treating chronic conditions such as rheumatoid arthritis. It is a rare cause of myasthenia gravis.

A2. **D.** Reflexes are normal or brisker than normal in myasthenia gravis.

A3. **D.** Thyroid antibodies may be found in myasthenia gravis but the thyroid functions are usually normal. Tensilon test or other investigations are not needed to confirm the diagnosis if the anti–acetylcholine receptor antibody test is positive.

A negative anti–acetylcholine receptor antibody test does not exclude the diagnosis of myasthenia gravis. Negative acetylcholine receptor antibody test usually occurs in patients with ocular myasthenia.

A4. **E.** Diarrhoea is a side effect of pyridostigmine.

TAKE-HOME MESSAGE

- The symptoms and signs of myasthenia gravis include (i) weakness of ocular muscles – ptosis and diplopia (ocular myasthenia); (ii) proximal muscle weakness (weakness of elbow and finger extension is common); (iii) facial changes – difficulty with eye closure and weakness of jaw closure (difficulty in chewing); (iv) bulbar symptoms – nasal speech, nasal regurgitation and dysphagia; (v) respiratory muscle involvement causing life-threatening respiratory difficulties on lying flat; (vi) trunk involvement; and (vii) weakness of neck muscles → head drooping.
- Myasthenia gravis characteristically affects proximal muscles in upper and lower limbs. However, no muscle wasting occurs and the reflexes are normal but may be increased or brisker.

- Patients may have slow ventilator recovery from general anaesthesia (curare-like muscle relaxants).
- Myasthenia gravis is associated with autoimmune diseases including thyrotoxicosis, systemic lupus erythematosus, rheumatoid arthritis and myocarditis.
- Patients have an increased risk of developing cancer, lymphoma and diseases associated with a thymoma (blood cytopenias, hypogammaglobulinaemia, polymyositis and the POEMS syndrome).
- The differential diagnosis of myasthenia gravis includes brainstem gliomas, multiple sclerosis, polymyositis, drug-induced myasthenia-like syndrome, Eaton–Lambert syndrome, basilar artery thrombosis, Tolosa–Hunt syndrome and chronic myelogenous leukemia.
- Investigations include (i) anti-AChR antibodies, (ii) EMG, (iii) the Tensilon test, (iv) serum skeletal muscle antibodies and (v) chest CT or MR scans – to assess thymic pathology.
- The management of myasthenia gravis includes (i) symptomatic management – acetylcholinesterase inhibition leads to symptomatic improvement; (ii) immunoactive therapy to limit the progression of the disease; (iii) support to help the patient accommodate to these changes; (iv) providing patient education; (v) management of myasthenia gravis crisis; and (vi) monitoring the progression of the disease and any complications.

FURTHER READINGS

Dalakas MC. Intravenous immunoglobulin in autoimmune neuromuscular diseases. *JAMA*. 2004;291(19): 2367-2375. Review.

Drachman DB. Myasthenia gravis. *N Engl J Med*. 1994;330(25):1797-1810. Review.

Fonseca V, Havard CW. The natural course of myasthenia gravis. *BMJ*. 1990;300(6737):1409-1410. Review.

Gilhus NE. Myasthenia gravis. *N Engl J Med*. 2016;375(26):2570-2581. Review.

Gilhus NE, Verschuuren JJ. Myasthenia gravis: subgroup classification and therapeutic strategies. *Lancet Neurol*. 2015;14(10):1023-1036. Review.

Meriggioli MN, Sanders DB. Autoimmune myasthenia gravis: emerging clinical and biological heterogeneity. *Lancet Neurol*. 2009;8(5):475-490. Review.

Richman DP. The future of research in myasthenia. *JAMA Neurol*. 2015;72(7):812-814. Review.

Scherer K, Bedlack RS, Simel DL. Does this patient have myasthenia gravis? *JAMA*. 2005;293(15): 1906-1914. Review.

Spillane J, Higham E, Kullmann DM. Myasthenia gravis. *BMJ*. 2012;345:e8497. Review.

Vincent A, Bowen J, Newsom-Davis J, McConville J. Seronegative generalised myasthenia gravis: clinical features, antibodies, and their targets. *Lancet Neurol*. 2003;2(2):99-106. Review.

Vincent A, Palace J, Hilton-Jones D. Myasthenia gravis. *Lancet*. 2001;357(9274):2122-2128. Review.

CASE 3.6

In the Intensive Care Unit

Amina Belouizdad, a 53-year-old woman from Algeria, has been in Saudi Arabia for religious Umra for about a week. She is brought by an ambulance to the emergency department of a local hospital in Medina because she is suffering from dizziness, fever, generalised fatigue and changes in her conscious state. Her husband, who accompanies her, provides a detailed history to the examining doctor and informs him that Amina has diabetes and has been diagnosed with high blood pressure for about 10 years. On examination, she is semiconscious. Her pulse rate is 120/min, blood pressure 130/90 mm Hg, respiratory rate 22/min and temperature (per rectum) 42.0°C. Her skin is dry and body mass index is 33. Neurological examination shows no localisation and a lumbar puncture shows normal opening fluid and clear cerebrospinal fluid. Computed tomography (CT) of the head and CT angiography did not show pathology. Liver transaminases, blood urea and creatinine are raised. She was admitted to the intensive care unit for further management. One hour later, she falls into a coma.

CASE DISCUSSION

Q1. On the basis of Mrs Belouizdad's presentation, what is your diagnosis?

Q2. What is your differential diagnosis?

Q3. What are the key clinical features of this disease? What are the scientific bases for these features?

Q4. What is the pathophysiology underlying these changes?

Q5. What are your management goals and management options?

ANSWERS

1. The findings of dizziness, changes in her conscious state (semiconscious, and then coma) and temperature per rectum 42.0°C, together with no pathology in her head CT scans and lumbar puncture, are consistent with the diagnosis of heat stroke. The patient is obese, hypertensive and diabetic, and these comorbidities may have placed her at a higher risk to develop heat stroke.
2. The differential diagnosis includes the following:
   - Meningitis
   - Encephalitis
   - Stroke

- Hepatic encephalopathy
- Uraemic encephalopathy
- Hyponatraemia
- Cerebral malaria
- Closed head trauma
- Diabetic ketoacidosis
- Malignant hypertension

The following are essential for the diagnosis of heat stroke:
- Hyperthermia (core body temperature >41°C)
- Dry skin
- Cerebral nervous system dysfunction (semiconscious, or coma)

3. Symptoms and signs:
   - Cardinal symptoms: The following are usually present: (i) hyperthermia; (ii) dry skin; (iii) cerebral nervous system dysfunction including behavioural changes, impairment of judgment, delirium or frank coma; (iv) seizures, which may occur during cooling; and (v) tachycardia, hypertension and hyperventilation.
   - Complications: Patients with heat stroke usually show a number of serious complications including rhabdomyolysis, acute renal failure, acute respiratory distress syndrome, intestinal ischaemia or intestinal infarction, haemorrhagic complications, disseminated intravascular coagulation, thrombocytopenia and hepatic dysfunction.

4. Laboratory findings:
   - Full blood count: Haemoconcentration and thrombocytopenia. The white blood cells are raised up to 40,000/μL.
   - Arterial blood gases: Respiratory alkalosis and metabolic acidosis (due to increased lactic acid), and hypoxaemia are present; arterial carbon dioxide tension is less than 20 mm Hg.
   - Blood glucose: Hypoglycaemia may occur in severe cases with fulminant hepatic failure.
   - Hypernatraemia: It occurs due to reduced fluid intake and dehydration. Also, it may be due to diabetic insipidus (secondary to central nervous system damage).
   - Hypokalaemia: It is usually present in the early phases. However, with the development of muscle damage (rhabdomyolysis), hyperkalaemia occurs.
   - Hyperphosphataemia: It may be secondary to excessive loss of phosphate in urine. It occurs with the development of rhabdomyolysis and renal failure.
   - Hypomagnesaemia may occur.
   - Liver function tests: Liver injury may result in raised transaminases (AST and ALT) to high levels in the early phases. Hyperbilirubinaemia occurs.
   - Kidney function tests: These show raised blood urea and creatinine. Also decreased glomerular filtration rate and increased uric acid levels are reported.
   - Urinalysis: Proteinuria is usually present. Microscopic examination of urine may be needed to differentiate between the presence of red blood cells and their absence (urine dipstick cannot differentiate between haemoglobin and myoglobin).

- CT scan of the brain is done in all patients with consciousness state deterioration.
- Chest radiograph is done to detect lung pathology (pneumonia, atelectasis and pulmonary oedema).
- Electrocardiogram: It detects sinus tachycardia with or without ischaemic changes, arrhythmias or conduction defects.
- Lumbar puncture: Examination of the cerebrospinal fluid is necessary to exclude meningitis.

5. Pathology and pathogenesis:
   - In the early phases: The hot environment stimulates the peripheral and hypothalamic heat receptors → stimulation of the hypothalamic thermoregulatory centre → increased blood flow to the peripheral circulation, and vasodilation → stimulation of sweating (but this is limited by the hot environment which interferes with evaporation and cooling mechanisms).
   - Elevated body temperature → stimulation of heart rate (tachycardia) and increased cardiac output and decreased renal perfusion.
   - The excessive loss of fluids and electrolytes in the sweat → reduced blood volume (reduced renal blood flow and more strain on cardiovascular haemodynamics) and impairment of the thermoregulation.
   - The cells of different body organs respond to sudden exposure to heat by producing heat shock proteins. The production of these proteins aims at stabilising the cellular situation and correction of microdamage at cellular levels.
   - The continuation of heat exposure → thermoregulatory failure, and alteration in the heat shock proteins → failure of the physiological mechanisms to correct the situation → more damage at body system organ levels including the central nervous system and the development of heat stroke.
   - Heat stroke is a multiorgan dysfunction due to failure of normal physiological mechanisms associated with exposure of the body to high temperature → direct cytotoxicity of heat, cell necrosis, inflammatory changes, failure of regulatory mechanisms and coagulopathy.
   - These changes result in circulatory failure, hypoxia, cardiopulmonary dysfunction, increased metabolic demands and dysfunction/damage at cellular, organ and body system levels.
   - Inflammatory cytokines play a role in the pathogenesis of heat stroke: Tumour necrosis factor (TNF)-alpha, IL-1β, IL-6, IL-10 and TNF receptors p55 and p75 are involved → imbalance between inflammatory and anti-inflammatory cytokines plus changes in the intracranial pressure and decreased cerebral blood flow and haemodynamic instability/failures.
   - These changes also contribute to cellular, organ and body system failures.

6. Management goals:
   - Immediate cooling of the body
   - Support of organ system functions, stabilisation of the haemodynamic changes and correction of any biochemical or haematological abnormalities

BACK TO BASIC SCIENCES

Q1. What are the main differences between heat exhaustion (heat stress) and heat stroke?

Table 3.6.1 summarises the differences between heat exhaustion and heat stroke.

Table 3.6.1 Differences between heat exhaustion and heat stroke

Heat exhaustion (heat stress)	Heat stroke
Mild, physiological changes to heat exposure in the environment	Severe illness; can cause multiorgan failure and death
Associated with excessive sweating, headaches, muscle fatigue, tiredness and body temperature <40°C	Core body temperature 40–47°C, no sweating (dry skin), and deterioration of consciousness state, delirium and coma
No organ failure	Multiorgan failure, circulatory failure, renal failure, damage of thermoregulatory mechanisms and coagulopathy occur
Nearly all patients recover unless their conditions progress to heat stroke	Prognosis not good. Nearly 50% of patients die or end with neurological damage and other complications

Q2. What are heat shock proteins?

Heat shock proteins are expressed when cells are stressed by heat, a lack of oxygen, a lack of blood flow, an influx of heavy metals or other stressors. Because of these stresses, some cellular proteins denature. Heat shock proteins on the contrary are protective and restorative of body functions. In such situations, heat shock proteins bind to the denatured proteins, and prevent them from causing damage. They also refold other denatured proteins and push them into the degradation pathways within the cells to protect the body from their damaging effects.

Q3. How would you explain death in the majority of patients with heat stroke?

1. Heat stroke usually causes neurological damage.
2. Heat stroke causes thermoregulatory failure and altered expression of heat shock proteins.
3. There is usually exaggerated acute-phase response, cytotoxic effects of heat and coagulopathy.
4. Multiorgan failure and failure of the normal physiological mechanisms occur.

Q4. What are the types of heat stroke?

Heat stroke could be (i) a classic or nonexertional heat stroke, due to exposure to a high environmental temperature and (ii) an exertional heat stroke from strenuous exercise.

However, in both types, the pathogenesis is related to the development of hyperthermia, systemic inflammatory response, failure of pathophysiological defence mechanisms, multiorgan dysfunction, encephalopathy and failure of thermoregulatory mechanisms.

Q5. What is the role of genetics in heat stroke?

Genetics may determine the susceptibility to heat stroke and may explain why heat exhaustion may progress to heat stroke in some people and not in others. The suscepti-bility genes may include encoding cytokines, coagulation proteins, heat shock proteins and adaptation to high temperature.

REVIEW QUESTIONS

Q1. Which *one* of the following is responsible for the impairment of thermoregulation in heat stroke?
A. Cutaneous vasodilation
B. Dehydration and salt loss
C. Tachycardia and increased cardiac output
D. Decreased perfusion of the kidney and intestines

Q2. Which *one* of the following physiological changes is *not part* of the acclimatisation to heat?
A. Activation of renin–angiotensin–aldosterone axis
B. Salt conservation by the sweat glands
C. Decreased capacity to excrete sweat
D. Expansion of the plasma volume
E. Increased glomerular filtration rate

Q3. Which *one* of the following statements about heat shock proteins is correct?
A. They have cytotoxic effects.
B. They exaggerate the damage caused by heat.
C. They cause cerebral ischaemia.
D. They are protective and restorative of cellular functions.

Q4. Which *one* of the following mechanisms is *not responsible* for the progression from heat stress (exhaustion) to heat stroke?
A. Thermoregulatory failure
B. Exaggeration of the acute-phase response
C. Excessive production of heat shock proteins
D. Alteration in the expression of heat shock proteins
E. Lack of acclimatisation

ANSWERS

A1. **B.** Dehydration and salt depletion are responsible for the impairment of the thermoregulatory mechanisms.

A2. **C.** All of the changes mentioned are correct and they are part of the physiological changes in the acclimatisation to heat except item C. There is an increase in the capacity to secrete sweat to help the body in the cooling effects (for further reading, check Bouchama and Knochel, 2003).

A3. **D.** Heat shock proteins have protective and restorative cellular functions.

A4. **C.** The excessive production of heat shock proteins is protective and protects cells from damage by heat, stress, ischaemia or hypoxia. However, because of poor production of heat shock proteins as in aging, lack of acclimatisation to heat and certain genetic polymorphism, there is a strong association to progression from heat stress to heat stroke. Also altered expression of heat shock proteins contributes to their inability to function normally.

TAKE-HOME MESSAGE

- Heat stroke is a life-threatening condition in which the core body temperature is >40°C, the skin is dry and the patient has delirium or is semiconscious or in coma.
- Heat exhaustion (heat stress) is a mild form of illness with no complications.
- The pathogenesis of heat stroke is related to failure of physiological mechanisms, thermoregulatory regulation, acute-phase responses, altered heat shock proteins, multiorgan failure and coagulopathy.
- Heat shock proteins are produced in response to exposure to heat, hypoxia and decreased blood flow. These proteins aim at restoration of cellular functions and they are protective proteins.
- Acclimatisation to heat comprises a number of physiological mechanisms that prepare the body to face high temperature and protect the body.
- The aims of management of heat stroke are (i) immediate cooling of the body and (ii) support of organ system functions, stabilisation of the haemodynamic changes and correction of any biochemical or haematological abnormalities.

FURTHER READINGS

Bouchama A, Knochel JP. Heat stroke. *N Engl J Med*. 2002;346(25):1978-1988. Review.
Heled Y, Fleischmann C, Epstein Y. Cytokines and their role in hyperthermia and heat stroke. *J Basic Clin Physiol Pharmacol*. 2013;24(2):85-96. Review.
Kosgallana AD, Mallik S, Patel V, Beran RG. Heat stroke induced cerebellar dysfunction: a "forgotten syndrome." *World J Clin Cases*. 2013;1(8):260-261.
Leon LR, Bouchama A. Heat stroke. *Compr Physiol*. 2015;5(2):611-647. Review.
Rikkert MG, Melis RJ, Claassen JA. Heat waves and dehydration in the elderly. *BMJ*. 2009;339:b2663.

CASE 3.7

Things Are Spinning Around Me

Diana McArthur, a 30-year-old housewife, comes in to see her general practitioner accompanied by her husband because she is suffering from a sudden sense of rotation of the surroundings induced by a change in the head position, turning over in the bed or any sudden changes in body position for the past 2 days. She has nausea and vomited twice. She gives no history of recent upper respiratory tract infection. She does not drink alcohol and gives no history of head trauma. On examination, there is no neurological deficit and eardrums are normal. The Dix–Hallpike manoeuvre is positive. Audiometry indicates normal hearing bilaterally.

CASE DISCUSSION

Q1. On the basis of Diana's presentation, what is your diagnosis?

Q2. What is your differential diagnosis?

Q3. What are the key clinical features of this disease? What are the scientific bases for these features?

Q4. What is the pathophysiology underlying these changes?

Q5. What are your management goals and management options?

ANSWERS

1. The findings of sudden vertigo induced by a change in the position of the head together with a positive Dix–Hallpike manoeuvre are supportive of the diagnosis of benign paroxysmal positional vertigo. The absence of neurological deficit excludes central causes of vertigo and the absence of hearing loss excludes Meniere disease.
2. The differential diagnosis:
   * Meniere disease
   * Migraine headache
   * Acute vestibular neuronitis
   * Benign paroxysmal positional vertigo
   * Labyrinthitis (inflammation of the labyrinthine organs caused by infection)
   * Alcohol intoxication
   * Vertebrobasilar artery insufficiency
   * Anxiety disorder
   * Acute anaemia

- Acute subdural haematoma in the elderly
- Acoustic neuroma (schwannoma)
- Orthostatic hypotension

The following are essential for the diagnosis of benign paroxysmal positional vertigo:
- Sudden-onset vertigo triggered by a change in the head position
- Positive Dix–Hallpike manoeuvre

3. **Symptoms:**
   - Spinning sensation of less than 1 minute
   - Usually noticed by the patient on changing the head position with respect to gravity
   - Also noticed when the patient gets in or out of bed, rolls over in bed or tilts the head forward or backward
   - Possibility of occurrence of nausea and vomiting
   - No cause known to the patient but may occur after head trauma or a visit to the dentist
   - More common in females (female-to-male ratio is 3:1)
   - Peak incidence between 50 and 60 years old but it occurs in younger people as well

4. **Signs:**
   - The aim of examination is to differentiate between benign paroxysmal positional vertigo and central causes of vertigo such as stroke and vestibular neuronitis.
   - The diagnosis is based on history together with the demonstration from examination that changes in the position of the head with respect to gravity provoke the symptoms and the sense of rotation.
   - Nystagmus in peripheral vertigo (benign paroxysmal positional vertigo) is positional and usually horizontal and rotational. It lessens or disappears when the patient focuses the gaze.
   - The Dix–Hallpike manoeuvre is positive in benign paroxysmal positional vertigo with a positive predictive value of 83% in this diagnosis.
   - Table 3.7.1 identifies key differences between peripheral and central vertigo.

   Laboratory investigations:
   - Audiometry helps in the diagnosis of Meniere disease and acoustic neuroma.
   - MRI scan of the brain helps in the diagnosis of cerebellopontine angle tumour (acoustic neuroma) and stroke.

5. **Pathogenesis:**
   - The pathogenesis of benign paroxysmal positional vertigo is related to dislodgement of otoconia from the macula of the utricle affecting the semicircular canal function.
   - With the changes in the head position, the otolithic debris moves to a new position in the semicircular canals, giving a false sense of rotation of the surroundings.

Table 3.7.1 Differences between peripheral vertigo and central vertigo

Item	Peripheral vertigo	Central vertigo
Example	Benign paroxysmal positional vertigo	Stroke
Nausea and vomiting	May be severe	Usually not present or less severe
Onset and course	Recurrent, transient occurs with the changes in the head position with respect to gravity or getting in and out of bed	Usually sustained Worsened by changing position
Balance	Mild to moderate imbalance, still able to walk	Severe imbalance Unable to stand or walk
Hearing loss	No hearing loss	Varies
Tinnitus	No tinnitus	Varies
Other neurological symptoms and signs	No other neurological symptoms or signs	Several other neurological symptoms and signs are usually elicited
Nystagmus	Positional	Spontaneous
	Lessens or disappears when the patient focuses the gaze	Observed in various directions Changing directions
	It is usually horizontal nystagmus or mixed vertical	It does not disappear when the patient focuses the gaze
Other aspects in history	Patient may give a history of recumbent position (visited the dentist office) or give a history of head trauma or being in bed for some time Patient may give a history of previous similar attacks	History of headache may be present Patient may give a history of high blood pressure, diabetes, dyslipidaemia or other vascular risk factors

6. Management goals:
   - Improve the clinical symptoms – sense of rotation.
   - Ameliorate nausea and vomiting.
   - Educate the patient.

Benign paroxysmal positional vertigo resolves without treatment within 7–17 days (it takes a longer duration to resolve when the posterior canal is affected).

Medications are mainly to relieve nausea and vomiting.

Canalith repositioning procedure is effective treatment in benign paroxysmal positional vertigo.

BACK TO BASIC SCIENCES

Q1. What is dizziness? What are the types of dizziness?

Dizziness has a broad meaning and describes a range of sensations. It includes the following three types:

1. Vertigo (a false sense of motion or a feeling that the surroundings are moving)

2. Light-headedness (feeling faint)
3. Disequilibrium (unsteadiness or loss of balance)

Clinically the doctor has to work out to differentiate between vertigo and light-headedness. This can be achieved by asking the patient, 'When you feel dizzy, do you feel that you are going to faint or do you feel like the surroundings are rotating?'

Q2. What are the causes of vertigo?

The commonest causes of vertigo are as follows:
1. Benign paroxysmal positional vertigo
2. Acute vestibular neuronitis
3. Meniere disease

   Following are the other causes of vertigo:
- Alcohol
- Aminoglycosides
- Salicylates
- Diuretics
- Antihypertensives
- Nitrates
- Antidepressants
- Anticonvulsants
- Sedatives
- Cocaine
- Cerebrovascular disorders
- Migraine
- Multiple sclerosis
- Intracranial tumours
- Eighth cranial nerve schwannoma

Q3. What are peripheral and central causes of vertigo?

The peripheral causes of vertigo include the following:
- Benign paroxysmal positional vertigo
- Acute labyrinthitis
- Herpes zoster (Ramsay Hunt syndrome)
- Meniere disease
- Otosclerosis
- Acute vestibular neuronitis

   The central causes of vertigo include the following:
- Cerebrovascular disease stroke
- Migraine
- Cerebellopontine angle tumour (acoustic neuroma)

   The differentiation between the two groups can be accomplished from the history and clinical examination. The Dix–Hallpike manoeuvre helps in the diagnosis of benign paroxysmal positional vertigo (the test has a positive predictive value of 83%).

Q4. How does history taking help in the diagnosis of the cause of vertigo?

1. A sense that the surroundings are moving, felt on changing the head position, raises the following possibilities: benign paroxysmal positional vertigo, acute labyrinthitis, cerebellopontine angle tumour, perilymphatic fistula and multiple sclerosis.
2. A recent history of upper respiratory tract infection raises the following possibilities: acute vestibular neuronitis and acute labyrinthitis.
3. The patient gives a history of stress or panic attacks, which raises the possibilities of psychological factors or migraine.
4. Episodes that are spontaneous and not triggered by specific cause raise the following possibilities: Meniere disease, migraine, multiple sclerosis, cerebrovascular disease and transient ischaemic attacks.
5. A history of trauma and loud noises heard by the patient raises the possibility of perilymphatic fistula.
6. Old age and being on immunosuppressive medication raise the possibility of herpes zoster.
7. A history of diabetes mellitus, hypertension, dyslipidaemia and other risk factors for cerebrovascular disease raises the possibility of transient ischaemic attack, stroke or drug-related vertigo.

Q5. What are the roles of investigations in the diagnosis of a patient with vertigo?

1. Dix–Hallpike is a useful clinical manoeuvre used in the diagnosis of benign paroxysmal positional vertigo.
2. Audiometry can help in the diagnosis of Meniere disease and acoustic neuroma.
3. MRI scan (coronal section) can help in the diagnosis of cerebellopontine angle tumour (acoustic neuroma) and stroke.

REVIEW QUESTIONS

Q1. Which *one* of the following is the commonest cause of vertigo?
A. Acute vestibular neuronitis
B. Benign paroxysmal positional vertigo
C. Meniere disease
D. Stroke
E. Acoustic neuroma

Q2. Which *one* of the following is related to the pathogenesis of benign paroxysmal positional vertigo?
A. Upper respiratory tract infection
B. Head trauma
C. Stress/panic attacks
D. Migraine
E. Otolithic debris in the semicircular canals

Q3. Which *one* of the following structures is commonly involved in benign paroxysmal positional vertigo?
A. Posterior semicircular canal
B. Anterior semicircular canal
C. Horizontal semicircular canal
D. All semicircular canals
E. Middle ear

Q4. Which *one* of the following clinical signs helps in the diagnosis of benign paroxysmal positional vertigo?
A. Hennebert sign
B. Romberg sign
C. Valsalva manoeuvre
D. Dix–Hallpike manoeuvre
E. Tullio phenomenon

ANSWERS

A1. **B.** Benign paroxysmal positional vertigo is the most common cause of vertigo.

A2. **E.** The movement of the otolithic debris in the semicircular canals leads to a false sense of rotation of the surroundings.

A3. **A.** The posterior semicircular canal is gravity dependent and is the most commonly affected in benign paroxysmal positional vertigo.

A4. **D.** The Dix–Hallpike manoeuvre has a positive predictive value of 83% in the diagnosis of benign paroxysmal positional vertigo.

Hennebert sign (vertigo or nystagmus caused by pushing on the tragus of the affected aide) indicates the presence of perilymphatic fistula.

Valsalva manoeuvre causes vertigo in patients with perilymphatic fistula.

Tullio phenomenon: Nystagmus and vertigo caused by loud noises/sounds are suggestive of a peripheral vertigo.

TAKE-HOME MESSAGE

- Dizziness has a broad meaning and describes the following three symptoms: vertigo, light-headedness and disequilibrium.
- Vertigo (a false sense of motion or the feeling that the surroundings are moving) is commonly caused by benign paroxysmal positional vertigo.
- Other causes of vertigo are acute vestibular neuronitis, Meniere disease, alcohol, drugs, stroke, migraine, multiple sclerosis and acoustic neuroma.
- Drugs causing vertigo include alcohol, aminoglycosides, anticonvulsants, antidepressants, cocaine, diuretics, nitroglycerine, salicylates and sedatives.

- The causes of vertigo can be grouped into two groups: central vertigo (e.g. stroke, migraine and acoustic neuroma) and peripheral vertigo (e.g. benign paroxysmal positional vertigo, labyrinthitis).
- Benign paroxysmal positional vertigo is diagnosed from history and clinical examination (the Dix–Hallpike manoeuvre has a positive predictive value of 83% and a negative predictive value of 52%).
- Investigations commonly used in the diagnosis include audiometry and MRI scan of the brain.
- Benign paroxysmal positional vertigo commonly resolves within 7–17 days. Medications are used to relieve nausea and vomiting.

FURTHER READINGS

Baloh RW. Vertigo. *Lancet*. 1998;352(9143):1841-1846. Review.

Furman JM, Cass SP. Benign paroxysmal positional vertigo. *N Engl J Med*. 1999;341(21):1590-1596.

Kanagalingam J, Hajioff D, Bennett S. Vertigo. *BMJ*. 2005;330(7490):523. Review.

Kim JS, Zee DS. Clinical practice. Benign paroxysmal positional vertigo. *N Engl J Med*. 2014;370(12): 1138-1147.

Labuguen RH. Initial evaluation of vertigo. *Am Fam Physician*. 2006;73(2):244-251. Review.

Ludman H. Vertigo and imbalance. *BMJ*. 2014;348:g283. Review.

Sajjadi H, Paparella MM. Meniere's disease. *Lancet*. 2008;372(9636):406-414. Review.

Post RE, Dickerson LM. Dizziness: a diagnostic approach. *Am Fam Physician*. 2010;82(4):361-368, 369. Review.

Swartz R, Longwell P. Treatment of vertigo. *Am Fam Physician*. 2005;71(6):1115-1122. Review.

CASE 3.8

My Feet Are Painfully Hot

Jamal Hussein, a 69-year-old retired army soldier, comes in to see his general practitioner because he is suffering from burning and tingling pain in his feet. Mr Hussein has been diagnosed with diabetes mellitus about 3 years ago; he is also on treatment for hypertension and high blood cholesterol for the past 10 years. Mr Hussein has smoked two packs of cigarettes per day for the past 20 years. He does not drink alcohol. On examination, his pulse rate is 95/min, blood pressure 145/90 mm Hg, temperature 36.8°C and respiratory rate 17/min. He has no goitre. Examination of the lower limbs reveals hyperaesthesia of both feet, and decreased vibration and proprioception sensations. Fasting blood glucose level is 7.6 mmol/L, and his haemoglobin A_{1c} is 8.0%.

CASE DISCUSSION

Q1. On the basis of Mr Hussein's presentation, what is your diagnosis?

Q2. What is your differential diagnosis?

Q3. What are the key clinical features of this disease? What are the scientific bases for these features?

Q4. What is the pathophysiology underlying these changes?

Q5. What are your management goals and management options?

ANSWERS

1. The findings of being diagnosed with type 2 diabetes and having burning and tingling pain in the feet, together with hypertension, high cholesterol for the past 10 years and the findings on examination of hyperaesthesia in the feet and decreased vibration and proprioception sensations, are consistent with the diagnosis of symmetrical distal diabetic polyneuropathy. Although he does not drink alcohol, he gives a history of heavy smoking for the past 20 years. Other causes of neuropathy including vitamin B12 deficiency, renal disease, inherited neuropathy, vasculitis and chronic inflammatory demyelinating polyneuropathy should be investigated and excluded. Further assessment including nerve conduction studies and skin biopsy is indicated.
2. The differential diagnosis includes the following:
   - A: Acquired immunodeficiency syndrome and amyloidosis
   - B: Vitamin B6 deficiency and vitamin B12 deficiency
   - C: Carcinoma and chronic liver disease

- D: Diabetes mellitus
- D: Drugs such as amiodarone, chloroquine, digoxin, isoniazid, lithium, phenytoin, vincristine, B6 excess and statins
- D: Diphtheria toxins
- E: Ethanol – chronic consumption
- F: Factory toxins (lead, arsenic and chemicals)
- G: Genetic disorders such as Charcot–Marie–Tooth disease type 1 and type 2, and Guillain–Barré syndrome
- H: Hypothyroidism and heavy metals (lead, arsenic, mercury, gold)
- I: Idiopathic
- K: Kidney failure
- L: Lyme disease and lymphoma
- M: Multiple myeloma and other monoclonal gammopathy
- N: Neurosarcoidosis and nutritional neuropathy
- O: Organophosphates and other causes such as tic paralysis, syphilis and vasculitic neuropathy

3. Clinical picture:

   Symptoms:
   - Sensory changes: (i) sensory loss → numbness or burning sensations; (ii) paraesthesia; (iii) temperature and pinprick (pain) sensation; (iv) vibration sensory loss; (v) proprioception loss; and (vi) loss of sensation in a 'glove and stocking distribution'.
   - Motor changes: (i) mild distal weakness and (ii) atrophy may be present.
   - Autonomic changes: (i) postural hypotension, (ii) disturbance of sweating, (iii) disturbance of cardiac rhythm and (iv) disturbance of gastrointestinal, bladder and sexual functions.
   - It is important to identify the chronicity of symptoms, the pattern and extent of involvement and the type of nerve fibres involved (sensory, motor or autonomic).
   - In diabetic neuropathy, sensory symptoms are predominant (tingling, burning and stabbing); sensory loss, weakness and numbness also occur. Motor symptoms are less common. They usually occur later in the disease. Sensory loss may result in the development of foot ulcers or gangrene. Loss of proprioception can result in unsteadiness in gait and increased likelihood of a fall.

   Signs:
   - There is a loss of sensations in a 'glove and stocking distribution' in the upper and lower limbs.
   - There is a loss of vibration sense (using a 128-Hz tuning fork).
   - There is a loss of proprioception, temperature and pinprick sensations.
   - Muscular wasting may be present in chronic cases.
   - Fasciculations may be present.
   - Flaccid tone of the muscles is present.
   - A distal-to-proximal gradient of reflex elicitation is present (decreased ankle reflex on both sides compared to knee reflex).
   - Plantar reflex is flexor.

Laboratory investigations: The following investigations may be needed in patients presenting with symmetrical peripheral polyneuropathy:

- Full blood count, blood film and erythrocyte sedimentation rate
- Fasting blood glucose level and haemoglobin A_{1c} level
- Vitamin B12
- Thyroid function tests
- Paraneoplastic panel evaluation (occult malignancy)
- Antibodies: Antimyelin-associated glycoprotein antibodies and antiganglioside antibodies
- Cryoglobulins
- CSF examinations: In the diagnosis of Guillain–Barré syndrome and chronic inflammatory demyelinating neuropathy (CSF proteins are elevated)
- Electromyography (EMG) needed if there is no clue found from the history, examination and biochemical tests; can help in differentiating axonal damage, myelin damage or mixed damages
- Nerve biopsy: Rarely needed; usually indicated in cases not diagnosed from history, examination and other investigations; sural and superficial peroneal nerves preferred for biopsy

In diabetic neuropathy, the following investigations may be recommended: full blood count, haemoglobin A_{1c}, fasting blood glucose, vitamin B12 and thyroid function tests, skin biopsy (recently introduced instead of nerve biopsy) and nerve conduction studies.

4. Pathology:
   - Nerve fibres of different types (sensory, motor or autonomic) and of different sizes may be involved.
   - The disorder may be directed to the axon, the myelin sheath or the vasa nervosa.
   - Diabetic neuropathy has the following subtypes: (i) small fibre neuropathy, (ii) painful symmetrical polyneuropathy, (iii) diabetic lumbosacral radiculoplexus neuropathy (asymmetrical pain and weakness in the proximal lower limb), (iv) mononeuropathy (carpal tunnel syndrome is the commonest mononeuropathy in diabetes, ulnar mononeuropathy, lateral cutaneous neuropathies), (v) treatment-induced neuropathy and (vi) mononeuritis multiplex (progressive neuropathy of the ulnar or peroneal nerves).
   - Sural nerve biopsy in diabetic patients with polyneuropathy shows (i) decreased myelinated nerve fibre density, (ii) swelling of axons and (iii) segmental demyelination.

5. Management goals:
   - Controlling the underlying disease process (e.g. controlling the blood glucose level)
   - Treating symptoms (e.g. pain)
   - Lifestyle interventions (diet, exercise, help to improve balance and decrease falls)
   - Patient education and improving quality of life
   - Pharmacological treatment in controlling pain in diabetic neuropathy, which includes the following:
     - Anticonvulsants: Gabapentin and pregabalin

    – Tricyclic antidepressants
    – Serotonin–norepinephrine reuptake inhibitors

BACK TO BASIC SCIENCES

Q1. What is the definition of diabetic sensorimotor polyneuropathy?

According to the Toronto Consensus Panel, the definition is 'a symmetrical length-dependent sensorimotor polyneuropathy attributable to metabolic and micro-vascular alterations as a result of chronic hyperglycaemia exposure and cardiovascular risk covariates'.

Q2. How different is diabetic neuropathy in patients with type 1 diabetes mellitus compared to in those with type 2 disease?

- Diabetic neuropathy is more prevalent in type 2 diabetes mellitus than in type 1 disease.
- Symptoms of diabetic sensorimotor polyneuropathy typically manifest earlier in type 2 diabetes mellitus than in type 1 disease – 8% have neuropathy at the time of the diagnosis of type 2 diabetes.
- The mechanism and pathogenesis of neuropathy in the two types of diabetes are not the same.
- The metabolic syndrome in type 2 diabetes is responsible for the pathogenesis of neuropathy, whereas in type 1 diabetes hyperglycaemia is responsible.
- Therefore, the enhanced glucose control is much more effective at preventing neuropathy in patients with type 1 diabetes than in those having type 2 disease.
- There is greater involvement of myelinated fibres in patients with type 1 diabetes than in those with type 2 disease.
- Patients should be screened for diabetic sensorimotor polyneuropathy at the diagnosis of type 2 diabetes and in 5 years after the diagnosis of type 1 disease.

Q3. What are the subtypes of diabetic neuropathy?

The subtypes of diabetic neuropathy are (i) small fibre neuropathy, (ii) painful symmetrical polyneuropathy, (iii) diabetic lumbosacral radiculoplexus neuropathy (asymmetrical pain and weakness in the proximal lower limb), (iv) mononeuropathy (carpal tunnel syndrome is the commonest mononeuropathy in diabetes, ulnar mononeuropathy, lateral cutaneous neuropathies), (v) treatment-induced neuropathy and (vi) mononeuritis multiplex (progressive neuropathy of the ulnar or peroneal nerves).

Q4. What are the essential parameters for the diagnosis of neuropathy in a patient with diabetes mellitus?

At least two out of the following three parameters should be present to give the diagnosis of probable neuropathy:

  (i) Presence of neuropathy symptoms
  (ii) Presence of neuropathic sensory examination findings
  (iii) Presence of abnormal reflexes

In order to confirm the diagnosis of neuropathy, you will need to perform nerve conduction studies or skin biopsy.

Q5. Discuss the drugs used in the management of neuropathic pain.

Table 3.8.1 summarises the drugs used to treat neuropathic pain.

Table 3.8.1 Drugs used to treat neuropathic pain

Group	Examples	Mechanisms of action	Advantages	Side effects
Antiepileptic drugs	Pregabalin Gabapentin Carbamazepine Lamotrigine Lacosamide	Both pregabalin and gabapentin have a similar mechanism – bind to calcium channels in the dorsal horn containing the α2δ subunit and decrease neurotransmitter release.	Both pregabalin and gabapentin have similar efficacy. Other drugs in this group show conflicting results. Generally, drugs in this group are less effective in diabetic neuropathy.	Pregabalin and gabapentin may cause peripheral oedema, dizziness, drowsiness, headache, weight gain, tremor, diplopia.
Antidepressants Tricyclic antidepressants	Amitriptyline Nortriptyline Imipramine	Inhibition of the membrane pump mechanisms responsible for uptake of norepinephrine and serotonin in adrenergic and serotonergic neurons.	Have consistently shown benefit in treating painful diabetic neuropathy. Have the advantages of once-daily dose and being available at a reasonable cost.	May have serious side effects including orthostasis, constipation, somnolence and erectile dysfunction. Are not recommended in patients with heart diseases.
Antidepressants Serotonin–norepinephrine reuptake inhibitors (SNRIs)	Duloxetine Venlafaxine	Inhibition of neuronal serotonin and norepinephrine reuptake and to a less extent inhibition of dopamine reuptake.	Have consistently shown benefit in treating painful diabetic neuropathy.	Syncope, hepatotoxicity, serotonin syndrome, abnormal bleeding, angle-closure glaucoma and seizure.
Opioid-based drugs	Oxycodone Morphine sulphate Tramadol Tapentadol	Opioids decrease intracellular cAMP by inhibiting adenylate cyclase. Thus, the release of neurotransmitters, such as substance P, GABA and dopamine, is inhibited. Opioids close N-type voltage-operated calcium channels and open calcium-dependent inwardly rectifying potassium channels. This results in reduced neuronal excitability.	Have consistently shown benefit in treating painful diabetic neuropathy.	Tolerance. Withdrawal symptoms on discontinuation. Risk of misuse.

REVIEW QUESTIONS

Q1. Which *one* of the following sensations is affected in demyelinating neuropathy?
A. Vibration and proprioception
B. Touch
C. Pain
D. Touch and pain

Q2. Which *one* of the following drugs *does not* cause peripheral neuropathy?
A. Statins
B. Vincristine
C. Telmisartan
D. Phenytoin
E. Metronidazole

Q3. All of the following cause neuropathy with autonomic features *except*
A. Diabetes mellitus.
B. Leprosy.
C. Amyloidosis.
D. Chemotherapy-related neuropathy.
E. Paraneoplastic syndrome.

Q4. The following drugs are used in managing pain in patients with distal symmetrical polyneuropathy. Which *one* of the following should be *avoided* in patients with cardiac diseases?
A. Gabapentin
B. Pregabalin
C. Amitriptyline
D. Topiramate
E. Duloxetine

ANSWERS

A1. **A.** Vibration and proprioception sensations are particularly affected in demyelinating neuropathy.

A2. **C.** Telmisartan is an angiotensin II receptor antagonist used in the management of hypertension. It is not known to cause peripheral neuropathy.

A3. **B.** Leprosy can cause chronic mononeuropathy multiplex without autonomic features. All others – diabetes mellitus, amyloidosis, chemotherapy, paraneoplastic syndrome, vitamin B12 deficiency, porphyria, heavy metal toxicity and alcoholism – can cause neuropathy with autonomic features.

A4. **C**. Tricyclic antidepressants such as amitriptyline, though used in the management of pain of patients, should be avoided in patients with cardiac disorders such as QT-interval prolongation or rhythm disturbances.

TAKE-HOME MESSAGE

- Polyneuropathy may be caused by acquired immune deficiency syndrome, amyloidosis, vitamin B12 or B6 deficiencies, carcinoma, chronic liver disease, diabetes mellitus, drugs, ethanol, toxins, genetic disorders, hypothyroidism, kidney failure, multiple myeloma and vasculitis, and could be idiopathic.
- Diabetic neuropathy is more prevalent in type 2 diabetes than in type 1 disease.
- Symptoms of diabetic sensorimotor polyneuropathy typically manifest earlier in type 2 diabetes than in type 1 disease.
- Hyperglycaemia appears to play a role in the pathogenesis of type 1 diabetes–related neuropathy, whereas in type 2 diabetes other factors such as metabolic syndrome and risks of cardiovascular changes are involved.
- Enhanced glucose control is much more effective at preventing neuropathy in patients with type 1 diabetes. In type 2 disease control, blood glucose is not effective in preventing neuropathy.
- Several subtypes of diabetic sensorimotor neuropathy have been identified. They can be summarised as follows: (i) small fibre neuropathy, (ii) painful symmetrical polyneuropathy, (iii) diabetic lumbosacral radiculoplexus neuropathy (asymmetrical pain and weakness in the proximal lower limb), (iv) mononeuropathy (e.g. carpal tunnel syndrome, ulnar mononeuropathy, lateral cutaneous neuropathies), (v) treatment-induced neuropathy and (vi) mononeuritis multiplex (progressive neuropathy of the ulnar or peroneal nerves).
- The commonest cause of diabetic mononeuropathy is carpal tunnel syndrome.
- The diagnosis of diabetic neuropathy is based on the presence of two of the following parameters:
  - **(i)** The presence of neuropathy symptoms
  - **(ii)** The presence of neuropathic sensory examination findings
  - **(iii)** The presence of abnormal reflexes

  Nerve conduction studies or skin biopsy should be carried out to confirm the diagnosis of neuropathy.
- The treatment of diabetic neuropathy in type 1 diabetes mellitus is glycaemic control, control of pain and patient education, whereas in type 2 diabetes the management of the metabolic changes and cardiovascular risk factors is important together with control of pain, patient education and exercise.

FURTHER READINGS

Callaghan BC, Cheng HT, Stables CL, Smith AL, Feldman EL. Diabetic neuropathy: clinical manifestations and current treatments. *Lancet Neurol.* 2012;11(6):521-534. doi:10.1016/S1474-4422(12)70065-0. Review.

Gandhi RA, Marques JL, Selvarajah D, Emery CJ, Tesfaye S. Painful diabetic neuropathy is associated with greater autonomic dysfunction than painless diabetic neuropathy. *Diabetes Care*. 2010;33(7):1585-1590.

Gwathmey KG, Burns TM, Collins MP, Dyck PJ. Vasculitic neuropathies. *Lancet Neurol*. 2014;13(1):67-82. doi:10.1016/S1474-4422(13)70236-9. Review.

Peltier A, Goutman SA, Callaghan BC. Painful diabetic neuropathy. *BMJ*. 2014;348:g1799. Review.

Tesfaye S, Boulton AJ, Dyck PJ, et al. Diabetic neuropathies: update on definitions, diagnostic criteria, estimation of severity, and treatments. *Diabetes Care*. 2010;33(10):2285-2293.

Valencia WM, Florez H. How to prevent the microvascular complications of type 2 diabetes beyond glucose control. *BMJ*. 2017;356:i6505. Review.

Vinik AI. Clinical Practice. Diabetic sensory and motor neuropathy. *N Engl J Med*. 2016;374(15):1455-1464.

Rheumatology and Immune System

CASE 4.1

'Stiffness in the Morning . . . '

Anna William, a 32-year-old secretary, gradually develops swollen fingers and painful wrists. She also noticed morning stiffness for more than 1 hour. She was seen, a few weeks ago, by her general practitioner and treated with ibuprofen. However, the pain, stiffness and swelling of her hands persisted and a few weeks later her knees became swollen and painful. Because her symptoms persisted for over 6 weeks, the general practitioner refered her to a rheumatologist. On examination, her wrists and metacarpophalangeal joints are found to be swollen and tender. She also has two subcutaneous nodules on the right elbow. The results of her investigations are summarised as follows:

X-rays of the hands show bony erosions in the metacarpal heads.

Table 4.1.1 summarises the blood test results.

She is treated with a weekly low dose of methotrexate.

CASE DISCUSSION

Q1. On the basis of Anna's presentation, what is your diagnosis?

Q2. What is your differential diagnosis?

Q3. What are the key clinical features of this disease? What are the scientific bases for these features?

Q4. What is the pathophysiology underlying these changes?

Q5. What are your management goals and management options?

ANSWERS

1. The findings of joint swelling, pain and morning stiffness (more than 1 hour) affecting small joints of the hands and the wrists together with the involvement of the large joints (the knees), the presence of rheumatoid nodules (two subcutaneous nodules on the right elbow) and the persistence of her symptoms for over 6 weeks are all suggestive of the diagnosis of rheumatoid arthritis.

   The C-reactive protein and erythrocyte sedimentation rate (ESR) may be raised during disease activity but they are not specific for rheumatoid arthritis. C3 and C4 levels are usually normal in rheumatoid arthritis.

   Although positive rheumatoid factor (RF) is consistent with rheumatoid arthritis, the positive results cannot differentiate between non-rheumatoid and rheumatoid arthritis. This is because 15% of patients with rheumatoid arthritis have a nonreactive titre. Again RF is not specific for the diagnosis – patients with chronic conditions

Table 4.1.1 Blood test results

Blood test	Anna's results	Range
C-reactive protein (CRP)	47	Normal <5 mg/L
Erythrocyte sedimentation rate (ESR)	55	Normal <20 mm/h
Complement C3	1.2	Normal 0.73–1.4 g/L
Complement C4	0.12	Normal 0.12–0.30 g/L
Rheumatoid factor	Negative	Normal <15 IU/mL
Antinuclear (ANA) test	Not detected	Negative <1 0 unit Positive 3.0–5.9 units Strongly positive >6.0 units

may have positive RF including systemic lupus erythematosus, polymyositis, syphilis, tuberculosis and viral hepatitis.

2　The differential diagnosis may include the following:
- Rheumatic fever
- Systemic lupus erythematosus
- Fibromyalgia
- Lyme disease
- Osteoarthritis
- Paraneoplastic syndrome
- Relapsing polytendinitis
- Psoriatic arthritis
- Sarcoidosis
- Sjögren syndrome
- Polymyalgia rheumatica
- Viral and other self-limited arthritis

The following are essential for the diagnosis of rheumatoid arthritis (American Rheumatism Association, 1988, revised version):
- Morning stiffness more than 1 hour
- Arthritis of hand joints
- Symmetrical arthritis
- Rheumatoid nodules
- Positive RF
- Radiological changes
- Duration more than 6 weeks

3. Symptoms and signs:
- Cardinal symptoms: (i) pain, joint swelling and stiffness affecting the small joints of hands, feet and wrists; (ii) involvement of large joints may occur (e.g. knees); (iii) the symptoms persist for more than 6 weeks: this helps in differentiating rheumatoid arthritis from viral and self-limited arthritis (usually the symptoms persist for 1–2 weeks); (iv) systematic symptoms (anorexia, weight loss, fatigue); and (v) extra-articular features, which are more common in patients with long-standing seropositive erosive disease.

They may occur at presentation. The pathophysiology of these extra-articular features is related to serositis, granuloma formation or vasculitis. The extra-articular features can be summarised as follows:

- Systemic: Fever, weight loss and fatigue
- Ocular: Episcleritis, scleromalacia, scleritis and keratoconjunctivitis sicca
- Vasculitis: Ulcers, pyoderma gangrenosum and mononeuritis multiplex
- Haematological: Anaemia, thrombosis and eosinophilia
- Cardiac: Pericarditis, myocarditis, endocarditis, conductive defects and coronary vasculitis
- Respiratory: Nodules, pleural effusion, fibrosing alveolitis and Caplan syndrome
- Musculoskeletal: Muscle wasting, bursitis and tenosynovitis
- Neurological: Peripheral neuropathy, mononeuritis multiplex, cervical cord compression and compression neuropathy

- Clinical examination shows the following:
  - Symmetrical swelling of metacarpophalangeal joints and proximal interphalangeal joints of the hands
  - Joints inflamed and tender to touch
  - Characteristic deformities in long-standing diseases (swan neck deformity, the boutonniere or buttonhole deformity, a Z deformity of the thumb)
  - Distal subluxation of the ulna at the distal radioulnar joints
  - Possibility of occurrence of triggering of fingers (due to nodules on the flexor tendon sheath)
  - Feet 'cock-up toe' deformity, calcaneovalgus (eversion) deformity and loss of the longitudinal arch of feet (flat foot)
  - Popliteal (Backer's) cysts and knee synovitis

Clinical characteristics of rheumatoid arthritis are summarised in Table 4.1.2.

4. Pathological features:
   - The disease is related to genetic and environmental factors.
   - Severity is related to genetic factors; particularly DR4 positive is commonly associated with severe erosive disease.
   - Cigarette smoking is a risk factor and is associated with severe disease.
   - The trigger point in the pathogenesis of rheumatoid arthritis is the synovial membrane (increased lymphocytes, plasma cells, macrophages and CD4 T-cells).
   - Activated T-cells stimulate B-cells to produce immunoglobulins including RF. Macrophages are stimulated to produce cytokines.
   - Several cells are involved in the pathogenesis (endothelial cells, bone cells, synovial cells and chondrocytes) to produce swelling and congestion of the synovial membrane, bone destruction and destruction of the cartilage and soft tissues.
   - Cytokines and in particular TNF-alpha are vital in the pathogenesis.
   - The B-cells release immunoglobulins and RF forming immune complexes and development of vasculitis.
   - Lymphoid tissues in the synovial membrane develop inflammatory granuloma, which plays a role in the destruction of the cartilage.

Table 4.1.2 Clinical characteristics of rheumatoid arthritis

Articular
Morning stiffness, 'gelling'
Symmetrical joint swelling
Predilection for wrists and proximal interphalangeal, metacarpophalangeal and metatarsophalangeal joints
Erosions of bone and cartilage
Joint subluxation and ulnar deviation
Inflammatory joint fluid
Carpal tunnel syndrome
Baker's cyst
Nonarticular
Rheumatoid nodules: Subcutaneous, pulmonary, scleral
Lung disease
Vasculitis, especially skin and peripheral nerves
Pleuropericarditis
Scleritis and episcleritis
Leg ulcers
Felty syndrome

Source: Andreoli TE, Benjamin IJ, Griggs RC, Wing EJ. Andreoli and Carpenter's Cecil Essentials of Medicine. 8th ed. Philadelphia, PA: Elsevier; 2010.

- Muscles adjacent to the affected joints are inflamed and atrophied.
- Rheumatoid nodules may be found in the lungs, pleura, pericardium and sclera.

5. Management goals:

The aims of management are to relieve the patient's symptoms, suppress inflammation and conservative restoration of function in the affected joints and early detection of any complications.

Therefore, the goals are as follows:

- Physical rest
- Anti-inflammatory therapy
- Passive exercise
- Follow-up

BACK TO BASIC SCIENCES

Q1. State examples of seronegative spondyloarthritis.

Seronegative spondyloarthritis shares association with HLA-B27 antigen and may include the following diseases:

- Ankylosing spondylitis
- Reactive arthritis

- Psoriatic arthritis
- Arthropathy associated with inflammatory bowel disease

Q2. What are the main differences between rheumatoid arthritis and seronegative spondyloarthritis?

Table 4.1.3 summarises the main differences between rheumatoid arthritis and seronegative spondyloarthritis.

Table 4.1.3 Main differences between rheumatoid arthritis and seronegative spondyloarthritis

Issue/point	Rheumatoid arthritis	Seronegative spondyloarthritis
Rheumatoid factor (RF)	Mostly positive (expect in 15%)	All negative
What does it comprise?	Rheumatoid arthritis	• Ankylosing spondylitis • Reactive arthritis • Psoriatic arthritis • Arthropathy associated with inflammatory bowel disease
Symptoms and clinical picture	As described earlier	Depend on the disease under this category

Q3. What are the indications for disease-modifying antirheumatic drugs (DMARDs)?

- Persistence of inflammatory synovitis for more than 6 weeks
- Systemic vasculitis
- Systemic lupus erythematosus with cardiac, renal or nervous system involvement
- As an adjunct to corticosteroid therapy

Q4. Discuss the DMARDs showing drug examples, mechanism of action, indications, side effects and monitoring required/frequency.

These drugs include the following:

- Azathioprine
- Cyclophosphamide
- Cyclosporine
- D-Penicillamine
- Gold
- Hydroxychloroquine
- Methotrexate

Q5. Discuss DMARDs.

Table 4.1.4 summarises DMARDs used in rheumatoid arthritis.

Table 4.1.4 Disease-modifying antirheumatic drugs (DMARDS) used in rheumatoid arthritis

Drug group	Mechanism of action	Disease indication	Adverse effects	Monitoring/frequency
Azathioprine	• Antagonises purine metabolism and inhibits the synthesis of DNA and RNA • Interferes with cellular metabolism • Inhibits mitosis	• Rheumatoid arthritis • Renal homotransplantations • Inflammatory bowel disease	• Cytopenia – leukopenia, thrombocytopenia, anaemia • Serious infections – viral, fungal, bacterial, protozoal • Temporary suppression of spermatogenesis • Pregnancy – Category D	• Complete blood test • Thiopurine methyltransferase (TPMT) testing • Watch for drug interactions, e.g. allopurinol
Cyclophosphamide	• Attachment of alkyl groups to DNA • Direct damage to DNA • Mispairing of nucleotides resulting in mutations	• Antirheumatic agent • Immunosuppressant agent • Antineoplastic agent (malignant lymphoma, multiple myeloma, leukaemia, neuroblastoma, adenocarcinoma of ovary, retinoblastoma, breast cancer) • Mutagens – increase rate of mutation	• Hepatotoxicity – mild rise in transaminases • Carcinogenic risk • Dizziness, diarrhoea, nausea, vomiting, abdominal pain • Haemorrhagic cystitis • Cardiac toxicity • Infections	• Monitor for leukopenia, thrombocytopenia regularly during treatment • Urine examination for RBCs • Watch for drug interactions
Cyclosporine	• Inhibits immunocompetent lymphocytes in G0 or G1 phase cell cycle – mainly T1 helper cells • Inhibits lymphokine production and release including IL-2	• Treatment of transplantation of kidney, liver and heart rejection • Rheumatoid arthritis • Psoriasis	• Hepatotoxicity • Carcinogenic risk • Drug interactions • Renal damage may occur	• Liver function tests • Cyclosporine level in blood • Watch for drug interactions

Drug	Mechanism	Indications	Side effects	Monitoring
D-Penicillamine	• Reduces number of T-lymphocytes • Inhibits macrophage functions • Decreases IL-1 • Decreases rheumatoid factor • Acts as chelating agent (Wilson disease) and immunosuppressant agent	• Treatment of Wilson disease • Reduces cysteine excretion in cystinuria • Treatment of severe and active rheumatoid arthritis	• Hepatotoxicity • Autoimmune disorders (lupus-like syndrome, autoimmune hepatitis) • Drug interactions	• Liver function tests • Watch for drug interactions
Gold	• Inhibition of the activity of atypical protein kinase Ciota (PKCiota), resulting in inhibition of tumour cell proliferation • Induction of cancer cell apoptosis • Immunosuppression	• Treatment of rheumatoid arthritis • Antineoplastic activities	• Pruritus, dermatitis • Stomatitis • Gastrointestinal symptoms • Albuminuria (e.g. nephrotic syndrome) • Haematuria • Agranulocytosis • Thrombocytopenia • Purpura • Aplastic anaemia	• Full blood count • Urinalysis • Clinical assessment
Hydroxychloroquine	Unknown	• Antimalarial • Treatment of lupus erythematosus • Acute and chronic rheumatoid arthritis	• Hepatotoxicity • Headache, drowsiness • Visual disturbances • Arrhythmias, bradycardia • Sudden cardiorespiratory arrest	• Liver function test • Watch for drug interactions
Methotrexate	• Antineoplastic • Antimetabolite • Blocks DNA • Inhibits the activation of helper cells • Cytotoxic immunosuppressant	• Antirheumatic agent • Immunosuppressant agent • Antimetabolite • Antineoplastic • Abortifacient	• Hepatotoxicity • Fatty liver • Liver fibrosis • Carcinogenesis	• Liver function tests • Liver biopsy every 1- to 2-year intervals • Watch for drug interactions • Folate supplements

REVIEW QUESTIONS

Q1. A 68-year-old patient who has been on treatment for rheumatoid arthritis for several years presents today because of calf pain and swelling of the calf region. The most likely diagnosis is
A. Knee effusion.
B. Baker's cyst.
C. Rupture of popliteal cyst.
D. Local bleeding in calf muscles.
E. Knee infection.

Q2. Loss of the longitudinal arch of the foot in patients with rheumatoid arthritis is most likely related to
A. Development of callosities.
B. Inflammation of the ankle joint.
C. Cock-up toe deformity.
D. Rupture of the tibialis posterior tendon.
E. Development of adventitious bursae.

Q3. A 26-year-old university graduate presented with pain and swelling of the small joints of the hands together with stiffness of 10–15 minutes. His symptoms continued for 2 weeks and he recovered in the third week. He was treated with ibuprofen three times a day. Which *one* of the following was the most likely diagnosis?
A. Rheumatoid arthritis
B. Polymyalgia rheumatica
C. Fibromyalgia
D. Viral arthritis

Q4. Which *one* of the following is *not* an extra-articular feature of rheumatoid arthritis?
A. Gynaecomastia
B. Endocarditis
C. Eosinophilia
D. Cervical cord compression

Q5. All of the following occur more commonly in patients with seropositive rheumatoid arthritis *except*
A. Vasculitis.
B. Erythema of small joints.
C. Extra-articular features.
D. Rheumatoid nodules.

Q6. A male patient with long-standing rheumatoid arthritis presents with occipital headache, paraesthesia in the arms and sometimes electric shock–like sensation along his upper limbs. Which *one* of the following is the most likely diagnosis?

A. Atlantoaxial subluxation

B. Osteoporosis of the cervical vertebrae

C. Cervical vasculitis

D. Increased intracranial pressure

Q7. A 60-year-old patient with long-standing seropositive rheumatoid arthritis presents with splenomegaly, lymphadenopathy and weight loss. Which *one* of the following is the best action in managing this patient?

A. Manage as Felty syndrome

B. Check the neutrophil count

C. Perform biopsy of the lymph nodes

D. Start DMARDs therapy

ANSWERS

A1. **C.** Rupture of a large cyst by knee flexion in the presence of large knee effusion results in severe calf pain and swelling of the calf region.

A2. **D.** The rupture of the tibialis posterior tendon is a complication that may occur in patients with rheumatoid arthritis and results in loss of the longitudinal arch of the foot.

A3. **D.** The short duration of the stiffness (10–15 minutes) and the continuation of arthritis for 2 weeks are not consistent with the diagnosis of rheumatoid arthritis. The presentation is most likely viral arthritis.

A4. **A.** Gynaecomastia is not part of extra-articular features of rheumatoid arthritis.

A5. **B.** Erythema is not a feature of rheumatoid arthritis. If present, it may suggest sepsis.

A6. **A.** Cervical cord compression as a result of subluxation of the cervical spine at the atlantoaxial joint is common in patients with long-standing rheumatoid arthritis, usually due to erosion and dysfunction of the ligament located posterior to the odontoid peg.

A7. **C.** Perform biopsy of lymph nodes to exclude lymphoma because patients with rheumatoid arthritis are at a higher risk of developing lymphoma.

TAKE-HOME MESSAGE

- The differential diagnosis of rheumatoid arthritis may include rheumatic fever, systemic lupus erythematosus, fibromyalgia, Lyme disease, osteoarthritis, paraneoplastic syndrome, relapsing polytendentitis, psoriatic arthritis, sarcoidosis, Sjögren syndrome, polymyalgia rheumatica and viral and other self-limited arthritis.

- Cardinal symptoms of rheumatoid arthritis are (i) pain, joint swelling and stiffness affecting the small joints of hands, feet and wrists; (ii) involvement of large joints may occur (e.g. knees); (iii) the symptoms persist for more than 6 weeks: this helps in differentiating rheumatoid arthritis from viral and self-limited arthritis (usually the symptoms persist for 1–2 weeks); (iv) systematic symptoms (anorexia, weight loss, fatigue); and (v) extra-articular features, which are more common in patients with long-standing seropositive erosive disease.
- The extra-articular features may occur at presentation.
- The extra-articular features may include (i) systemic: fever, weight loss and fatigue; (ii) ocular changes: episcleritis, scleromalacia, scleritis and keratoconjunctivitis sicca; (iii) vasculitis: ulcers, pyoderma gangrenosum and mononeuritis multiplex; (iv) haematological changes: anaemia, thrombosis and eosinophilia; (v) cardiac pathology: pericarditis, myocarditis, endocarditis, conductive defects and coronary vasculitis; (vi) respiratory: nodules, pleural effusion, fibrosing alveolitis and Caplan syndrome; (vii) musculoskeletal: muscle wasting, bursitis and tenosynovitis; and (viii) neurological: peripheral neuropathy, mononeuritis multiplex, cervical cord compression and compression neuropathy.
- The disease is related to genetic and environmental factors.
- Severity is related to genetic factors; particularly DR4 positive is commonly associated with severe erosive disease.
- Cigarette smoking is a risk factor and is associated with severe disease.
- The use of DMARDs is indicated mainly in the following conditions: (i) persistence of inflammatory synovitis for more than 6 weeks; (ii) systemic vasculitis; (iii) systemic lupus erythematosus with cardiac, renal or nervous system involvement; and (iv) as an adjunct to corticosteroid therapy.

FURTHER READINGS

Burmester GR, Pope JE. Novel treatment strategies in rheumatoid arthritis. *Lancet.* 2017;389(10086): 2338-2348. Review.

Choy EH, Panayi GS. Cytokine pathways and joint inflammation in rheumatoid arthritis. *N Engl J Med.* 2001;344(12):907-916. Review.

Dinarello CA. The role of the interleukin-1-receptor antagonist in blocking inflammation mediated by interleukin-1. *N Engl J Med.* 2000;343(10):732-734. Review.

McInnes IB, Schett G. The pathogenesis of rheumatoid arthritis. *N Engl J Med.* 2011;365(23):2205-2219. Review.

McInnes IB, Schett G. Pathogenetic insights from the treatment of rheumatoid arthritis. *Lancet.* 2017; 389(10086):2328-2337. Review.

O'Dell JR. Therapeutic strategies for rheumatoid arthritis. *N Engl J Med.* 2004;350(25):2591-2602. Review.

Olsen NJ, Stein CM. New drugs for rheumatoid arthritis. *N Engl J Med.* 2004;350(21):2167-2179. Review.

Scott DL, Kingsley GH. Tumor necrosis factor inhibitors for rheumatoid arthritis. *N Engl J Med.* 2006; 355(7):704-712. Review.

Smolen JS, Aletaha D, McInnes IB. Rheumatoid arthritis. *Lancet.* 2016;388(10055):2023-2038. Review.

CASE 4.2

'Progressive Pain in My Knees'

Mrs Kim Oliver, a 55-year-old kindergarten manager, comes in to see her general practitioner because of a 4-year history of progressive pain in both knees particularly during walking. She always feels stiffness in her knees for about 20–30 minutes when she continues in the same position for too long. She also has difficulties in walking because of pain. Sometimes she feels as if one of her knees would 'give out'. On examination her pulse is 95/min, blood pressure 130/80 mm Hg, her temperature is 37.0°C and the respiratory rate is 20/min. Her BMI is 41. Examination of the knees shows tenderness over the joint line, and patellofemoral crepitus is heard on flexion of her knees. Examination of the hands reveals enlargement of two of the proximal interphalangeal joints (PIP; Bouchard's nodes) and some of the distal interphalangeal joints (DIP; Heberden's nodes). Similar changes are noted in her feet.

CASE DISCUSSION

Q1. On the basis of Kim's presentation, what is your diagnosis?

Q2. What is your differential diagnosis?

Q3. What are the key clinical features of this disease? What are the scientific bases for these features?

Q4. What is the pathophysiology underlying these changes?

Q5. What are your management goals and management options?

ANSWERS

1. The findings of progressive pain in both knees particularly during walking and stiffness in the knees when she continues in the same position for too long in a female patient, 55 years old, who has a BMI of 41 and Bouchard's and Heberden's nodes in her hands and feet are consistent with the diagnosis of osteoarthritis.

2. The differential diagnosis includes the following:
   - Gout
   - Pseudogout
   - Fibromyalgia
   - Rheumatoid arthritis
   - Avascular necrosis

The following are essential for the diagnosis of osteoarthritis:

- Age of the patient is >50 years.
- The onset of pain is insidious, over months or years (commonly affected joints: knees and hips; or others: elbow, ankle, small joints of hands, interphalangeal joints and back).
- Pain is mainly related to movement in weight-bearing joints, relieved on rest.
- Morning stiffness is brief (<15 minutes).
- Usually one or a few joints are affected.
- Palpable and sometimes audible crepitus is present (sometimes absent).
- Bony swelling (osteophytes) around the joint margin may be present (Heberden's, distal interphalangeal and Bouchard's nodules on proximal interphalangeal nodes).

3. Clinical picture:

Symptoms:

- Slowly progressive pain in joints over months or years in individuals older than 50 years
- Functional restriction (decreased activity)
- Patients usually obese with high BMI
- Morning stiffness and stiffness during rest, usually lasting <15 minutes (brief compared to rheumatoid arthritis)
- Pain usually relieved by rest and simple analgesics but in advanced cases, the joint becomes unstable, as the pain may not respond to analgesics

Signs:

- Reduced range of movement of affected joints and the presence of crepitus.
- Malalignment with a bony enlargement, but no inflammatory changes (no erythema).
- Muscle wasting around severely affected joints.
- In osteoarthritis of the hands, the DIP are more affected than the PIP and bony nodules. Heberden's and Bouchard's nodules may be present in the DIP and PIP joints, respectively.

4. Pathological features:

- The risk factors of osteoarthritis are mainly related to age, genetics (primary osteoarthritis) or trauma, occupation and usage (secondary osteoarthritis).
- Osteoarthritis pathogenesis involves the following:
  1. Destruction and breakdown of the cartilage matrix
  2. Fissuring of the cartilage surface (fibrillation) and focal damages
  3. Erosion of cartilage fragments and release of proteoglycan and collagen fragments into the synovial fluid
  4. Progressive loss of function, pain and progression
- Differences between rheumatoid arthritis and osteoarthritis are summarised in Fig. 4.2.1.

5. Management goals:

- Explain the condition and educate the patient.
- Improve the strength of muscles around the affected joints.

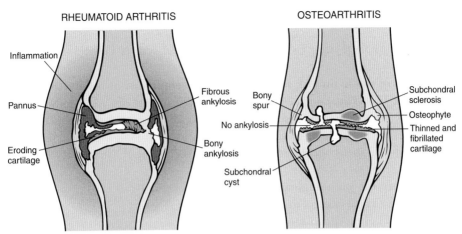

Figure 4.2.1 Morphological differences between rheumatoid arthritis and osteoarthritis. (*Source: Kumar V, Abbas AK, Fausto N, Mitchell R. Robbins Basic Pathology, 8th Edition. London, UK: Elsevier; 2007.*)

- Reduce the adverse mechanical pressure on the affected joints (weight loss if obese, use of walking stick).
- Relieve pain.

Management options:

A. Physiotherapy: Aim is to strengthen muscles around the joint.

B. Drug treatment: Paracetamol, topical NSAIDs and opiates may be needed in severe pain not responding to other analgesics and intra-articular injection of corticosteroids.

C. Surgery: It is recommended in patients with osteoarthritis when pain and stiffness are severe and there is reduction in function making an impact on the quality of life and failure of medical treatment to help.

The options are as follows:
- – Osteotomy
- – Joint replacement
- – Total joint replacement

BACK TO BASIC SCIENCES

Q1. What is osteoarthritis?

Osteoarthritis is the most common type of arthritis and the major cause of disability and pain in older people. It is associated with progressive loss of joint function and pain because of focal loss of articular hyaline cartilage and proliferation of new bone causing joint malalignment. The disease commonly affects the knee and hip, and can affect small joints (DIP and PIP), the lower back, cervical region and clavicular joints.

Q2. Do genetic factors play a role in the development of osteoarthritis?
Several studies showed that genetics plays a significant role in hand, hip and knee osteo-arthritis (for further reading, check Eyre et al., 2017 and, Warner and Valdes, 2017).

Q3. What are the main risk factors for the development of osteoarthritis?
Known risk factors may include (i) age >50 years; (ii) genetic and family history; (iii) obesity, gender (more in females) and hormonal factors; (iv) trauma (secondary osteoarthritis); (v) occupation (secondary osteoarthritis); (vi) joint alignment; (vii) joint stability and (viii) metabolic disorders (for further reading, check Chen et al., 2017).

Q4. What are the pathological changes in osteoarthritis?
The key pathological changes in osteoarthritis are as follows:
- Destruction of the articular cartilage
- Thickening of the subchondral bone
- Formation of osteophytes
- Variable degrees of chronic inflammation of the synovium (less than in rheumatoid arthritis)
- Degeneration of ligaments and menisci
- Formation of osteophytes
- Hypertrophy of the joint capsule
- Atrophy of the muscles around the affected joint (for further reading, check Chen et al., 2017)

Q5. What are the radiographic hallmark changes in osteoarthritis?
- Loss of joint space (reflecting thinning of the articular cartilage)
- Meniscal cartilage lesions
- The narrowing of the joint space usually asymmetrical in appearance (in inflammatory conditions such as rheumatoid arthritis, the joint space is usually symmetrical)
- Subchondral bone showing cystic formation
- New bone formation producing osteophytes at the joint margin
- Thickening and sclerosing of subchondral bone (appears as sharp white on plain X-ray)
- Collapse, subluxation and bone remodelling resulting in abnormal alignment (for further reading, check Brown, 2013)

REVIEW QUESTIONS

Q1. Which *one* of the following is *not* among the joints commonly affected in osteoarthritis?
A. Knee
B. Hip
C. Elbow
D. Distal interphalangeal
E. Cervical

Q2. Which *one* of the following is a primary point in the pathogenesis of osteoarthritis?
A. Infiltration of the synovial membrane with lymphocytes and plasma cells
B. Stimulation of B-cells to produce immunoglobulin
C. Turnover of aggrecan component in the articular cartilage
D. Production of TNF-alpha, which regulates cytokine production

Q3. In a patient with osteoarthritis of the hip, which *one* of the following is *not* among the clinical findings?
A. Anterior groin tenderness lateral to the femoral pulse
B. Jerky asymmetric gait
C. Weakness and wasting of the quadriceps muscles
D. Fixed extension and internal rotation deformity of the hip

Q4. Which *one* of the following is *not* a radiological change in osteoarthritis of the knee?
A. Symmetrical narrowing of the joint space
B. New bone formation producing ostephytes at the joint margins
C. Sclerosing of the subchondral bone
D. Normal bone density

Q5. In a patient with hip osteoarthritis, which *one* of the following tests should be ordered?
A. Erythrocyte sedimentation rate (ESR)
B. C-reactive protein (CRP)
C. Uric acid level
D. Plain X-ray
E. Full blood count

Q6. In osteoarthritis, which *one* of the following nonpharmacological treatments may have relatively good outcomes?
A. Therapeutic ultrasound
B. Weight loss
C. Aerobic exercise
D. Water-based exercise

ANSWERS

A1. **C.** The elbow and the ankle may be affected in osteoarthritis but they are not among the commonly affected joints.

A2. **C.** The primary changes are mainly in the articular cartilage.

A3. **D.** Usually there is fixed flexion and external rotation deformity of the hip.

A4. **A.** The narrowing of the joint space in osteoarthritis is characteristically asymmetrical.

A5. **D.** Plain X-ray of the hip may reveal one or more of the typical features of osteo-arthritis. All other tests, full blood count, ESR, CRP and uric acid level, are normal in osteoarthritis.

A6. **B.** Weight loss improves outcomes. A meta-analysis of weight reduction and knee osteoarthritis concluded that weight loss of 5% from the baseline was sufficient to reduce disability and reduce pain and disability if the patient lost more than 6 kg. Other nonpharmacological treatments were of limited value and did not have strong evidence to support their effectiveness (for further reading, check Christensen et al., 2017).

TAKE-HOME MESSAGE

- The differential diagnosis of osteoarthritis may include gout, pseudogout, fibromy-algia, rheumatoid arthritis and avascular necrosis.
- Osteoarthritis is the most common type of arthritis and the major cause of disability and pain in older people.
- It is associated with progressive loss of joint function and pain because of focal loss of articular hyaline cartilage and proliferation of new bone causing joint malalignment.
- The disease commonly affects the knee and hip, and can affect small joints (DIP and PIP), the lower back, cervical region and clavicular joints.
- The elbow and the ankle may be affected in osteoarthritis but they are not among the commonly affected joints.
- The primary pathological changes are mainly in the articular cartilage.
- Several studies showed that genetics plays a significant role in hand, hip and knee osteoarthritis.
- Known risk factors for the development of osteoarthritis may include (i) age >50 years; (ii) genetic and family history; (iii) obesity, gender (more in females) and hormonal factors; (iv) trauma (secondary osteoarthritis); (v) occupation (secondary osteoarthritis); (vi) joint alignment; (vii) joint stability; and (viii) metabolic disorders.

FURTHER READINGS

Brown AK. How to interpret plain radiographs in clinical practice. *Best Pract Res Clin Rheumatol.* 2013;27(2):249-269. Review.
Chen D, Shen J, Zhao W, et al. Osteoarthritis: toward a comprehensive understanding of pathological mechanism. *Bone Res.* 2017;5:16044. Review.
Christensen R, Bartels EM, Astrup A, Bliddal H. Effect of weight reduction in obese patients diagnosed with knee osteoarthritis: a systematic review and meta-analysis. *Ann Rheum Dis.* 2007;66(4):433-439. Review.
Eyre S, Orozco G, Worthington J. The genetics revolution in rheumatology: large scale genomic arrays and genetic mapping. *Nat Rev Rheumatol.* 2017;13(7):421-432. Review.
Felson DT. Clinical practice. Osteoarthritis of the knee. *N Engl J Med.* 2006;354(8):841-848. Review.
Hamerman D. The biology of osteoarthritis. *N Engl J Med.* 1989;320(20):1322-1330. Review.
Lane NE. Clinical practice. Osteoarthritis of the hip. *N Engl J Med.* 2007;357(14):1413-1421. Review.
Sinusas K. Osteoarthritis: diagnosis and treatment. *Am Fam Physician.* 2012;85(1):49-56.
Warner SC, Valdes AM. Genetic association studies in osteoarthritis: is it fairytale? *Curr Opin Rheumatol.* 2017;29(1):103-109. Review.

CASE 4.3

'After My Fall . . . '

Smith Kennelly, an 80-year-old farmer, comes in to see his general practitioner for a check-up. A month ago, Mr Kennelly had undergone a surgery for a fracture of the neck of the left femur following his fall in the bathroom. Mr Kennelly has smoked two packs of cigarettes daily for the past 30 years and has increased his smoking after the death of his wife 6 months ago. The results of his investigations are as follows:

Vitamin D [1,25-$(OH)_2$D] is 12 pmol/L (normal 20–120 pmol/L).

Bone mineral density (BMD) test T-score of the hip is −1.8 and of the spine is −2.7.

CASE DISCUSSION

Q1. On the basis of Smith's presentation, what is your diagnosis?

Q2. What is your differential diagnosis?

Q3. What are the key clinical features of this disease? What are the scientific bases for these features?

Q4. What is the pathophysiology underlying these changes?

Q5. What are your management goals and management options?

ANSWERS

1. The findings from this case show that Smith, aged 80 years, is a heavy smoker and gives a history of fracture of the neck of the left femur following a fall that required surgery and has reduced scores of BMD test T-scores. These findings are consistent with the diagnosis of osteoporosis.
2. The differential diagnosis includes the following:
   - Osteomalacia (bones are soft due to decreased mineral-to-collagen ratio)
   - Other diseases that cause pathological fracture (leukaemia, lymphoma, metastasis, renal osteodystrophy)
   - Homocystinuria/homocystinaemia
   - Hyperparathyroidism
   - Sickle cell disease
   - Mastocytosis (mast cell proliferation and accumulation in the various body organs)
   - Multiple myeloma
   - Paget disease
   - Scurvy

The following are essential for the diagnosis of osteoporosis:
- Osteoporosis is usually asymptomatic until a fracture occurs.
- Patients may give a history of chronic back pain, gradual height loss and kyphosis.
- Osteopenia is detected on X-ray.
- Patients have a history of acute vertebral fracture, peripheral osteoporotic fracture or hip fracture.
- BMD test T-score of the lumbar spine or hip is −2.5.

3. Clinical picture:

Symptoms:
- The disease is usually asymptomatic, more common in females, with progressive decrease in height and kyphotic deformity.
- Patients usually present with a low trauma or fragility fracture, usually vertebrae or hips.
- Common bones that are prone to fracture in osteoporosis are (i) proximal femur; (ii) distal forearm, (iii) spine (thoracic 11 to lumbar 2) and (iv) proximal humerus. Other bones susceptible are the ribs, pelvis, proximal tibia and ankle (not all schools are in agreement with the inclusion of ankle fractures).
- Patients with lumbar fracture present with sharp midline pain radiating to the flanks. It may be asymptomatic.
- Hip fractures generally occur following falls.

Signs:
- Evidence of osteopenia and fractures
- Height loss
- Kyphotic deformity of the upper thoracic spine
- Spinal tenderness
- Reduced rib–pelvis and increased wall–occiput distances

Radiological investigations:
- Plain X-ray bone loss, osteopenia, bone mass density loss, kyphosis of thoracic spine and changes in vertebrae
- CT scan: Compression fractures of vertebrae
- MRI scans: May reveal vertebral fractures with localised swelling/oedema (T2)

4. Pathological features:
- Genetic and environmental factors play a role in the development of osteoporosis. The compromised bone strength predisposing to an increased risk for fractures in osteoporosis is related to increased bone loss by osteoclasts and decreased new bone formation by osteoblasts.
- Osteoporosis could be primary or secondary.
- Common causes of secondary osteoporosis are as follows:
  - Hormonal causes: Hypogonadism (decreased estrogen in females and decreased androgens in males), increased growth hormone, increased parathyroid hormone and hyperthyroidism

> – Gastrointestinal causes: Chronic liver diseases (interference with the hydroxylation of vitamin D), malabsorption (lack of calcium and vitamin D) and inflammatory bowel disease
> – Sedentary lifestyle, smoking, alcohol in excess and poor diet
> – Medications: Corticosteroids, gonadotrophin-releasing hormone (GnRH)., heparin, thyroxin, sedatives and anticonvulsants
> – Medical conditions: Multiple myeloma, cystic fibrosis, homocystinaemia, homocystinuria, anorexia nervosa, HIV infection, systemic mastocytosis and rheumatoid arthritis

5. Management goals:
- Prevention
- Improving the clinical presentation
- Pain control and management of fractures
- Lifestyle changes and patient education

Management options:
- Calcium supplementation
- Vitamin D supplementation
- Physical activity
- Medications: (i) Bisphosphonates, (ii) selective estrogen receptor modulators, (iii) estrogen and (iv) anabolic agents

Drugs used in the prevention and treatment of osteoporosis are summarised in Table 4.3.1.

Table 4.3.1 Drugs used for prevention and treatment of osteoporosis

Agent	Prevention	Treatment	Dose	Vertebral fracture reduction	Hip fracture reduction	Cost per year ($)
Alendronate	Yes	Yes	Prevention: 5 mg PO daily, 35 mg PO weekly Treatment: 10 mg PO daily, 70 mg PO weekly	Yes	Yes	965 (but is now generic)
Risedronate	Yes	Yes	Prevention and treatment: 5 mg PO daily, 35 mg PO weekly, 150 mg PO monthly	Yes	Yes	965
Ibandronate	Yes	Yes	2.5 mg PO daily, 150 mg PO monthly, 3 mg IV every 3 months	Yes	No	1043–2000

Continued

Table 4.3.1 Drugs used for prevention and treatment of osteoporosis—cont'd

Agent	Prevention	Treatment	Dose	Vertebral fracture reduction	Hip fracture reduction	Cost per year ($)
Zoledronic acid	No	Yes	5 mg IV (in infusion) yearly	Yes	Yes	~100
Raloxifene	Yes	Yes	60 mg PO daily	Yes	No	1082
Hormone replacement therapy	Yes	Management	0.625 mg PO daily conjugated estrogen or equivalent (0.45, 0.3 mg also available)	Yes	Yes	65–522
Calcitonin	No	Yes	200 IU daily intranasal	Yes	No	1148
Teriparatide (PTH [1–34])	No	Yes	20 mcg SC daily	Yes	No	8528

Source: Andreoli TE, Benjamin IJ, Griggs RC, Wing EJ. Andreoli and Carpenter's Cecil Essentials of Medicine. 8th ed. Philadelphia, PA: Elsevier; 2010.
PO, orally; PTH, parathyroid hormone; SC, subcutaneously.

BACK TO BASIC SCIENCES

Q1. What is osteoporosis?
According to the National Institutes of Health, osteoporosis is defined as 'skeletal disorder characterised by compromised bone strength predisposing to an increased risk for fractures. The outcomes of the disorder include fractures, bone pain, height loss, and physical deformity.'

Q2. What are the factors that significantly influence fracture risk?
- Falls and traumatic injuries
- Skeletal microarchitecture
- Bone turnover
- Damage caused by microfractures
- Pattern and degree of mineralisation
- No BMD threshold for fracture has been identified yet.
- The Fracture Risk Assessment Tool (FRAX) looks promising. It is based on individual patient models that integrate the risk associated with clinical risk factors as well as BMD at the femoral neck.

Q3. Briefly discuss the biology of bone.
- Heritable factors, gender and ethnicity account for 60%–80% of the development of the skeletal system.
- Nutrition, lifestyle and exercise also have a significant impact on peak bone mass.
- The cells involved in bone biology are mainly osteocytes, osteoblasts and osteoclasts.
- Bone remodelling and bone resorption is important for repair and redistribution of the skeleton to adapt to mechanical stresses to provide calcium in the circulation.

- Osteocytes are the main cells in the bone forming 90%–95% of bone cells. They are derived from osteoblasts.
- Mature osteocytes within a bone contain dendritic processes and regulate osteoblast recruitment and bone formation.
- Osteocytes have several important physiological functions including (i) production of proteins that regulate mineralisation including PHEX, DMP-1 (positive effect) and FGF-23 (negative effect); and (ii) regulation of bone resorption through direct and indirect mechanisms.
- Cytokines critical to the process of recruitment of osteoclasts include IL-1, IL-6, osteoprotegerin (OPG) and receptor activator of nuclear factor κβ ligand (RANKL).

Q4. Which patients are at a higher risk of osteoporosis and are recommended for BMD test?
- Family history of osteoporotic fracture
- Low body weight, BMI < 19
- Early menopause
- Osteopenia on plain X-ray
- Low trauma fracture
- Having one of the diseases associated with osteoporosis

Q5. What are the diseases associated with secondary osteoporosis?
Endocrine disorders:
- Hypogonadism
- Increased cortisol levels
- Hyperthyroidism
- Hyperparathyroidism
- Diabetes mellitus

Haematological and oncological disorders:
- Sickle cell anaemia
- Thalassemia
- Multiple myeloma
- Haemolytic anaemia
- Myeloproliferative disorders
- Skeletal metastasis
- Mastocytosis

Metabolic disorders:
- Gaucher disease
- Homocystinuria
- Pompe disease

Nutritional deficiencies and gastrointestinal disorders:
- Vitamin D
- Pancreatic insufficiency

- Cirrhosis
- Cholestasis
- Malabsorption
- Inflammatory bowel disease
- Bile salt disorders
- Cystic fibrosis
- Anorexia nervosa

Medications:
- Heparin
- Chemotherapy
- Glucocorticoids
- Thyroxin
- Alcohol
- Proton pump inhibitors
- Gonadotropin-releasing hormone agonists
- Antiepileptics

Other conditions:
- Pregnancy-associated osteoporosis
- Immobilisation
- Rheumatoid arthritis
- Marfan syndrome
- Ehlers–Danlos syndrome

Q6. What are the key differences between osteoporosis and osteomalacia?

Table 4.3.2 summarises the differences between osteoporosis and osteomalacia.

Table 4.3.2 Differences between osteoporosis and osteomalacia

Item	Osteoporosis	Osteomalacia
Definition	Compromised bone strength predisposing to an increased risk for fractures	Defective mineralisation of bone due to vitamin D deficiency, vitamin D resistance or hypophosphataemia
Mineral-to-collagen ratio	Within normal	Decreased
Mineral content	Normal	Low
Causes	Primary or secondary	Mainly related to vitamin D deficiency, vitamin D malabsorption, impaired hydroxylation of vitamin D and hypophosphataemia

Q7. What are the mechanisms underlying the development of osteoporosis with advancing age?

- Reduction of bone formation and failure to keep pace with bone resorption
- Bone resorption not increased

- Accumulation of fat in bone marrow space → inhibition of bone marrow stem cells to differentiate to osteoblasts → failure of bone formation

REVIEW QUESTIONS

Q1. Which *one* of the following endocrine disorders is *not* associated with secondary osteoporosis?
A. Hypoparathyroidism
B. Hyperthyroidism
C. Hypogonadism
D. Increased cortisol levels
E. Diabetes mellitus

Q2. Which *one* of the following haematological disorders is *not* associated with secondary osteoporosis?
A. Multiple myeloma
B. Sickle cell anaemia
C. Thalassemia
D. Polycythaemia
E. Mastocytosis

Q3. Which *one* of the following medicines is *not* associated with secondary osteoporosis?
A. Antiepileptics
B. Gamma globulins
C. Alcohol
D. Chemotherapy
E. Proton pump inhibitors

Q4. Which *one* of the following is *not* among bones commonly prone to fractures in osteoporosis?
A. Spine
B. Proximal femur
C. Ankle bones
D. Proximal humerus
E. Distal forearm

Q5. Which vertebrae are commonly prone to fractures in osteoporosis?
A. C1–C5
B. T1–T5
C. L5–S5
D. T11–L2
E. T12–L5

Q6. Regarding DXA scores, which *one* of the following is considered osteopenia?

A. T-score of -2.5 to -3.0

B. T-score of -1.0 to -2.5

C. T-score of $+ 2.00$ to 0.0

D. T-score of $+ 2.5$ to $+ 3.0$

E. T-score of 0.0 to -1.0

ANSWERS

A1. **A.** Hyperparathyroidism is associated with osteoporosis and not hypothyroidism.

A2. **D.** Polycythaemia is not associated with osteoporosis.

A3. **B.** Gamma globulins are not among the drugs associated with osteoporosis.

A4. **C.** The ankle is not among the bones/regions known to be commonly prone to fractures in osteoporosis.

A5. **D.** The vertebrae commonly prone to fracture in osteoporosis are typically thoracic 11 to lumbar 2.

A6. **B.** A T-score of -1.0 to -2.5 is consistent with osteopenia.

TAKE-HOME MESSAGE

- According to the National Institutes of Health, osteoporosis is defined as 'skeletal disorder characterised by compromised bone strength predisposing to an increased risk for fractures. The outcomes of the disorder include fractures, bone pain, height loss and physical deformity.'
- The differential diagnoses of osteoporosis include osteomalacia (bones are soft due to decreased mineral-to-collagen ratio), other diseases that cause pathological fracture (leukaemia, lymphoma, metastasis, renal osteodystrophy), homocystinuria/homocysti-naemia, hyperparathyroidism, sickle cell disease, mastocytosis (mast cell proliferation and accumulation in the various body organs), multiple myeloma, Paget disease and scurvy.
- Genetic and environmental factors play a role in the development of osteoporosis. The compromised bone strength predisposing to an increased risk for fractures in osteoporosis is related to increased bone loss by osteoclasts and decreased new bone formation by osteoblasts.
- Osteoporosis could be primary or secondary.
- The management goals and options are prevention, pain control, management of fractures, lifestyle changes and patient education.

FURTHER READINGS

Black DM, Rosen CJ. Clinical Practice. Postmenopausal osteoporosis. *N Engl J Med*. 2016;374(3):254–262. Review.

Canalis E, Giustina A, Bilezikian JP. Mechanisms of anabolic therapies for osteoporosis. *N Engl J Med.* 2007;357(9):905-916. Review.

Ebeling PR. Clinical practice. Osteoporosis in men. *N Engl J Med.* 2008;358(14):1474-1482. Review.

Favus MJ. Bisphosphonates for osteoporosis. *N Engl J Med.* 2010;363(21):2027-2035. Review.

Holick MF. Vitamin D deficiency. *N Engl J Med.* 2007;357(3):266-281. Review.

Raisz LG. Clinical practice. Screening for osteoporosis. *N Engl J Med.* 2005;353(2):164-171. Review.

Seeman E, Delmas PD. Bone quality—the material and structural basis of bone strength and fragility. *N Engl J Med.* 2006;354(21):2250-2261. Review.

Weinstein RS. Clinical practice. Glucocorticoid-induced bone disease. *N Engl J Med.* 2011;365(1):62-70.

CASE 4.4

'Is It Serious?'

Mary Eisenhower, a 35-year-old assistant teacher, presents to her general practitioner with acute pleurisy and arthralgia of her hands. The results of her investigations are summarised in Table 4.4.1.

Mary was treated with prednisolone and her pleurisy was resolved. The doctor gradually reduced the dose of prednisolone over days and arranged for a follow-up.

CASE DISCUSSION

Q1. On the basis of Mary's presentation, what is your diagnosis?

Q2. What is your differential diagnosis?

Q3. What are the key clinical features of this disease? What are the scientific bases for these features?

Q4. What is the pathophysiology underlying these changes?

Q5. What are your management goals and management options?

ANSWERS

1. The findings in a 35-year-old female of pleurisy and arthralgia of her hands together with positive tests for antinuclear antibody (ANA), double-stranded DNA (dsDNA) antibodies of IgG, low C4, low haemoglobin and normocytic, normochromic anaemia, raised C-reactive protein (CRP), raised erythrocyte sedimentation rate (ESR) and the response of symptoms to prednisolone treatment are all suggestive of the diagnosis of systemic lupus erythematosus (SLE).
2. The differential diagnosis includes the following:
   - Drug-induced lupus (procainamide, isoniazid, hydralazine)
   - Fibromyalgia
   - Infectious mononucleosis
   - Epstein–Barr virus (EBV)
   - Mixed connective tissue disease
   - Rheumatoid arthritis
   - Scleroderma
   - Sjögren syndrome
   - Dermatomyositis
   - Polyarteritis nodosa
   - Endocarditis

Table 4.4.1 Blood test results

Blood test	Mary's results	Range
Haemoglobin (Hb)	11.0	123–157 g/L (in females)
Blood film	A blood film shows microcytic normochromic anaemia	
Antinuclear antibody (ANA) test	6.5	Negative <1.0 unit Positive 3.0–5.9 units Strongly positive >6.0 units
Double-stranded DNA (dsDNA) antibodies, IgG	90 IU/mL	Negative <30.0 IU/mL Positive >75.0 IU/mL
Complement C4	0.08	Normal 0.12–0.30 g/L
C-reactive protein (CRP)	41	Normal <5 mg/L
Erythrocyte sedimentation rate	38	Normal <20 mm/h

- Hepatitis C
- Antiphospholipid syndrome
- Pneumonitis
- Other causes of pleuritic chest pain

3. Clinical picture:

Symptoms:

- Most patients have fever, malaise and tiredness with the exacerbation of the disease. But the symptoms do not correlate with the disease activity or severity.
- Symmetrical small joint arthralgia of hands resembling rheumatoid arthritis is common. There is no joint deformity or erosion of bones in most cases.
- A vascular necrosis of the hip or knee joints may occur due to the disease or treatment with corticosteroids.
- Erythema in the 'butterfly' distribution of the cheeks. The skin is affected in 85% of patients and characteristically across the bridge of the nose.
- Other skin manifestations may include the following:
  - Vasculitis of fingertips and nail folds
  - Purpura and urticaria
  - Photosensitivity
  - Livedo reticularis
  - Palmar and plantar rash
  - Pigmentation
  - Alopecia
  - Raynaud phenomenon
  - Discoid lupus (a benign form)
- Recurrent pleurisy and pleural effusions, usually bilateral, are seen in 50%–60% of patients (effusion is exudate).
- Other pulmonary manifestations include pneumonitis, atelectasis and restrictive lung disease.

- The heart and vascular system are involved in 20%–25% of patients. These include the following:
  - Pericarditis
  - Pericardial effusion
  - Cardiomyopathy (rare)
  - Myocarditis
  - Aortic valve lesion
  - Ischaemic heart disease (patients are at a higher risk)
- Vasculitis and Raynaud disease and arterial and venous thrombosis (usually associated with anti-phospholipid syndrome)
- Nervous system is involved in 60%–65% of patients including the following:
  - Stroke
  - Depression
  - Psychotic changes
  - Epilepsy
  - Migraine
  - Cerebellar ataxia
  - Aseptic meningitis
  - Cranial nerve lesions
  - Cerebrovascular disease
  - Polyneuropathy
- The kidneys are involved in only 20% of patients. Proteinuria is seen in the early stages of lupus nephritis and treatment should be started to delay the proteinuria of renal involvement.
- Renal biopsy is recommended if urinary casts or fragmented red blood cells are present. This will help in the assessment of glomerulonephritis and severity of the disease.
- Other organs/structures involved:
  - Eyes (retinal vasculitis = cytoid bodies)
  - Episcleritis
  - Conjunctivitis
  - Optic neuritis
  - Secondary Sjögren
  - Mouth ulcers
  - Small bowel infarction/perforation
  - Pancreatic involvement
  - Liver involvement

4. Laboratory changes (Table 4.4.2):
   - High ESR, high anti-dsDNA and low C3 indicate a herald of SLE.
   - PCR is normal in SLE. If raised, the patient may have pleurisy, arthritis or infection.
   - ANA is positive in other conditions including rheumatoid arthritis, scleroderma, autoimmune thyroiditis and Sjögren syndrome.

Table 4.4.2 Blood tests recommended in a patient presenting with a clinical picture suggestive of systemic lupus erythematosus

Blood test	Results	Interpretation
Full blood count and blood film	• Haemoglobin – low • White blood cell count – low • Lymphocytes – low • Platelet count – low • Erythrocyte sedimentation rate – raised • C-reactive protein (CRP) – raised • Normocytic normochromic anaemia	Chronic inflammatory disease, with possible suppression of bone marrow. CRP is high in pleuritis, infection and arthritis.
Antibodies • ANA	Raised	Sensitive but not specific for SLE.
• dsDNA	Positive in 60%	Not sensitive. May remain high during the remission.
• Anti-Ro (SS-A)	Positive in 30%–40%	Also positive in primary Sjögren in 60%–90% of cases.
• Anti-La (SS-B)	Positive in 13%	Also positive in primary Sjögren.
• Anti-Sm	Positive in 10%	Not sensitive for SLE.
• Anti-UI-RNP	Positive in 15%	Not specific for SLE.
Serum complement • C3 • C4	Low Low	Suggest disease activity.
Antiphospholipid antibodies	• False-positive test for syphilis • Lupus anticoagulant • Anticardiolipin antibodies +++	These tests return to normal levels as the disease flare improves.
Urea Creatinine Serum albumin Urinary albumin/creatinine	Raised Raised Low High	The disease is advanced. All indicate lupus nephritis.

- C4 is decreased in autoimmune disorders, in the active phase of lupus erythematosus and in rheumatoid arthritis.
- Undetectable C4 level but normal C3 in patients suggests a congenital C4 deficiency. Levels of C4 are increased in patients with autoimmune haemolytic anaemia.

Pathological features:

- SLE is an autoimmune disorder with several systemic/organ involvement.
- Characteristically IgG and complement deposition are observed in the biopsies of the kidney and skin.
- The pathogenesis of SLE is related to interactions between genetic, hormonal and some environmental factors that trigger the production of antibodies and consequently systemic inflammation.

- The genetic factors have been widely studied recently and more than 40 loci have been identified. One of the chromosomal regions related to SLE is the HLA locus, especially class II region (HLA-DRB1, -DOA1 and -DQB1).
- Hormonal factors include oestrogen and hormone replacement therapy.
- Environmental factors include infection with EBV, cytomegalovirus (CMV), ultraviolet light, cigarette smoking and some drugs such as hydralazine, d-penicillamine and TNF-alpha blockers.

5. Management goals:
   - Educating the patient about the nature of the disease
   - Symptomatic treatment of arthralgia, fever and serositis
   - Management of disease flare
   - Early detection of renal, nervous and haemolytic anaemia
   - Use of corticosteroids and immunosuppressive drugs

BACK TO BASIC SCIENCES

Q1. What is SLE?

SLE is a chronic multisystem autoimmune disorder with a heterogeneous pattern of clinical and serological manifestations. The disease affects the skin (e.g. solar malar rash), oral cavity (e.g. buccal or tongue ulcer), synovitis (e.g. synovitis of the small joint of hands) and serositis (e.g. pleurisy, pleural effusion, pleural rub, pericardial pain, pericardial effusion), and haematological changes (e.g. anaemia, leukopenia, haemolytic anaemia, lymphopenia, thrombocytopenia), together with neurological changes (e.g. seizures, mononeuritis multiplex, peripheral and cranial neuropathy) and renal involvement (glomerulonephritis).

Q2. Briefly comment on the epidemiology of SLE.

- The incidence of SLE is approximately 1–10 per 100,000.
- It is relatively common in African, Hispanic, Chinese and Asian descendants. It is usually associated with poor social support.
- It is relatively more common in females, with a ratio of approximately 1:10 (males:females).

Q3. Briefly discuss the pathogenesis of SLE.

- The pathogenesis of SLE is related to interactions between genetic, hormonal and some environmental factors that trigger the production of antibodies and consequently systemic inflammation.
- The genetic factors have been widely studied recently and more than 40 loci have been identified. One of the chromosomal regions related to SLE is the HLA locus, especially class II region (HLA-DRB1, DOA1 and DQB1).
- Hormonal factors include oestrogen and hormone replacement therapy.
- Environmental factors include infection with EBV, CMV, ultraviolet light, cigarette smoking and some drugs such as hydralazine, D-penicillamine and TNF-alpha blockers.

Q4. What is the prognosis of SLE?

- The prognosis of SLE has significantly improved in the past 60 years. The 5-year survival rate used to be 50% in 1950, but currently is 90%.
- The change is usually due to better diagnostic approaches and advances in immunosuppressive therapy, diagnosis and transplantation.

Q5. How can you explain the high cardiovascular morbidity in patients with SLE?

The high cardiovascular morbidity is related to classic cardiovascular risks including smoking, hypertension and dyslipidaemia, together with chronic inflammation associated with the autoimmune disorders, adding to the accelerated atherosclerosis. The thrombotic events are also known to be involved in SLE cardiovascular mortality.

Q6. Briefly discuss the use of ANA in the diagnosis of SLE.

ANA is not specific for any autoimmune rheumatic disease including SLE. It may be positive in other disorders such as primary biliary cirrhosis, subacute bacterial endocarditis, viral infections and lymphoproliferative disease, e.g. Waldenström macroglobulinaemia.

If positive and clinically you suspect SLE, other more specific tests such as dsDNA should be ordered.

REVIEW QUESTIONS

Q1. In the pathogenesis of SLE, which *one* of the following is responsible for the release of proinflammatory cytokines and increased vascular permeability?
A. T-lymphocytes
B. B-lymphocytes
C. Thrombocytes
D. Complement fragment C3a
E. Plasma cells

Q2. Which *one* of the following is *not* raised in active SLE?
A. ESR
B. CRP
C. dsDNA antibody titre
D. ANAs

Q3. Which *one* of the following pairs of antibodies correlates well with primary Sjögren syndrome diagnosis?
A. dsDNA and anti-Sm
B. Anti-Ro and anti-La
C. Anti-Sm and ANA
D. Anti-U1-RNP and anti-Sm

Q4. Which *one* of the following is less likely a haematological feature of SLE?
A. Normocytic normochromic anaemia
B. Leukopenia
C. Lymphopenia
D. Thrombocytosis

Q5. Which *one* of the following laboratory tests is most specific for SLE?
A. ANA
B. dsDNA
C. Anti-U1-RNP
D. Anti-La

Q6. In mild SLE with skin and small joint involvement not responding to NSAIDs, which *one* of the following medications should be used next?
A. Corticosteroids
B. Azathioprine
C. Methotrexate
D. Hydroxychloroquine

ANSWERS

A1. **D.** Complement C3 and C4 are usually consumed during the flare of SLE. Complement fragment C3a is responsible for the release of proinflammatory cytokines and the increased vascular permeability.

A2. **B.** CRP is usually not raised in active SLE, whereas ESR is usually raised. The rise of CRP may necessitate a search for any source of infection.

A3. **B.** Both anti-Ro (SS-A) and anti-La (SS-B) are positive in primary Sjögren syndrome in 60%–70% and 35%–85% of patients, respectively.

A4. **D.** Thrombocytopenia occurs in about 20% of patients due to autoimmunity, and usually responds to corticosteroid therapy and/or splenomegaly.

A5. **B.** dsDNA antibodies are positive in 60%–70% of patients with SLE, which together with low C3 usually indicates flare of the disease. Both tests are very specific markers for SLE. On the other hand, ANA is highly sensitive but not specific to SLE. Other antibodies are not as specific for SLE as dsDNA.

A6. **D.** Next to the use of NSAIDs, the patient should be treated with hydroxychloroquine (antimalarial). Because of ocular toxicity, the patient should undergo ophthalmic review on commencement of the treatment.

TAKE-HOME MESSAGE

- SLE is a chronic multisystem autoimmune disorder with a heterogeneous pattern of clinical and serological manifestations.

- The disease affects the skin (e.g. solar malar rash), oral cavity (e.g. buccal or tongue ulcer), synovitis (e.g. synovitis of the small joint of hands) and serositis (e.g. pleurisy, pleural effusion, pleural rub, pericardial pain, pericardial effusion), and haematological changes (e.g. anaemia, leukopenia, haemolytic anaemia, lymphopenia, thrombocytopenia), together with neurological changes (e.g. seizures, mononeuritis multiplex, peripheral and cranial neuropathy) and renal involvement (glomerulonephritis).
- The incidence of SLE is approximately 1–10 per 100,000.
- It is relatively common in African, Hispanic, Chinese and Asian descendants. It is usually associated with poor social support.
- It is relatively more common in females, with a ratio of approximately 1:10 (males:females).
- The pathogenesis of SLE is related to interactions between genetic, hormonal and some environmental factors that trigger the production of antibodies and consequently systemic inflammation.
- ANA is not specific for any autoimmune rheumatic disease including SLE.
- ANA may be positive in other disorders such as primary biliary cirrhosis, subacute bacterial endocarditis, viral infections and lymphoproliferative disease, e.g. Waldenström macroglobulinaemia.
- C4 is decreased in autoimmune disorders, in the active phase of lupus erythematosus and in rheumatoid arthritis.
- Undetectable C4 level but normal C3 in patients suggests a congenital C4 deficiency. Levels of C4 are increased in patients with autoimmune haemolytic anaemia.
- anti-dsDNA antibodies are positive in 60-70% of cases of SLE.
- CRP is usually not raised in active SLE, whereas ESR is usually raised. The rise of CRP may necessitate a search for any source of infection.
- Both anti-Ro (SS-A) and anti-La (SS-B) are positive in primary Sjögren syndrome in 60%–70% and 35%–85% of patients, respectively.
- Next to the use of NSAIDs, the patient should be treated with hydroxychloroquine (antimalarial). Because of ocular toxicity, the patient should undergo ophthalmic review on commencement of the treatment.

FURTHER READINGS

D'Cruz DP. Systemic lupus erythematosus. *BMJ*. 2006;332(7546):890-894. Review.

Hahn BH. Antibodies to DNA. *N Engl J Med*. 1998;338(19):1359-1368. Review.

Hahn BH. Belimumab for systemic lupus erythematosus. *N Engl J Med*. 2013;368(16):1528-1535. Review.

Mackillop LH, Germain SJ, Nelson-Piercy C. Systemic lupus erythematosus. *BMJ*. 2007;335(7626):933-936. Review.

Madhok R. Systemic lupus erythematosus: lupus nephritis. *BMJ Clin Evid*. 2015;2015:1123.

Madhok R, Wu O. Systemic lupus erythematosus. *BMJ Clin Evid*. 2007;2007:1123. Review.

Madhok R, Wu O. Systemic lupus erythematosus. *BMJ Clin Evid*. 2009;2009:1123. Review.

Rahman A, Isenberg DA. Systemic lupus erythematosus. *N Engl J Med*. 2008;358(9):929-939. Review.

Tsokos GC. Systemic lupus erythematosus. *N Engl J Med*. 2011;365(22):2110-2121. Review.

CASE 4.5

'I Have Pain in My Heels . . . '

Thomas Blackwell, a 22-year-old policeman, presents to his general practitioner because he is suffering from photophobia, painful hot left ankle and painful micturition for the past few days. On examination, his pulse is 100/min, blood pressure is 120/80 mm Hg, temperature is 37.5°C and respiratory rate is 22/min.

He has bilateral conjunctivitis, aphthous–like mouth ulcers and several ulcers around the glans penis. The doctor takes a biopsy from the urethral discharge. The results of his investigations are shown as follows:

Table 4.5.1 summarises blood test results.

X-ray of the left ankle: It is normal.

Biopsy of the urethral discharge: No organisms are detected, gonococci negative and *Chlamydia* DNA is detected by polymerase chain reaction (PCR).

Thomas is treated with diclofenac for the tendonitis and ankle pain. His chlamydial urethritis was treated with doxycycline. The doctor examined and investigated him for other sexually transmitted diseases.

CASE DISCUSSION

Q1. On the basis of Thomas' presentation, what is your diagnosis?

Q2. What is your differential diagnosis?

Q3. What are the key clinical features of this disease? What are the scientific bases for these features?

Q4. What is the pathophysiology underlying these changes?

Q5. What are your management goals and management options?

ANSWERS

1. The findings of arthritis, hot and tender left ankle, dysuria and urethral discharge for a few days together with signs of inflammation of the left ankle (swollen and hot skin), aphthous–like mouth ulcers, ulcers around the glans penis and the findings by PCR that a biopsy of urethral discharge is positive for chlamydial DNA, are all suggestive of the diagnosis of reactive arthritis.
2. The differential diagnosis includes the following:
   - Gonococcal arthritis
   - Enteropathic arthritis associated with inflammatory bowel disease (IBD)

Table 4.5.1 Blood test results

Blood test	Thomas' results	Range
Haemoglobin (Hb)	150	130–180 g/L (males)
White blood cell count	5.5	4.0–11.0 × 10⁹/L
Erythrocyte sedimentation rate (ESR)	60	Normal <20 mm/h
Rheumatoid factor	Negative	Normal <15 IU/mL

- Gouty arthritis
- Rheumatic fever
- Psoriatic arthritis
- Rheumatoid arthritis
- Still disease

3. Clinical picture:

Symptoms and signs:

- Arthritis (symptomatic, oligoarticular, affecting the lower extremity more and may be associated with sacroiliitis) may occur.
- Genitourinary (nonspecific urethritis, cervicitis in females, cystitis, haematuria, urethral discharge) may occur.
- Skin changes (keratoderma blennorrhagica, balanitis circinata and ulceration on the tongue and buccal cavity) may occur.
- Ocular changes may occur (e.g. conjunctivitis).
- Fever and weight loss may occur.

Arthritis in this disease follows nongonococcal urethritis or infectious dysentery. The arthritis usually occurs 1–3 weeks following the infection. The presentation may be acute or insidious.

The urethritis is usually symptomatic presenting with mucopurulent urethral discharge and haematuria may be present. The disease may be asymptomatic.

Enthesitis is common causing plantar fasciitis or Achilles tendon enthesitis.

4. Laboratory investigations (Table 4.5.2):

5. Pathological features:

- The trigger for reactive arthritis could be any of the following organisms: (i) genitourinary infection: *Chlamydia trachomatis* is a common cause of nongonococcal urethritis; and (ii) enteritis (e.g. *Salmonella, Shigella, Campylobacter, Yersinia*).
- Patients are usually genetically susceptible. Over two-thirds are HLA-B27 positive. Others may be positive for cross-reacting antigen – B7, B22, B40 and B42.
- Reactive arthritis is a self-limited condition. However, approximately 10%–20% of patients may have persistent symptoms and the disease may relapse.

6. Management goals:

- Treat infection with antibiotics (doxycycline 100 mg twice daily for 3 months if *Chlamydia* infection is suspected or confirmed).
- Screen the sexual partner, take cultures and treat accordingly.

Table 4.5.2 Investigations recommended in a patient presenting with a picture suggestive of reactive arthritis

Investigation	Why is it needed?
Culture from urethra or cervix in females	May detect *C. trachomatis* or *N. gonorrhoeae*, but may be sterile at the onset of urethritis
Stool culture	May detect *Salmonella*, *Shigella*, *Campylobacter* or *Yersinia* infection
Direct immunofluorescence antibody test and enzyme immunoassay using monoclonal antibodies	Usually not required, as their role in the diagnosis is uncertain
Radiology of peripheral joints	May show soft-tissue swelling, juxta-articular osteopenia, areas of periostitis and new bone formation

- Relieve pain – NSAIDs and local or oral corticosteroids.
- Relapsing cases should be managed with sulfasalazine or methotrexate.
- Resistant cases can be treated with TNF-alpha-blocking agent.
- Educate the patient.

BACK TO BASIC SCIENCES

Q1. What does postinfectious arthritis mean?
It refers to arthritis that follows an identifiable infection but does not have the characteristics of joint sepsis. Examples of postinfectious arthritis may include (i) reactive arthritis, (ii) rheumatic fever and (iii) meningococcal arthritis.

Q2. Give examples of infectious agents that trigger reactive arthritis.
Reactive arthritis occurs particularly in outbreaks caused by *Salmonella typhimurium*, *Shigella flexneri*, *Campylobacter jejuni* and *Yersinia enterocolitica*. Nongonococcal urethritis and *C. trachomatis* are also trigger factors of reactive arthritis.

Other microbial agents that have been linked with reactive arthritis may include *Cryptosporidium*, *Giardia lamblia* and *Shigella sonnei*.

Q3. Briefly discuss the role of genetic factors in the development of reactive arthritis.
The HLA-B27 gene increases the risk of reactive arthritis approximately 40-fold. It is associated with a longer duration of episodes and recurrence.

Q4. What do we mean by undifferentiated spondyloarthropathy?
Reactive arthritis may be indistinguishable from psoriatic arthritis and enteropathic enteritis. In these situations, the term 'undifferentiated spondyloarthropathy' is used as they share common ground.

Q5. Briefly discuss eye changes in patients with reactive arthritis.
- Painful red eye
- Conjunctivitis
- Iritis

The patients presenting with a painful red eye should be reviewed by an ophthalmologist immediately.

Q6. What are the skin changes associated with reactive arthritis?
- Keratoderma blennorrhagica (painless, red, raised plaques on hands and feet)
- Balanitis circinata (painless superficial ulcerations on the glans penis)
- Nail dystrophy

REVIEW QUESTIONS

Q1. Which *one* of the following is *not* postinfective arthritis?
A. Reactive arthritis
B. Rheumatic fever
C. Meningococcal arthritis
D. Psoriatic arthritis

Q2. In the chronic severe form of reactive arthritis, the drug of choice is
A. Hydroxychloroquine
B. Anti-TNF-alpha
C. Corticosteroids
D. Methotrexate

Q3. Which *one* of the following is *not* among the skin lesions characteristic of reactive arthritis?
A. Keratoderma blennorrhagica
B. Balanitis circinata
C. Erythema nodosum
D. Nail dystrophy

Q4. Which *one* of the following microorganisms is *not* related to reactive arthritis?
A. *Chlamydia trachomatis*
B. *Yersinia enterocolitica*
C. *Borrelia burgdorferi*
D. *Salmonella typhimurium*
E. *Campylobacter jejuni*

Q5. Which *one* of the following is *not* among the presenting symptoms of reactive arthritis?
A. Lower limb oligoarthritis
B. Enthesitis

C. Sinusitis

D. Acute sacroiliitis

E. Urethritis

ANSWERS

A1. **D.** Psoriasis arthritis is not a postinfective arthritis.

A2. **B.** Inhibition of TNF-alpha may be much more effective in patients with chronic severe reactive arthritis when other disease-modifying anti-rheumatic drugs (DMARDs) have failed.

A3. **C.** Erythema nodosum may occur with conditions such as sarcoidosis, tuberculosis, IBD, streptococcal infection and cancer, and with the intake of certain medications.

A4. **C.** *B. burgdorferi* is a bacterial species responsible for Lyme disease transmitted by infected ticks.

A5. **C.** Sinusitis is not among the presenting features of reactive arthritis.

TAKE-HOME MESSAGE

- Postinfectious arthritis means arthritis that follows an identifiable infection but does not have the characteristics of joint sepsis. Examples of postinfectious arthritis may include (i) reactive arthritis, (ii) rheumatic fever and (iii) meningococcal arthritis.
- Reactive arthritis occurs particularly in outbreaks caused by *S. typhimurium*, *S. flexneri*, *C. jejuni* and *Y. enterocolitica*.
- Nongonococcal urethritis and *C. trachomatis* are also trigger factors of reactive arthritis.
- Reactive arthritis may be indistinguishable from psoriatic arthritis and enteropathic enteritis. In these situations, the term 'undifferentiated spondyloarthropathy' is used as they share common ground.
- The clinical picture of reactive arthritis includes (i) arthritis (symptomatic, oligoarticular, affecting the lower extremity more and may be associated with sacroiliitis); (ii) genitourinary (nonspecific urethritis, cervicitis in females, cystitis, haematuria, urethral discharge); (iii) skin changes (keratoderma blennorrhagica, balanitis circinata and ulceration on the tongue and buccal cavity); (iv) ocular changes may occur (e.g. conjunctivitis); and (v) fever and weight loss may occur.
- The urethritis is usually symptomatic presenting with mucopurulent urethral discharge and haematuria may be present. The disease may be asymptomatic.
- Enthesitis is common causing plantar fasciitis or Achilles tendon enthesitis.
- The goals and options of management are (i) treat infection with antibiotics (doxycycline 100 mg twice daily for 3 months if *Chlamydia* infection is suspected or confirmed); (ii) screen the sexual partner, take cultures and treat accordingly;

(iii) relieve pain – NSAIDs and local or oral corticosteroids; (iv) relapsing cases should be managed with sulfasalazine or methotrexate; (v) resistant cases can be treated with TNF-alpha-blocking agent; and (vi) educate the patient.

FURTHER READINGS

Barth WF, Segal K. Reactive arthritis (Reiter's syndrome). *Am Fam Physician*. 1999;60(2):499-503, 507. Review.

Dougados M, Baeten D. Spondyloarthritis. *Lancet*. 2011;377(9783):2127-2137. Review.

Kataria RK, Brent LH. Spondyloarthropathies. *Am Fam Physician*. 2004;69(12):2853-2860. Review.

Keat A. Reiter's syndrome and reactive arthritis in perspective. *N Engl J Med*. 1983;309(26):1606-1615. Review.

Mäki-Ikola O, Granfors K. Salmonella-triggered reactive arthritis. *Lancet*. 1992;339(8801):1096-1098. Review.

Miller KE. Diagnosis and treatment of Chlamydia trachomatis infection. *Am Fam Physician*. 2006;73(8):1411-1416. Review.

CASE 4.6

'Red and Tender . . . '

Michael Norman, a 49-year-old man, comes in to see his general practitioner because he is suffering from severe pain in his left big toe. He denies trauma or pain in other joints. Mr Norman drinks alcohol and last night he drank a few beers with his friends. He gives a history of recent urinary colic and he passed two small urinary stones 2 years ago. On examination, his pulse is 85/min, his blood pressure is 120/80 mm Hg, temperature is 36.8°C and respiratory rate is 18/min. His left toe is swollen, warm, red and tender. The remainder of the examination is normal. The results of his investigations are summarised as follows:

Table 4.6.1 summarises blood test results.

A 24-hour serum uric acid execretion = 446 mg/dL. A synovial fluid taken from the joint shows needle-shaped crystals with negative birefringence under polarised microscopy.

CASE DISCUSSION

Q1. On the basis of Michael's presentation, what is your diagnosis?

Q2. What is your differential diagnosis?

Q3. What are the key clinical features of this disease? What are the scientific bases for these features?

Q4. What is the pathophysiology underlying these changes?

Q5. What are your management goals and management options?

ANSWERS

1. The findings of severe pain in his big toe, with no history of trauma and the clinical examination which reveals that the left big toe is swollen, warm, red and tender together with the presence of needle-shaped crystals with negative birefringence under polarised microscopy of the synovial fluid aspirated from the affected joint are all consistent with the diagnosis of acute gout.

2. The differential diagnosis includes the following:
   - Pseudogout
   - Trauma/fracture
   - Septic arthritis
   - Cellulitis

Table 4.6.1 Blood test results

Blood test	Michael's results	Normal range
Haemoglobin (Hb)	14	13.5–17.5 g/dL
White blood cell count	8.5	3.5–10.5 × 10⁹/L
Erythrocyte sedimentation rate (ESR)	95	Normal <20 mm/h
Random blood glucose	7.0	Fasting: 3.6–5.8 mmol/L
Serum urate	0.60	0.12–0.42 mmol/L
Serum calcium	2.4	2.1–2.6 mmol/L
Serum phosphate	1.2	0.8–1.4 mmol/L

- Reactive arthritis
- Haemarthritis
- Osteoarthritis
- Chronic lead poisoning
- Sarcoidosis
- Psoriatic arthritis
- Bursitis (inflamed bunion)

The following are essential for the diagnosis of acute gout:

- It is monoarticular, usually affecting the metatarsophalangeal joint of the big toe (70% of patients).
- It presents suddenly, and may wake the patient from sleep.
- The affected joint is red, hot, swollen, painful and tender.
- The patient may be feverish, with leukocytosis and raised erythrocyte sedimentation rate (ESR). High serum uric acid may be present in 60% of patients. However, serum uric acid may be normal or low during an acute attack.
- Patients may give a history of risk factors, e.g. thiazide diuretics, alcohol consumption and myeloproliferative disorders.
- Joint aspiration shows needle-shaped, negative birefringent crystals of monosodium urate by polarising light microscopy. Gram stain of the synovial fluid is negative.
- The gold standard that offers definitive diagnosis is joint aspiration analysis of the synovial fluid. However, if the joint aspiration is not feasible, the diagnosis is usually based on clinical findings alone.
- There is usually a dramatic response to treatment with anti-inflammatory drugs.

3. Clinical picture:

Symptoms:

- Cardinal symptoms: (i) sudden-onset monoarticular pain, usually metatarsophalangeal joint of the big toe, in 70% of patients; (ii) the affected joint is swollen, red, hot and tender; (iii) the patient may be feverish; and (iv) the patient may give a history of risk factors (e.g. alcohol consumption, thiazides diuretics, or myeloproliferative disorders, multiple myeloma, haemoglobinopathies, chronic renal disease, sarcoidosis, hypothyroidism, psoriasis).

Signs:

- The arthritis is monoarticular, commonly the metatarsophalangeal joint of the big toe (differential diagnosis is trauma, gout and pseudogout).
- The affected joint is swollen, red, hot and tender.
- The patient may be feverish.
- Examine the patient for tophi on the external ears, hands, feet, olecranon, tendons, bones and cartilage.

4. Pathological features:

- Uric acid is the end product of the purine metabolism in humans.
- Approximately two-thirds of uric acid is excreted by the kidneys and the remaining one-third is eliminated via the gastrointestinal tract.
- The kidney handles uric acid: The renal clearance of urate is a bidirectional transport model. In the first phase, reabsorption of uric acid takes place (98%–100%); in the second phase, uric acid is secreted (50%); in the third phase, postsecretory reabsorption occurs (40%–44%); and in the final phase, 6%–10% of uric acid is eliminated in the urine.
- It is important to note here that low-dose aspirin blocks urate secretion resulting in hyperuricaemia.
- However, a dose of aspirin of 3–4 g/day blocks uric acid reabsorption resulting in a decrease of uric acid in the blood by eliminating most uric acid in the urine.
- Genetic and environmental factors may affect uric acid production and uric acid excretion resulting in hyperuricaemia.
- Factors that increase uric acid production may include myeloma, Hodgkin disease, leukaemia, polycythaemia rubra vera, Waldernström macroglobulinaemia, cytotoxic drugs and secondary polycythaemia.
- The increase in uric acid production may be idiopathic such as in hypoxanthine-guanine phosphoribosyltransferase (HGPRT) deficiency and in glucose-6-phosphatase deficiency with glycogen storage disease type 1.
- Factors that decrease renal excretion of uric acid include hypertension, myxoedema, increased alcohol consumption, ketoacidosis, sarcoidosis, thiazide diuretics, beta-blockers, angiotensin-converting enzyme inhibitors, salicylates (low doses), cyclosporine A and chronic renal disease (Figure 4.6.1 shows the molecular bases involved in the pathogenesis of acute gout.

5. Management goals:

- Relieve the patient's pain.
- Handle the inflammation.
- Stop any factor that may affect uric acid excretion/production.
- Educate the patient.

In acute attack:

- Administer nonsteroidal anti-inflammatory drugs.
- Stop aspirin if the patient is on aspirin.
- Administer intra-articular corticosteroids.
- Taper off corticosteroids – orally or intravenously – over 7–10 days.

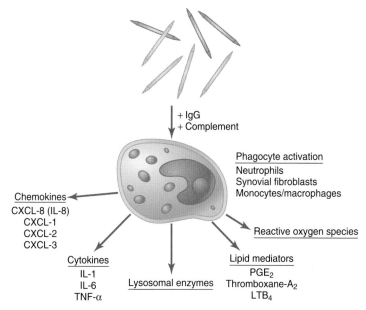

Figure 4.6.1 Pathogenesis of acute gout. *(Source: Andreoli TE, Benjamin IJ, Griggs RC, Wing EJ. Andreoli and Carpenter's Cecil Essentials of Medicine. 8th ed. Philadelphia, PA: Elsevier; 2010.)*

BACK TO BASIC SCIENCES

Q1. What are the main differences between gout and pseudogout?

Table 4.6.2 summarises the main differences between gout and pseudogout.

Table 4.6.2 Main differences between gout and pseudogout

Item	Gout	Pseudogout
Distribution	Lower extremities – metatarsophalangeal, metatarsal, knee joints	Knee, wrist or first metatarsophalangeal joints
Synovial fluid 　WBC counts 　Gram stain 　Synovial crystals	3000–50,000/mm³ Negative Negative birefringence under polarised microscopy	2000–50,000/mm³ Negative Sharp, weakly positive birefringence under polarised microscopy
Plain X-ray	Asymmetric swelling	Soft-tissue swelling plus chondrocalcinosis (calcification of the cartilage)

Q2. Can we use serum uric acid as a screening test for gout in an asymptomatic patient?

No, measurement of the serum uric acid in asymptomatic patients is not a useful screening test for gout.

Q3. What is the role of C-reactive protein, ESR and serum uric acid in the diagnosis of acute gouty arthritis?

A high C-reactive protein and a high ESR support inflammation but both tests are not specific. A high serum uric acid may support gout, but most patients with hyperuricaemia do not have gout and patients presenting with acute gout may have low serum urate during an acute attack.

Q4. What is the gold standard for the diagnosis of gout?

The gold standard that offers definitive diagnosis is joint aspiration analysis of the synovial fluid. However, if the joint aspiration is not feasible, the diagnosis is usually based on clinical findings alone.

Q5. What are the findings of the synovial fluid analysis that can confirm the diagnosis of gout?

- Under polarised light, monosodium urate crystals are needle shaped and negatively birefringent.
- Synovial fluid count of white blood cells is 2000–50,000/mm³.
- Gram stain and culture of the synovial fluids are negative.

Q6. What could the presence of crystals within neutrophils mean?

The presence of the crystals within the neutrophils indicates acute gout. The presence of the crystals extracellularly may indicate that gout is chronic.

Q7. What is the role of radiology (plain X-ray) in a patient presenting with a red, hot, warm, painful big toe?

There is no role of X-ray in the diagnosis of acute gout. However, plain X-ray may help in the exclusion of fracture and other non-gout etiologies.

REVIEW QUESTIONS

Q1. Which *one* of the following medications is *not* a risk factor for hyperuricaemia?
A. Low-dose aspirin
B. High-dose aspirin
C. Beta-blockers
D. Angiotensin-converting enzyme inhibitor

Q2. Which *one* of the following statements about acute gout is *not* correct?
A. The metatarsophalangeal joint of the big toe is affected in two-thirds of patients.
B. The pain wakes up the patient from sleep.
C. The patient responds dramatically to anti-inflammatory drugs.
D. High blood uric acid concentration is necessary for the diagnosis.

Q3. Which *one* of the following conditions is *not* a cause of hyperuricaemia?
A. Multiple myeloma
B. Sarcoidosis
C. Haemoglobinopathies
D. Glucose-6-phosphate dehydrogenase deficiency
E. Psoriasis

Q4. Which *one* of the following statements about the pathogenesis of acute gouty arthritis is correct?
A. IL-26 receptor is implicated in crystal-triggered inflammation.
B. Activation of IL-1β and IL-8 leads to cellular activation and influx of neutrophils.
C. The sodium urate crystal production is dependent on the serum uric acid concentration.
D. Proinflammatory mediators are released in response to direct irritation caused by sodium urate crystals.

Q5. Which *one* of the following is the drug of choice for treating a patient presenting with acute gouty arthritis?
A. Allopurinol
B. Febuxostat
C. Naproxen
D. Losartan

Q6. Which antihypertensive drug would you prescribe to a hypertensive patient with recurrent attacks of acute gouty arthritis over the past 2 years?
A. Beta-blockers
B. Angiotensin-converting enzyme inhibitor
C. Calcium channel blocker
D. Thiazide diuretics

ANSWERS

A1. **B.** A low-dose aspirin blocks urate secretion resulting in hyperuricaemia. Other drugs such as beta-blockers and angiotensin-converting enzyme inhibitor decrease renal excretion of uric acid. Only a high dose of aspirin 3–4 g/day blocks uric acid reabsorption and facilitates urinary excretion of uric acid and hence decreases uric acid levels in the blood.

A2. **D.** High blood uric acid is found in approximately 60% of patients with acute gouty arthritis. It is not a requirement for the diagnosis.

A3. **D.** Glucose-6-phosphate dehydrogenase deficiency is an X-linked recessive inborn error of metabolism that predisposes to haemolysis of red blood cells and jaundice in response to triggers including foods, infections and antimalarial drugs.

On the other hand, glucose-6-phosphatase deficiency is associated with glycogen storage disease type 1 and the increased production of uric acid.

A4. **B**. NLRP3 receptor is implicated in crystal-triggered inflammation in acute gouty arthritis. The activation of IL-1β triggers the activation of IL-8 and the latter causes cellular activation and influx of neutrophils.

The ingestion of polymorphonuclear leukocytes of sodium urate crystals causes the release of several proinflammatory cytokines, particularly IL-1β, and complement.

A5. **C**. Naproxen or any nonsteroidal anti-inflammatory drug in high dose should be prescribed to reduce the pain and swelling.

Allopurinol and febuxostat are recommended to reduce serum uric acid levels but both should not be used during an acute attack.

A6. **C**. Both losartan and calcium channel blockers are able to lower uric acid and any of them should be prescribed.

TAKE-HOME MESSAGE

- Cardinal symptoms of acute gout are (i) sudden-onset monoarticular pain, usually metatarsophalangeal joint of the big toe, in 70% of patients; (ii) the affected joint is swollen, red, hot and tender; (iii) the patient may be feverish; and (iv) the patient may give a history of risk factors (e.g. alcohol consumption, thiazide diuretics, or myeloproliferative disorders, multiple myeloma, haemoglobinopathies, chronic renal disease, sarcoidosis, hypothyroidism, psoriasis).
- The clinical signs of acute gout are (i) monoarticular arthritis, commonly the meta-tarsophalangeal joint of the big toe (differential diagnosis is trauma, gout and pseu-dogout); (ii) the affected joint is swollen, red, hot and tender; (iii) the patient may be feverish; and (iv) tophi may be present on the external ears, hands, feet, olecranon, tendons, bones and cartilage.
- Measurement of the serum uric acid in asymptomatic patients is not a useful screen-ing test for gout.
- A high C-reactive protein and a high ESR support inflammation but both tests are not specific.
- A high serum uric acid may support gout, but most patients with hyperuricaemia do not have gout and patients presenting with acute gout may have low serum urate during an acute attack.
- The gold standard that offers definitive diagnosis is joint aspiration analysis of the synovial fluid. However, if the joint aspiration is not feasible, the diagnosis is usually based on clinical findings alone.
- The goals of management are (i) relieve the patient's pain; (ii) handle the inflam-mation; (iii) stop any factor that may affect uric acid excretion/production; and (iv) educate the patient.

FURTHER READINGS

Choi HK, Soriano LC, Zhang Y, Rodríguez LA. Antihypertensive drugs and risk of incident gout among patients with hypertension: population-based case-control study. *BMJ*. 2012;344:d8190.

Dalbeth N, Merriman TR, Stamp LK. Gout. *Lancet*. 2016;388(10055):2039-2052. Review.

Emmerson BT. The management of gout. *N Engl J Med*. 1996;334(7):445-451. Review.

Richette P, Bardin T. Gout. *Lancet*. 2010;375(9711):318-328. Review.

Underwood M. Gout. *BMJ Clin Evid*. 2011;2011:1120. Review.

Underwood M. Gout. *BMJ Clin Evid*. 2015;2015:1120. Review.

'I Was Nearly Dead ...'

James Donald, a 35-year-old carpenter, injured his finger while trying to pull out a rusty nail. He was taken to the emergency department and was given first aid treatment including antitetanus immunoglobulin. Within a few minutes of getting the injection, he developed tightness in the chest, became grey and made gasping sounds, and lost consciousness for 2–3 minutes. The treating doctor immediately administered intramuscular epinephrine (adrenaline) and intravenous antihistamine and monitored his vital signs.

CASE DISCUSSION

Q1. On the basis of James' presentation, what is your diagnosis?

Q2. What is your differential diagnosis?

Q3. What are the key clinical features of this disease? What are the scientific bases for these features?

Q4. What is the pathophysiology underlying these changes?

Q5. What are your management goals and management options?

ANSWERS

1. The findings of tightness in the chest, loss of consciousness for 2–3 minutes, becoming grey and making gasping sounds for a few minutes following receiving antitetanus immunoglobulin together with being fully recovered after receiving intramuscular epinephrine (adrenaline) and intravenous antihistamine are suggestive of the diagnosis of anaphylaxis.
2. The differential diagnosis includes the following:
   - Hereditary angio-oedema
   - Other forms of shock (cardiogenic, septic, hypovolaemia)
   - Massive pulmonary embolism
   - Myocardial dysfunction
   - Pheochromocytoma
   - Malignant carcinoid syndrome
   - Angio-oedema caused by ACE inhibitor (ACE inhibitors alter the degradation of bradykinin)
   - Pulmonary oedema
   - Stridor (epiglottitis, croup, foreign body, tumour, smoke/toxin)
   - Wheezing (asthma, pulmonary oedema, chronic obstructive pulmonary disease)

The following are essential for the diagnosis of anaphylaxis:

- Acute allergic response with systemic changes involving (i) cutaneous – urticaria, angio-oedema and flushing; (ii) respiratory – laryngeal oedema, asthma and shortness of breath; (iii) cardiovascular – arrhythmias, hypotension, increased capillary permeability and extracellular fluid loss; and (iv) gastrointestinal – nausea, vomiting and loose bowel motions.
- The following questions are important in the diagnosis. (i) Is there a trigger? (ii) Is there a past history of atopy or similar reactions? (iii) Is there multisystem involvement? (iv) Is there any historical information about medications, foods, exposure to chemicals or insect bite within 1 hour of the reaction?

3. Clinical picture:

Symptoms:

Sudden changes including the following:

- – Shortness of breath
- – Anxiety
- – Palpitation
- – Chest discomfort
- – Dizziness
- – Difficulty in swallowing
- – Unable to talk or complete a short statement
- – Cyanosis
- – Loss of consciousness

Signs:

- Skin: Urticarial, angio-oedematous lesions and signs of atopic dermatitis
- Eye, ear, nose and throat: Periorbital swelling, croups and congestion of the mucous membranes of the nose
- Respiratory system: Increased respiratory rate, audible wheezes and cyanosis
- Cardiovascular system: Low blood pressure, tachycardia, cardiovascular collapse and hypoxia

This is an emergency situation and the patient should be managed immediately.

4. Laboratory investigations:

- Assessment of the presence of IgE antibody
- Assessment of allergen-specific IgE much more helpful in the evaluation than that of total IgE antibody

This is an emergency situation. The treatment should start immediately and rarely such tests are needed.

5. Management goals:

- Ensure airway patency and the patient is placed in Trendelenburg position.
- Ensure good oxygenation of tissues (oxygen via nasal cannula).
- Relax bronchial smooth muscles, improve vasomotor tone and stop vasopermeability (epinephrine (1:1000) 0.2–0.5 mg intramuscular in adults, repeated in 15–30 minutes).

- Patients on beta-blockers may not benefit from epinephrine administration (glucagon IV 1–5 mg/h in adults).
- Prevent the progression of symptoms and signs (antihistamine injection).
- Protect against the late phase of biphasic anaphylaxis and protracted reaction (start the patient on prednisone 20 mg orally).

BACK TO BASIC SCIENCES

Q1. How would you assess the severity of an anaphylaxis reaction?

The aim of the assessment is to decide whether adrenaline is needed and whether you need help from a doctor trained in airway and circulatory support.

The assessment may cover the following:
- Orofacial swelling
- Signs of stridor and laryngeal swelling
- Bronchospasm and wheezing
- Cyanosis
- Pulmonary oedema
- Shock
- Cardiovascular collapse, palpitations and arrhythmias
- Loss of consciousness
- Cardiac arrest

Q2. How would you manage a patient with anaphylaxis?

- Ensure airway patency. Place the patient in Trendelenburg position. Keep the patient in semirecumbent position if he or she has trouble with airway and you need to call an expert in airway management.
- Stop any cause. If the patient is given IV drug or blood products, stop immediately.
- Give oxygen via nasal cannula.
- Administer adrenaline (epinephrine) 0.2–0.5 mg intramuscular in adults; repeat in 15–30 minutes, if needed.
- Prevent the progression of symptoms and signs (antihistamine injection).
- Protect against the late phase of biphasic anaphylaxis and protracted reaction (start the patient on prednisone 20 mg orally).

Q3. Why should adrenaline be administrated? What are the pharmacological mechanisms of adrenaline?

Adrenaline is alpha-1-adrenergic agonist $\rightarrow$ vasoconstriction (increases blood pressure) + decreased capillary permeability (mucosal oedema).

Adrenaline acts on beta-1-adrenergic receptors $\rightarrow$ increase the force and rate of cardiac contractility + decrease mediator release.

Q4. Discuss the mechanisms underlying hypotension and circulatory collapse in patients with anaphylaxis.

- Vasodilatation caused by histamine, bradykinin and cytokines → nitric oxide production → relative hypovolaemia → hypotension.
- Capillary leakage (increased capillary permeability) → absolute hypovolaemia (plasma loss in the interstitial space) → adding to hypotension.
- Myocardial dysfunction occurs in anaphylaxis (anaphylaxis-induced myocardial ischaemia and Takotsubo cardiomyopathy) → these changes contribute to hypotension and circulating collapse (for further reading, check Cha et al., 2016).

Q5. What precautions/actions would you take in a patient presenting with anaphylaxis who has been on treatment with beta-blockers?

Patients on a beta-adrenoceptor blocker can be resistant to adrenaline treatment for their anaphylaxis. Glucagon should be considered. These patients need continuous monitoring in the hospital particularly in relation to their haemodynamics.

Q6. Give examples of drugs that are commonly associated with anaphylaxis.

- Penicillins
- Cephalosporins
- Nonsteroidal anti-inflammatory drugs (NSAIDs)
- Aspirin
- Radiocontrast media
- Narcotics
- Vancomycin

Note that anaphylaxis caused by aspirin, NSAIDs, radiocontrast media, narcotics and vancomycin is non-IgE-mediated.

Q7. Why are corticosteroids not the first line of treatment of anaphylaxis?

Compared to adrenaline, corticosteroids take significantly longer time to show their effects. Adrenaline works immediately via cell surface receptors, whereas corticosteroids must cross the cell wall, reach the nucleus and alter the protein synthesis before the resulting protein can act or mediate anti-inflammatory effects.

Comparing the effect of adrenaline with that of corticosteroids, corticosteroids take hours to act and are not suitable in managing emergency situations such as anaphylaxis.

REVIEW QUESTIONS

Q1. According to the National Institute for Health and Care Excellence (NICE) quality standards for anaphylaxis, which *one* of the following is *not* correct?

A. Patients with anaphylaxis should be given training to use an adrenaline autoinjector.

B. Patients with anaphylaxis should be referred to a specialist allergy service.

C. Patients with a systemic reaction for a wasp or bee sting should be referred for immunotherapy.

D. The risk of biphasic reaction in patients with anaphylaxis is less likely if adrenaline treatment is delayed.

Q2. Which *one* of the following is *not* correct in managing stridor in a patient with anaphylaxis?

A. Administration of adrenaline intramuscularly

B. Administration of corticosteroids

C. High concentration of humidified oxygen

D. Keeping patient in semirecumbent position

Q3. The mechanisms underlying hypotension and circulatory collapse in anaphylaxis include all of the following *except*

A. Vasodilation.

B. Capillary leakage.

C. Myocardial ischaemia.

D. Peripheral vasoconstriction.

E. Cardiomyopathy.

Q4. Which *one* of the following is *not* a pharmacological action of adrenaline?

A. Increased heart rate (SA node)

B. Eye mydriasis

C. Bronchi relaxation

D. Inhibition of histamine release from mast cells

E. Bladder sphincter relaxation

Q5. Regarding the location of H receptors, which *one* of the following is *not* correct?

A. H_1 receptors – smooth muscles

B. H_4 receptors – haematopoietic cells

C. H_3 receptors – myocardial cells

D. H_2 receptors – parietal cells

ANSWERS

A1. **D.** The risk of biphasic reaction is more likely to occur in these patients if adrenaline treatment is delayed.

A2. **B.** Corticosteroids are not effective in emergency situations such as stridor. Adrenaline (0.5 mL of 1:1000 solution) should be given IM. In some cases, it is given intravenously in a bolus of up to 50 μg. Delay of administration of adrenaline increases the risk of mortality. The patients in such a situation should not be placed flat (such position may precipitate respiratory arrest).

A3. **D.** Peripheral vasodilation, not vasoconstriction, occurs in anaphylaxis.

A4. **E.** The action of adrenaline on the bladder is constriction of its sphincter.

A5. **C.** H_3 receptors are present on CNS cells.

TAKE-HOME MESSAGE

- Anaphylaxis is an acute allergic response with systemic changes involving (i) cutaneous – urticaria, angio-oedema and flushing; (ii) respiratory – laryngeal oedema, asthma and shortness of breath; (iii) cardiovascular – arrhythmias, hypotension, increased capillary permeability and extracellular fluid loss; and (iv) gastrointestinal – nausea, vomiting and loose bowel motions.
- The following questions are important in the diagnosis. (i) Is there a trigger? (ii) Is there a past history of atopy or similar reactions? (iii) Is there multisystem involvement? (iv) Is there any historical information about medications, foods, exposure to chemicals or insect bite within 1 hour of the reaction?
- The goals of management are (i) ensure airway patency and the patient is placed in Trendelenburg position; (ii) ensure good oxygenation of tissues (oxygen via nasal cannula); (iii) relax bronchial smooth muscles, improve vasomotor tone and stop vasopermeability (epinephrine 0.2–0.5 mg intramuscular in adults, repeated in 15–30 minutes); (iv) patients on beta-blockers may not benefit from epinephrine administration (glucagon IV 1–5 mg/h in adults); (v) prevent the progression of symptoms and signs (antihistamine injection); and (vi) protect against the late phase of biphasic anaphylaxis and protracted reaction (start the patient on prednisone 20 mg orally).
- Compared to adrenaline, corticosteroids take significantly longer time to show their effects. Adrenaline works immediately via cell surface receptors, whereas corticosteroids must cross the cell wall, reach the nucleus and alter the protein synthesis before the resulting protein can act or mediate anti-inflammatory effects.

FURTHER READINGS

Centre for Clinical Practice at NICE (UK). Anaphylaxis: Assessment to Confirm an Anaphylactic Episode and the Decision to Refer After Emergency Treatment for a Suspected Anaphylactic Episode. Manchester, UK: National Institute for Health and Clinical Excellence (UK); 2011.

Cha YS, Kim H, Bang MH, et al. Evaluation of myocardial injury through serum troponin I and echocardiography in anaphylaxis. *Am J Emerg Med.* 2016;34(2):140-144.

Demoly P, Botros HG, Rabillon J, David B, Bousquet J. Anaphylaxis to antitetanus toxoid serum. *Allergy.* 2002;57(9):860-861.

Dzingina M, Stegenga H, Heath M, et al. Assessment and referral after emergency treatment of a suspected anaphylactic episode: summary of NICE guidance. *BMJ.* 2011;343:d7595.

Endocrine System

CASE 5.1

'The Trouble with My Vision . . . '

Mark Alan, a 49-year-old truck driver, presents to his general practitioner because he is suffering from a headache of 6-month duration, generalised tiredness and low back pain. Recently, he has had two accidents when he did not see cars on his left side and hit them while changing lanes. On examination, his pulse is 70/min, blood pressure 150/100 mm Hg and respiratory rate 15/min. He is afebrile. He has coarse facial features, large jaw and frontal bossing; when he smiles, his teeth appear to be widely spaced. His driving licence photo, issued 3 years ago, shows that his facial features have changed and he looked to have fine features in the photo. Visual field examination reveals bilateral hemianopia (loss of the lateral part of the visual field on both sides). His hands and feet are large and spade-like. Urine dipstick shows the presence of glucose ++.

Laboratory investigations are summarised in Table 5.1.1.

MRI scan shows enlarged pituitary gland and its fossa. A pituitary adenoma of approximately 17 mm is present within the gland.

CASE DISCUSSION

Q1. On the basis of Mark's presentation, what is your diagnosis?

Q2. What is your differential diagnosis?

Q3. What are the key clinical features of this disease? What are the scientific bases for these features?

Q4. What is the pathophysiology underlying these changes?

Q5. What are your management goals and management options?

ANSWERS

1. The findings of headaches for 6 months, generalised tiredness, low back pain, high blood pressure, coarse facial features, large jaw, frontal bossing, widely separated teeth and changes in his facial features compared to his own photo taken 3 years earlier, together with bilateral hemianopia, spade-like hands and feet, the presence of glucose in urine (glucose positive ++) and the changes in his laboratory investigations (increased growth hormone [GH], impaired glucose tolerance and increased insulin-like growth factor [IGF-1]) are all consistent with the diagnosis of acromegaly. The radiological changes as demonstrated by the MRI scan (enlarged pituitary gland and the presence of a pituitary adenoma of approximately 17 mm) together with

Table 5.1.1 Mark's blood test results

Blood test	Mark's results	Normal range
Growth hormone (GH) (μg/L)	11	<8
Glucose tolerance test (mmol/L)		
Fasting	8.8	3.3–5.8
60 minutes	13	6.7–9.4
90 minutes	13	5.6–7.8
120 minutes	11	3.9–6.7
Insulin-like growth factor (IGF-1) (ng/mL)	329	40–259 (males aged 46–50 years) 44–227 (females aged 46–50 years)
Serum prolactin (nmol/L)	0.97	<1.29
Thyroid-stimulating hormone (TSH) (μU/mL)	1.3	0.4–5.0

the biochemical/hormonal changes indicate that the cause of his presentation is an active pituitary adenoma predisposing to excessive amounts of the GH.

2. The differential diagnosis includes the following:
   - Familial
   - McCune–Albright syndrome
   - Hyperinsulinism
   - Carney complex (naevi, atrial myxoma, neurofibroma and ephelides) – a familial condition with multiple neoplasia and a GH-producing tumour

3. Clinical picture:
   Symptoms:
   - Headaches
   - Increased frequency of urination and feeling thirst
   - Weight gain
   - Shortness of breath
   - Muscle weakness
   - Joint pains
   - Arthropathy
   - Increased sweating
   - Multiple skin tags
   - Sleep apnoea
   - Amenorrhoea/oligomenorrhoea in females
   - Impotence/poor libido
   - Galactorrhoea
   Signs:
   - Hypertension
   - Changes in facial features
   - Prominent supraorbital ridge
   - Prognathism

- Interdental separation
- Large tongue
- Visual field defect - compression of the optic chiasm results in bitemporal hemianopia. However, any visual field defect can result from suprasellar extension of the tumour.
- Thick, greasy skin
- Multiple skin tags
- Excessive sweating
- Hirsutism
- Spade-like hands and feet
- Carpal tunnel syndrome
- Heart failure
- Proximal myopathy
- Glycosuria
- Recurrent colonic polyps

4. Laboratory investigations:
   - GH level: On its own, the GH level cannot be diagnostic. An undetectable GH may exclude acromegaly.
   - IGF-1 level: It is important in the diagnosis. It is usually raised in acromegaly.
   - A glucose tolerance test: Approximately 25% of patients with acromegaly have a positive glucose tolerance test.
   - Visual field defect: Bitemporal hemianopia is classically present.
   - MRI scan of the pituitary: It may reveal a pituitary adenoma or microadenoma.
   - Prolactin levels: Hyperprolactinaemia may be present in 30% of patients (some adenomas secrete GH and prolactin).

5. Management goals:
   - Control pituitary adenoma and its mechanical pressure effects.
   - Relieve symptoms.
   - Achieve a mean GH level below 2.5 μg/L (a safe GH level).
   - Achieve a normal IGF-1.
   - Delay the progress of comorbidities (hypertension, heart failure, coronary artery disease) and death.
   - Reduce the risk of colonic cancer.
   - Control hypertension and diabetes.
   - Educate the patient and assess whether surgery, radiotherapy or medical treatment is better for the patient treatment.

BACK TO BASIC SCIENCES

Q1. What are the key findings of the diagnosis of acromegaly?

- Clinical picture
- An elevated age-adjusted serum IGF-1 concentration
- A serum GH nadir greater than 0.4 μg/L following a 75-g oral glucose challenge

Q2. What is the prevalence of acromegaly?

The prevalence of acromegaly is approximately 40–60 per million.

Q3. What are the causes of acromegaly?

- More than 99% of cases are caused by GH-secreting pituitary microadenoma or macroadenoma.
- Ectopic secretion of GH-secreting hormone is rare.
- Multiple endocrine neoplasia (MEN type 1) is present.
- McCune–Albright syndrome and Carney complex, both are rare causes.

Q4. What are the investigations needed for the diagnosis of acromegaly?

- GH concentration
- IGF-1
- The 75-g oral glucose tolerance test
- Serum prolactin level
- Visual field defect
- MRI scan of the pituitary

Q5. What are the other investigations needed to assess a patient confirmed to have acromegaly?

- Serum thyroid-stimulating hormone and free thyroxin
- Serum cortisol
- Serum gonadotropins and sex hormones
- Fasting blood glucose level
- HbA_{1c}
- Serum calcium (for patients with MEN type 1)
- ECG/echocardiography
- Chest X-ray and X-ray of hands and large joints
- Sleep studies for sleep apnoea
- Colonoscopy (for any polyps and follow-up)

Q6. What is the physiological role of IGF-1?

IGF-1 mediates nearly all the physiological actions of the GH.

Q7. What is the role of surgery in acromegaly?

- It is the treatment of choice in most patients.
- Transsphenoidal surgery (surgical adenomectomy) has a cure rate of 90% in patients with a microadenoma and 40%–50% in those with a macroadenoma.

Q8. What are the comorbidities commonly found at the time of the diagnosis of acromegaly?

- Hypertension 35%–38%

- Carpal tunnel syndrome 20%–24%
- Arthritis 25%
- Sleep apnoea 25%–29%
- Diabetes mellitus, insulin resistant 18%–22%
- Headache 15%–22%
- Bitemporal hemianopia

REVIEW QUESTIONS

Q1. Which *one* of the following is diagnostic of acromegaly?
A. Karyotyping in females
B. Visual field examination
C. Glucose tolerance test with failure of GH suppression
D. GH level
E. MRI scan of the pituitary

Q2. Which *one* of the following is the best prognostic marker of surgical cure in acromegaly?
A. Patient age
B. Cavernous sinus invasion
C. Preoperative GH and IGF-1 level
D. Tumour size as per MRI scan
E. Prolactin level

Q3. Which *one* of the following is less likely among the presenting symptoms of acromegaly?
A. Headache
B. Visual disturbances
C. Goitre
D. Polymenorrhoea
E. Galactorrhoea

Q4. Which *one* of the following about somatostatin receptor agonists is correct?
A. Octreotide is a natural analogue of somatostatin.
B. Lanreotide acts selectively on somatostatin receptor subtypes SSTR2.
C. Octreotide is used as a long-term treatment to achieve the treatment target.
D. The main side effect of octreotide is urinary stones.

Q5. Which *one* of the following is the appropriate first line of treatment in acromegaly?
A. Transsphenoidal surgery
B. Pituitary radiotherapy
C. Pasireotide treatment
D. GH antagonists

ANSWERS

A1. **C.** The failure of suppression of GH in glucose tolerance test below 0.3 μg/L, or sometimes it shows a paradoxical rise is diagnostic of acromegaly.

Karyotyping is not indicated and the measurement of the GH may help in excluding acromegaly if levels are undetectable.

A2. **B.** Surgery (pituitary microadenectomy) will result in clinical remission in majority of patients (60%–90%). In macroadenoma, only 40%–50% of patients will have remission.

In some studies, preoperative GH and IGF-1 levels are shown to be useful prognostic markers of surgical cure. High preoperative levels are associated with low surgical cure. However, the best single preoperative predictor has been shown to be cavernous sinus invasion, followed by preoperative GH and IGF-1 levels.

A3. **D.** Oligomenorrhoea or amenorrhoea is among the symptoms of acromegaly, not polymenorrhoea.

A4. **B.** The main side effects of octreotide and lanreotide are nausea, vomiting, diarrhoea, steatorrhoea, bleeding, headache, development of gallstones/liver problems, weight gain, cold intolerance and worsening heart condition symptoms. Both octreotide and lanreotide can be used on a short-term basis in treating acromegaly, but they cannot help in achieving treatment targets. Both are synthetic analogues.

A5. **A.** GH antagonists are used in patients in whom GH and IGF-1 levels cannot be reduced to safe levels with somatostatin analogues alone or by surgery or radiotherapy.

Surgery is the first line of treatment, usually through the transsphenoidal approach. Rarely transfrontal surgery is required (in massive macroadenoma). Pasireotide is a new somatostatin receptor agonist and its role in the treatment of patients with acromegaly is still under exploration.

TAKE-HOME MESSAGE

- The prevalence of acromegaly is approximately 40–60 per million.
- The causes of acromegaly are (i) more than 99% of cases are caused by GH-secreting pituitary microadenoma or macroadenoma; (ii) ectopic secretion of GH-secreting hormone is rare; and (iii) MEN type 1, McCune–Albright syndrome and Carney complex.
- The presenting symptoms in acromegaly include headaches, increased frequency of urination, feeling thirst, weight gain, shortness of breath, muscle weakness, joint pains, arthropathy, increased sweating, multiple skin tags, sleep apnoea, amenorrhoea/oligomenorrhoea in females, impotence/poor libido and galactorrhoea.
- The diagnosis of acromegaly is based on the clinical picture and an elevated age-adjusted serum IGF-1 concentration and a serum GH nadir greater than 0.4 μg/L following a 75-g oral glucose challenge.

- Surgery is the first line of treatment, usually through the transsphenoidal approach. Rarely transfrontal surgery is required (in massive macroadenoma). Pasireotide is a new somatostatin receptor agonist and its role in the treatment of patients with acromegaly is still under exploration.
- Surgery (pituitary microadenectomy) will result in clinical remission in the majority of patients (60%–90%). In macroadenoma, only 40%–50% of patients will have remission.
- In some studies, young age and preoperative GH and IGF-1 levels are shown to be useful prognostic markers of surgical cure. High preoperative levels are associated with low surgical cure. However, the best single preoperative predictor has been shown to be cavernous sinus invasion, followed by preoperative GH and IGF-1 levels.
- The main side effects of octreotide and lanreotide are nausea, vomiting, diarrhoea, steatorrhoea, bleeding, headache, development of gallstones/liver problems, weight gain, cold intolerance and worsening heart condition symptoms. Both can be used on a short-term basis but they cannot help in achieving treatment targets. Both are synthetic analogues.
- GH antagonists are used in patients in whom GH and IGF-1 levels cannot be reduced to safe levels with somatostatin analogues alone or by surgery or radiotherapy.

FURTHER READINGS

Agrawal N, Ioachimescu AG. Prognostic factors of biochemical remission after transsphenoidal surgery for acromegaly: a structured review. *Pituitary*. 2020 Oct;23(5):582-594. doi: 10.1007/s11102-020-01063-x.

Danzig J. Acromegaly. *BMJ*. 2007;335(7624):824-825. Review.

Klibanski A, Zervas NT. Diagnosis and management of hormone-secreting pituitary adenomas. *N Engl J Med*. 1991;324(12):822-831. Review.

Lake MG, Krook LS, Cruz SV. Pituitary adenomas: an overview. *Am Fam Physician*. 2013;88(5):319-327. Review.

Lamberts SW, van der Lely AJ, de Herder WW, Hofland LJ. Octreotide. *N Engl J Med*. 1996;334(4):246-254. Review.

Maugans TA, Coates ML. Diagnosis and treatment of acromegaly. *Am Fam Physician*. 1995;52(1):207-213. Review.

Melmed S. Medical progress: acromegaly. *N Engl J Med*. 2006;355(24):2558-2573. Review. No abstract available. Erratum in: *N Engl J Med*. 2007;356(8):879.

Reddy R, Hope S, Wass J. Acromegaly. *BMJ*. 2010;341:c4189. Review.

CASE 5.2

'I Feel Too Hot ...'

Lily Thompson, a 36-year-old social worker at a secondary school, comes in to see her general practitioner because of anxiety and sleep disturbances. Her anxiety started 5 months ago following hearing the news that one of the students in her school has committed suicide. Lily always feels hot and she has to keep wiping her hands all the time. These symptoms started nearly at the same time.

Lily has noticed tremor in her hands. She lost 5 kg in body weight over the past 3 months, although her appetite has been increased and she is not exercising. At times she feels her heartbeats (palpitations) even at rest. On examination, her pulse rate is 110/min (regular), blood pressure 160/90 mm Hg, temperature 37.0°C and respiratory rate 22/min. She looks anxious and her BMI is 18. Eye examination shows exophthalmos and lid lagging on looking down, and a white rim of sclera is seen above and below the cornea. Her hands are soft and warm. Her palms are warm and wet and her outstretched hands show fine tremors. Neck examination shows a frontal swelling in the midline that moves up on swallowing. The swelling is smooth to palpation. No palpable lymph nodes are present. A bruit is heard over the neck swelling. Upper and lower limb examination shows shoulder and pelvic girdle weakness, respectively. All tendon reflexes are bilaterally symmetrical and brisk.

The results of Lily's blood tests are summarised in Table 5.2.1.

A thyroid scan shows homogenous uptake of the radioactive iodine.

CASE DISCUSSION

Q1. On the basis of Lily's presentation, what is your diagnosis?

Q2. What is your differential diagnosis?

Q3. What are the key clinical features of this disease? What are the scientific bases for these features?

Q4. What is the pathophysiology underlying these changes?

Q5. What are your management goals and management options?

ANSWERS

1. The findings of anxiety, sleep disturbance, feeling hot, wiping hands all the time, tremor of hands, loss of body weight although her appetite has been increased and she is not exercising, and palpitations, together with the clinical examination findings

Table 5.2.1 Lily's blood test results

Blood test	Lily's results	Normal range
Serum triiodothyronine (T3 free) (pmol/L)	13	3.5–6.5
Serum thyroxin (T4 free) (pmol/L)	36	8.5–15.2
Thyroid-stimulating hormone (TSH) (μU/mL)	0.04	0.4–5.0
TSH receptor IgG antibodies (TRAb)	Raised +++	Negative

including increased heart rate, elevated blood pressure and respiratory rate, exophthalmos, lid lagging on looking down, a white rim of the sclerae seen above and below the cornea, tremor of the outstretched hands, presence of goitre, a bruit heard over the thyroid, proximal weakness (shoulder and pelvic girdle muscles) and symmetrically brisk tendon reflexes on both sides are all supportive of the diagnosis of Graves disease.

The laboratory findings of high T3 and T4, low thyroid-stimulating hormone (TSH) and raised TSH receptor IgG antibodies together with homogenous increased uptake of radioactive iodine and the presence of exophthalmos are confirming the diagnosis of Graves disease.

2. The differential diagnosis includes the following:
   - Diffuse toxic goitre (Graves disease)
   - Subacute thyroiditis
   - Toxic multinodular goitre
   - Toxic adenoma
   - Factitious thyrotoxicosis
   - Iatrogenic thyrotoxicosis
   - Iodine-induced thyrotoxicosis
   - Thyrotropin-secreting pituitary adenoma
   - Anxiety disorders
   - Hashimoto thyroiditis
   - Papillary thyroid carcinoma
   - Pheochromocytoma
   - Struma ovarii
   - Radiation-induced thyroiditis

   The following are essential for the diagnosis of Graves disease:
   - Clinical picture, raised T3 and T4 and low TSH plus raised TSH receptor IgG antibodies
   - Homogenous uptake of radioactive iodine
   - Eye changes: Increased tear production, periorbital oedema, conjunctival oedema (chemosis), proptosis (5%–15% is unilateral), diplopia (extraocular muscle dysfunction) and corneal ulcer (Fig. 5.2.1)
   - Pretibial myxoedema

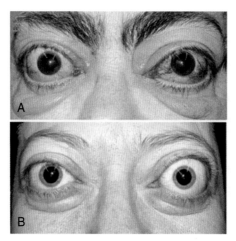

Figure 5.2.1 Eye changes in Graves ophthalmopathy. *(Source: Goldman L, Schafer Al. Goldman-Cecil Medicine. 25th ed. Elsevier; 2016.)*

- Autoimmune disorder: Presence of any of the following autoimmune disorders – vitiligo, pernicious anaemia, type 1 diabetes mellitus, celiac disease and myasthenia gravis
- Thyroid acropachy (clubbing, swelling of digits, periosteal reaction of long bones)

3. Clinical picture:

Symptoms:
- Anxiety
- Weight loss
- Increased appetite
- Heat intolerance
- Sweating
- Fatigue
- Tiredness
- Irritability
- Insomnia
- Tremor
- Depression
- Loss of libido
- Amenorrhoea
- Diarrhoea
- Pruritus
- Periodic paralysis

Signs:
- Tachycardia
- Atrial fibrillation
- Tremor
- Hyperreflexia

- Warm, moist hands
- Hair loss
- Onycholysis
- Lid retraction
- Lid lag

As stated earlier, Graves disease is a syndrome comprising thyrotoxicosis, goitre, orbitopathy (eye and orbit changes), dermatopathy, autoimmunity and/or thyroid acropathy. It is not necessary to have all these components to make the diagnosis. The presence of thyrotoxicosis together with eye changes or dermatopathy (pretibial myxoedema) is diagnostic of Graves disease.

4. Laboratory findings:
   - Serum TSH. In hyperthyroidism, TSH is suppressed <0.05 mU/L.
   - Raised free T3 and/or T4: T4 is almost always raised but T3 is more sensitive as there are occasional cases of isolated T3 thyrotoxicosis.
   - TSH receptor–stimulating antibodies: They should be measured routinely with T3, T4 and TSH. Although the second generations of assays for these antibodies have more than 95% sensitivity and specificity, the third-generation tests have 97%–99% specificity for primary hyperthyroidism.
   - Thyroid peroxidase and thyroglobulin antibodies: These are less specific for Graves disease.
   - Thyroid scintiscanning with technetium-99m or iodine-131: It may be needed in thyrotoxicosis without hyperthyroidism.

Pathological features:
- Environmental and genetic factors are involved in the pathogenesis of Graves disease.
- Environmental factors such as dietary iodine, smoking, infections and emotional stress are the contributing factors in the pathogenesis of Graves disease.
- Genetic and epigenetic determinants are the leading factors (genes encoding thyroglobulin, thyrotropin receptor, HLA-DR Beta-Arg74, cytotoxic T-lymphocyte-associated antigen 4, CD25, CD40 and hypermethylation of several genes are the contributing factors).
- Graves disease is associated with cytotoxic T-lymphocyte-associated antigen 4.
- Graves disease may be triggered by infection (Gram-negative organisms including *Escherichia coli* and *Yersinia enterocolitica* infections).
- Graves disease is associated with autoimmune diseases such as type 1 diabetes mellitus, vitiligo and myasthenia gravis.
- Therefore, Graves disease can be considered an autoimmune complex syndrome.
- Serum IgG antibodies bind to the TSH receptor in thyroid resulting in stimulation of thyroid hormone production (antibodies behave like TSH).
- The autoregulation (physiological regulation), controlled by the hypothalamic–pituitary–thyroid axis, is lost and the feedback cannot regulate the production of thyroxin (continuous production of thyroxin and the regulatory mechanisms are out of control).

Fig. 5.2.2 summarises immune mechanisms in Graves disease and Hashimoto thyroiditis.

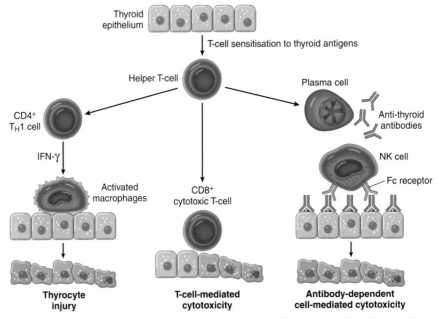

Figure 5.2.2 Immune mechanisms in Graves disease and Hashimoto thyroiditis. *(Source: Kumar V, Abbas AK, Fausto N, Mitchell R. Robbins Basic Pathology, 8th Edition. London, UK: Elsevier; 2007.)*

5. Management goals and options:
- Control the hypothyroidism and associated systemic changes.
- Relieve symptoms.
- Delay the progress of comorbidities (such as arrhythmias and heart failure).
- Educate the patient about the nature of their disease, the eye changes, the treatment options available and the advantages and disadvantages of each option.
- Provide medical therapy (antithyroid drugs).
- Provide radiotherapy.
- Perform surgery (thyroidectomy).

BACK TO BASIC SCIENCES

Q1. What are the key mechanisms underlying the pathogenesis of Graves disease?
Graves disease is an autoimmune disease. The activating thyrotrophin–receptor antibodies are responsible for inducing thyroid hormone overproduction.

Q2. What are the common presenting symptoms of hyperthyroidism in elderly persons?
- The common presenting symptoms of hyperthyroidism in the elderly are weight loss, decreased appetite and cardiac manifestations such as atrial fibrillations.

- The common presenting symptoms of hyperthyroidism in young persons are weight loss, increased appetite, sweating, fatigue, heat intolerance, tremors, anxiety and palpitations.

Q3. What are the clinical eye changes associated with the development of thyroid-associated ophthalmology?

A number of clinical changes may be observed with the development of thyroid-associated ophthalmology. The following changes may occur over 3 years: Proptosis, eyelid swelling, diplopia, increased tearing, ocular discomfort, periorbital oedema, chemosis, scleral injection, corneal ulcers and keratitis.

Other eye changes are as follows:
- Lid retraction (92%)
- Exophthalmos (65%)
- Ocular pain (25%–30%)
- Increased lacrimation (20%–25%)
- Optic neuropathy (6%)

Q4. What is the mechanism underlying lid retraction in Graves disease?

Increased sympathetic tone is responsible for lid retraction.

Q5. What are the other symptoms in patients with hyperthyroidism that mimic overstimulation of the sympathetic nervous system?

- Impaired concentration
- Anxiety
- Shortness of breath
- Tachycardia
- Tremor
- Sweating
- Insomnia
- Irritability
- Hypertension
- Hyperreflexia
- Eyelid retraction

Q6. What are the new developments in the pathogenesis of ophthalmopathy in Graves disease?

Orbital fibroblasts, lymphocytes, T- and B-cells and myofibroblasts appear to play a role in the pathogenesis of ophthalmopathy in Graves disease.

Insulin-like growth factor-1 receptor is overexpressed on orbital fibroblasts together with thyrotropin receptors and thyroid-stimulating antibodies appear to contribute to the pathogenesis of ophthalmopathy in Graves disease.

REVIEW QUESTIONS

Q1. A 20-year-old university student presents with symptoms suggestive of hyperthyroidism. She had a history of mild hypothyroidism (autoimmune thyroiditis) and she has been taking 100 μg of L-thyroxin daily. Clinically she is extremely thyrotoxic with a pulse rate of 190/min. The thyroid gland was not palpable. You suspect factious thyrotoxicosis. Which *one* of the following investigations can help you?

A. TSH measurement
B. T3 and T4 measurements
C. A technetium scintiscan of the thyroid
D. TSH receptor stimulation antibodies

Q2. A 52-year-old secretary presents to her general practitioner because of fatigue and aches for the past 12 months and menorrhagia. On examination, her BMI has increased from 25 to 32 kg/m², her voice has become hoarse and her skin is dry. Which *one* of the following is the most likely diagnosis?

A. Addison disease
B. Thyrotoxicosis
C. Acromegaly
D. Primary hypothyroidism
E. Cushing disease

Q3. A 55-year-old school manager presents with progressive unilateral proptosis of his left eye and increased tear production for the past 6 months. He is very concerned about his eye, looks anxious and has some tremors of the hands. He gives no history of upper respiratory tract or postnasal discharge but has loose bowel motions for the past 4–6 months. Which *one* of the following is the most likely diagnosis?

A. Orbital pseudotumour
B. Orbital cellulitis
C. Cavernous sinus thrombosis
D. Graves disease
E. Intraorbital neoplasm

Q4. In patients with Graves disease, the most likely cause of diplopia is
A. Periorbital oedema.
B. Conjunctival oedema.
C. Extraocular muscle dysfunction.
D. Proptosis.
E. Corneal ulcers.

Q5. The most diagnostic test of primary hyperthyroidism is
A. High serum T3 level.
B. High serum T4 level.
C. Raised TSH receptor–stimulating antibodies.
D. Low serum TSH level.
E. Raised thyroid peroxidase antibodies.

Q6. Which *one* of the following tests has high sensitivity and specificity for Graves disease?
A. Serum T3 and T4 levels
B. Serum thyroglobulin antibodies
C. Serum TSH level
D. Thyroid peroxidase antibodies
E. TSH receptor–stimulating antibodies

Q7. Which *one* of the following is the most common cause of hyperthyroidism?
A. Toxic multinodular goitre
B. Hashimoto thyroiditis
C. Toxic adenoma
D. Subacute thyroiditis
E. Graves disease

ANSWERS

A1. **C.** The patient is most likely taking an overdose of L-thyroxin possibly to keep her weight down. A technetium scintiscan of the thyroid can help in confirming factious thyrotoxicosis. The scan will show no thyroid trapping of $^{99m}TcO_4$ supporting the diagnosis of factious thyroiditis (excessive intake of thyroxin).

A2. **D.** The presence of tiredness, fatigue, increased BMI, changes in voice (harsh voice), menorrhagia and dry skin are suggestive of the diagnosis of primary hypothyroidism.

A3. **D.** Graves disease is the most common cause of bilateral and unilateral exophthalmos. Unilateral exophthalmos occurs in 5%–15% of patients with Graves disease. The presence of anxiety, tremor of hands and loose bowel motions are consistent with hyperthyroidism (Kamminga et al., 2003).

A4. **C.** Extraocular muscle dysfunction is the most likely cause of diplopia in the patients.

A5. **D.** Low TSH (<0.05 μU/L) has a high sensitivity and specificity for the diagnosis of primary hyperthyroidism.

A6. **E.** The third generation of TSH receptor–stimulating antibodies has 97%–99% specificity for Graves disease.

A7. **E.** The most common cause of hyperthyroidism is Graves disease.

TAKE-HOME MESSAGE

- The diagnosis of Graves disease is based on the following: (i) Clinical picture, raised T3 and T4 and low TSH plus raised TSH receptor IgG antibodies; (ii) homogenous uptake of radioactive iodine; (iii) eye changes: increased tear production, periorbital oedema, conjunctival oedema (chemosis), proptosis (5%–15% is unilateral), diplopia (extraocular muscle dysfunction) and corneal ulcer; (iv) pretibial myxoedema; (v) autoimmune disorder – any of the following autoimmune disorders may be present: vitiligo, pernicious anaemia, type 1 diabetes mellitus, celiac disease and myasthenia gravis; and (vi) thyroid acropachy (clubbing, swelling of digits, periosteal reaction of long bones).
- The laboratory investigations are as follows: (i) serum TSH: in hyperthyroidism, TSH is suppressed, <0.05 mU/L; (ii) raised free T3 and/or T4: T4 is almost always raised but T3 is more sensitive as there are occasional cases of isolated T3 thyrotoxicosis; (iii) TSH receptor–stimulating antibodies: should be measured routinely with T3, T4 and TSH (although the second generations of assays for these antibodies have more than 95% sensitivity and specificity, the third-generation tests have 97%–99% specificity for primary hyperthyroidism); (iv) thyroid peroxidase and thyroglobulin antibodies (less specific for Graves disease); and (v) thyroid scintiscanning with technetium-99m or iodine-131 (may be needed in thyrotoxicosis without hyperthyroidism).
- Graves disease is the most common cause of bilateral and unilateral exophthalmos. Unilateral exophthalmos occurs in 5%–15% of patients with Graves disease. The presence of anxiety, tremor of hands and loose bowel motions are consistent with hyperthyroidism.
- The management of Graves disease includes the following: (i) Control the hypothyroidism and associated systemic changes; (ii) relieve symptoms; (iii) delay the progress of comorbidities (arrhythmias, heart failure, etc.); and (iv) educate the patient about the nature of their disease, the eye changes and the treatment options available and the advantages and disadvantages of each option.
- The options of management are medical therapy (antithyroid drugs), radiotherapy or surgery (thyroidectomy).

FURTHER READINGS

Ajjan RA, Weetman AP. Techniques to quantify TSH receptor antibodies. *Nat Clin Pract Endocrinol Metab.* 2008;4(8):461–468. Review.

Anagnostis P, Adamidou F, Poulasouchidou M, Karras S. Severe eyelid oedema in Graves' ophthalmopathy. *BMJ Case Rep.* 2013;2013:bcr2013010305. Review.

Bahn RS. Graves' ophthalmopathy. *N Engl J Med.* 2010;362(8):726–738. Review.

Bartalena L, Tanda ML. Clinical practice. Graves' ophthalmopathy. *N Engl J Med.* 2009;360(10):994–1001. Review.

Brent GA. Clinical practice. Graves' disease. *N Engl J Med.* 2008;358(24):2594–2605. Review.

Cooper DS. Antithyroid drugs. *N Engl J Med.* 2005;352(9):905–917. Review.

Donangelo I, Braunstein GD. Update on subclinical hyperthyroidism. *Am Fam Physician.* 2011;83(8): 933–938. Review.

Gutch M, Sanjay S, Razi SM, Gupta KK. Thyroid acropachy: Frequently overlooked finding. *Indian J Endocrinol Metab.* 2014;18(4):590-591.

Kamminga N, Jansonius NM, Pott JW, Links TP. Unilateral proptosis: the role of medical history. *Br J Ophthalmol.* 2003;87(3):370-371.

Khalilzadeh O, Noshad S, Rashidi A, Amirzargar A. Graves' ophthalmopathy: a review of immunogenetics. *Curr Genomics.* 2011;12(8):564-575.

Kravets I. Hyperthyroidism: diagnosis and treatment. *Am Fam Physician.* 2016;93(5):363-370. Review.

Nygaard B. Hyperthyroidism in pregnancy. *BMJ Clin Evid.* 2015;2015:0611.

Reid JR, Wheeler SF. Hyperthyroidism: diagnosis and treatment. *Am Fam Physician.* 2005;72(4):623-630. Review.

Ross DS. Radioiodine therapy for hyperthyroidism. *N Engl J Med.* 2011;364(6):542-550. Review.

Smith TJ, Hegedüs L. Graves' disease. *N Engl J Med.* 2016;375(16):1552-1565. Review.

Vaidya B, Pearce SH. Diagnosis and management of thyrotoxicosis. *BMJ.* 2014;349:g5128. doi:10.1136/bmj.g5128. Review. No abstract available.

Weetman AP. Graves' disease. *N Engl J Med.* 2000;343(17):1236-1248. Review.

CASE 5.3

'Did Not Work ...'

Nardeen Ahmad, a 38-year-old pharmacist, comes in to see her general practitioner because she is suffering from facial hair and acne and progressive back pain for more than 1 year. She tried a range of methods to manage her facial hair with no success. She also noticed that her menstrual periods are not regular and sometimes she has no periods for 3 or more months.

On examination, Nardeen has a moon face, facial hair and acne. Her pulse rate is 85/min, blood pressure 160/95 mm Hg, temperature 36.8°C and respiratory rate 18/min. She has central obesity and thin extremities. Her body weight is 55 kg, height is 141 cm and BMI is 27.8. Her skin is thin and atrophied. Neurological examination reveals no neurological deficit. Cranial nerve examinations including visual field are all normal. She has proximal muscle weakness of the shoulder girdle and pelvic thigh muscles. Abdominal examination shows several purpura striae. Pelvic ultrasound is normal.

Urine test for glucose is positive.

Nardeen's blood test results are summarised in Table 5.3.1.

MRI scan of the upper abdomen shows a mass measuring 2 × 3 × 3.1 cm in the region of the right adrenal gland. The mass is located anterior and superior to the right kidney. There is no evidence of enlarged abdominal lymph nodes or other masses.

CASE DISCUSSION

Q1. On the basis of Nardeen's presentation, what is your diagnosis?

Q2. What is your differential diagnosis?

Q3. What are the key clinical features of this disease? What are the scientific bases for these features?

Q4. What is the pathophysiology underlying these changes?

Q5. What are your management goals and management options?

ANSWERS

1. The findings of moon face, facial hair and acne, central obesity and thin extremities, back pain, amenorrhoea, high blood pressure, thin skin, proximal muscle weakness, abdominal purpura striae and positive urine test for glucose together with upper limit of normal haemoglobin concentration, low serum potassium, raised fasting blood glucose level, raised blood lipids, loss of diurnal variation of the serum cortisol (at 8:00 a.m. compared to at 4:00 p.m.), elevated serum dehydroepiandrosterone

Table 5.3.1 Nardeen's blood test results

Blood test	Nardeen's results	Normal range
Haemoglobin (Hb) (g/L)	157	123–157 (female) 140–174 (male)
Serum sodium (mmol/L)	150	135–145
Serum potassium (mmol/L)	3.2	3.5–5.0
Fasting blood glucose (mmol/L)	7.9	3.3–5.8
Blood cholesterol (mmol/L)	7.5	<5.2
Serum triglyceride (mmol/L)	3.7	<2.20
Serum cortisol (nmol/L) 8:00 a.m. 4:00 p.m.	1250 1200	110–607 83–469
Serum dehydroepiandrosterone (mmol/L)	13.1	1.3–6.7
Serum testosterone (nmol/L)	5.6	<2.1 (female) 6.7–28.9 (male)
Adrenocorticotrophic hormone (ACTH) (pmol/L)	<1	1.3–16.7

sulphate (DHEAS), elevated serum testosterone and low serum adrenocorticotrophic hormone (ACTH) are suggestive of Cushing syndrome.

The MRI scan of the abdomen shows the presence of a mass (2 × 3 × 3.1 cm) in the region of the right adrenal gland. The mass is located anterior and superior to the right kidney. There is no evidence of enlarged abdominal lymph nodes or other masses. Pelvic ultrasound is normal. These radiological findings support the notion that the cause of Cushing syndrome is adenoma of the right adrenal gland.

2. The differential diagnosis includes the following:
   - Chronic alcoholism
   - Obesity
   - Primary hyperaldosteronism
   - Diabetes mellitus
   - Depression

3. Clinical picture:
   The diagnosis is based on clinical features and investigations.
   Symptoms:
   - Changes in facial appearance (facial hairs, acne)
   - Weight gain (central obesity)
   - Thin extremities
   - Thin skin and bruising
   - Depression
   - Psychosis

- Insomnia
- Back pain
- Amenorrhoea/oligomenorrhoea
- Loss of libido
- Polyuria

Signs:
- Moon face
- Plethora
- Hirsutism
- Acne
- Buffalo hump (a lump of fat at the top of the back between the shoulders)
- Central obesity
- Depression
- Psychosis
- Thin skin
- Skin infections
- Purple striae
- Pigmentation
- Osteoporosis
- Pathological fractures (vertebrae, ribs)
- Kyphosis
- Hypertension
- Proximal muscle weakness

Fig. 5.3.1 summarises major clinical manifestations of Cushing syndrome.

4. Laboratory investigations:
   - Loss of circadian rhythm: Cortisol levels are elevated at 8:00 a.m. and at 4:00 p.m.; there are no diurnal variations.
   - Midnight serum cortisol level >50 nmol/L asleep or 207 nmol/L awake is indicative of Cushing syndrome.
   - Plasma ACTH level: Low or undetectable ACTH levels <10 ng/L are indicators of non-ACTH-dependent Cushing syndrome (e.g. adrenal adenoma, adrenal carcinoma or exogenous treatment with glucocorticoids).
   - 24-hour urinary free cortisol measurement: It is a simple but not reliable test.
   - MRI scan of the adrenal: It is helpful in patients with adrenal adenoma and adrenal carcinoma. Adrenal carcinomas are usually larger and have an irregular outline, necrotic/bleeding changes and signs of infiltration or metastasis. Patients with adrenal hyperplasia will show bilateral enlargement of the adrenal glands.
   - Pituitary MRI: A pituitary adenoma may be present (Cushing disease).
   - Plasma potassium: This test should be carried out after stopping all diuretics. A low plasma potassium level is common in ectopic ACTH secretion.
   - High-dose dexamethasone suppression test: Failure of plasma cortisol suppression suggests ectopic secretion of ACTH or an adrenal tumour.

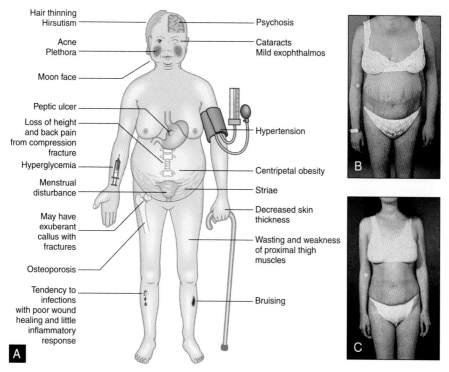

Figure 5.3.1 (A and B) Major clinical manifestations of Cushing syndrome. (C) The same patient before the development of Cushing syndrome. *(Source: Ralston S, Penman I, Strachan M, Hobson R. Davidson's Principles & Practice of Medicine. 23rd ed. UK: Elsevier; 2018.)*

- Chest X-ray: It may reveal carcinoma of the bronchus or bronchial carcinoid. Usually MRI scan of the whole lungs, mediastinum and abdomen is recommended.
- Selective catheterisation of the inferior petrosal sinus to take samples and measure ACTH together with blood samples taken from peripheral blood. A basal gradient of central ACTH:peripheral ACTH ratio of more than 2:1 is indicative of Cushing disease.

Pathological features.

Table 5.3.2 summarises the causes of Cushing and key differentiating points of each cause.

Fig. 5.3.2 summarises the possible causes of Cushing and underlying pathophysiological mechanisms.

5. Management goals:
   - Identify and manage the cause of excessive secretion of cortisol.
   - Manage the body changes caused by chronic secretion of corticosteroids such as osteoporosis.
   - Prescribe hormone replacement after surgical resection (e.g. pituitary adenoma, adrenalectomy).
   - Patients not suitable for surgical management are treated medically.
   - Provide patient education and symptomatic treatment as needed.

Table 5.3.2 Causes of Cushing and key differentiating points of each cause

Cause	Biochemical and hormonal changes	Radiological changes
1. Cushing disease[a] (pituitary adenoma)	Raised serum ACTH	MRI scan shows the pituitary adenoma
2. Ectopic secretion of ACTH[b]	Raised serum ACTH	MRI scan shows the lung or pancreatic tumour
3. Adrenal adenoma[b]	Serum ACTH is low	MRI scan shows the adrenal adenoma, the remaining adrenal gland is atrophied
4. Adrenal carcinoma[b]	Serum ACTH is low	MRI scan shows the adrenal carcinoma, the remaining adrenal gland is atrophied
5. Adrenal hyperplasia[b]	Serum ACTH is low	MRI scan shows adrenal hyperplasia
6. Chronic treatment with corticosteroids[b]	Serum ACTH is low	History of chronic treatment with corticosteroids

ACTH, adrenocorticotrophic hormone.
[a]Cushing disease.
[b]Cushing syndrome.

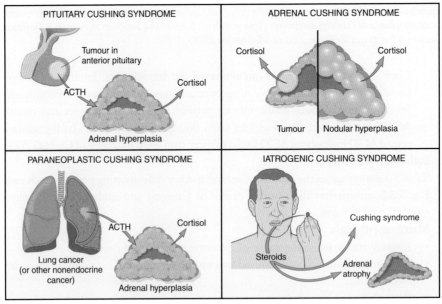

Figure 5.3.2 Possible causes of Cushing and underlying pathophysiological mechanisms. Cases due to a pituitary adenoma are known as Cushing disease. They represent the classic disease first described by Dr Harvey Cushing (1869-1939). Cushing disease is a form of Cushing syndrome. ACTH, adrenocorticotrophic hormone. *(Source: Ralston S, Penman I, Strachan M, Hobson R. Davidson's Principles & Practice of Medicine. 23rd ed. UK: Elsevier; 2018.)*

1. Surgical management:
   - Transsphenoidal resection of a pituitary adenoma in patients with Cushing disease
   - Laparoscopic adrenalectomy if remission occurs after pituitary surgery
   - Surgical resection of adrenal carcinoma
2. Medical management:
   - Hydrocortisone replacement after resection of pituitary adenoma or adrenal adenoma
   - Ketoconazole in patients with Cushing disease who are not suitable for surgical management
   - Can also use ketoconazole in patients with adrenal carcinoma who are not suitable for surgical management
   - Mitotane treatment for adrenal carcinoma
   - Bisphosphonates for the management of osteoporosis

BACK TO BASIC SCIENCES

Q1. Discuss briefly the adrenal anatomy and physiology.

The adrenal (suprarenal) glands are located superior to each kidney. Each adrenal has an outer cortex and an inner medulla. The adrenal cortex is composed of the following zones: (i) the zona glomerulosa (outer zone), (ii) the zona fasciculata (middle zone) and (ii) the zona reticularis (inner zone).

Corticosteroids are synthesised from cholesterol by the cytochrome P-450 enzymes in the adrenal gland.

1. The zona glomerulosa produces aldosterone, a mineralocorticoid hormone. Aldosterone is triggered by an increased extracellular potassium concentration and by the activation of the renin–angiotensin–aldosterone system. It promotes potassium loss and sodium retention.
2. The zona fasciculata is responsible for the synthesis of glucocorticoids. The process is controlled by the ACTH secretion from the anterior pituitary through the hypothalamic–pituitary–adrenal axis.
3. The zona reticularis is responsible for the synthesis of the dehydroepiandrosterone DHEA, DHEAS and androstenedione.

The adrenal medulla consists of the chromaffin cells, which synthesise catecholamine hormones from the amino acid tyrosine.

Q2. On the basis of the previous question, is the adrenal gland regulated only by the hypothalamic–pituitary–adrenal axis?

The different zones of the adrenal cortex are regulated by different mechanisms:

1. The zona glomerulosa is regulated by aldosterone and the renin–angiotensin–aldosterone system.
2. The zona fasciculata is regulated by the hypothalamic–pituitary–adrenal axis.

Q3. What are the key differences between Cushing disease and Cushing syndrome?
- Cushing disease refers to ACTH-dependent Cushing caused by a pituitary adenoma.
- Cushing syndrome refers to the following:
  1. Ectopic ACTH secretion
  2. Adrenal adenoma producing cortisol
  3. Adrenal carcinoma producing cortisol
  4. Excessive exogenous cortisol in patients on prolonged treatment with corticosteroids
- Cushing disease is the cause in 80% of women in ACTH-dependent cases. However, the commonest cause of all cases of Cushing is excessive exogenous treatment with corticosteroids.

Q4. Who should be referred for laboratory tests with a provisional diagnosis of Cushing?
- Patients with unusual features for their age (osteoporosis and livid striae in young men)
- Patients with multiple progressive features of Cushing syndrome
- Children with decreasing height percentile and increasing weight
- Patients with adrenal adenoma found incidentally on routine CT scan of the abdomen for other reasons

Q5. What are the diagnostic approaches for investigating such patients?
There are three important approaches:
1. It is important to confirm the diagnosis before attempting to search for the cause.
2. Factors affecting hypercortisolaemia and giving false-positive results should be considered while interpreting the results (e.g. acute intercurrent illness and intake of oral oestrogen).
3. The following tests are to be considered:
   - Low-dose dexamethasone suppression test (LDDST) or overnight dexamethasone suppression test
   - Urinary free cortisol
   - Midnight serum cortisol
   - Late-night salivary cortisol

Q6. What is the use of the high-dose dexamethasone suppression test?
This test is used to demonstrate the failure of plasma cortisol suppression in patients with ectopic ACTH secretion and patients with adrenal tumour. However, this test is no longer recommended and bilateral inferior petrosal sinus sampling is preferred instead.

Q7. What is the principle behind the bilateral inferior petrosal sinus sampling test?
The principle behind this test is to compare the ACTH gradient of the ACTH level in the petrosal sinus with the ACTH gradient in the peripheral blood. A gradient of central ACTH:peripheral ACTH of more than 2:1 is indicative of Cushing disease.

REVIEW QUESTIONS

Q1. Which *one* of the following biochemical tests can differentiate Cushing disease from ectopic ACTH production?
A. Plasma ACTH
B. Plasma potassium
C. High-dose dexamethasone suppression test
D. Urinary free cortisol

Q2. Which *one* of the following drugs *does not* interfere with the low-dose dexamethasone suppression test results?
A. Carbamazepine
B. Phenytoin
C. Phenobarbital
D. Rifampicin
E. Gentamicin

Q3. Which *one* of the following is *less likely* to be among the presenting picture of Cushing syndrome?
A. Thin skin
B. Osteoporosis
C. Hypokalemia
D. Polymenorrhoea
E. Proximal muscle atrophy

Q4. Which *one* of the following is *less likely* to be a sign of Cushing syndrome?
A. Avascular bone necrosis
B. Easy bruising
C. Buffalo hump
D. Diabetes insipidus

ANSWERS

A1. **B.** Plasma potassium is low in patients with ectopic ACTH secretion. But it is also low in 10% of patients with Cushing disease. Several procedures should be taken before conducting this test such as stopping diuretics before measuring potassium concentration. Repeated measures showing low serum potassium can be useful in such differentiation.

A2. **E.** Gentamicin is not metabolised and is excreted by the kidneys.

A3. **D.** Usually the patients have amenorrhoea or oligomenorrhoea.

A4. **D**. Diabetes mellitus, renal glycosuria, renal calculi, proximal muscle weakness, back pain and osteoporosis are more commonly seen in Cushing syndrome. Diabetes insipidus is not present.

TAKE-HOME MESSAGE

- Cushing disease refers to ACTH-dependent Cushing caused by a pituitary adenoma.
- Cushing syndrome refers to the following: (i) Ectopic ACTH secretion, (ii) adrenal adenoma producing cortisol, (iii) adrenal carcinoma producing cortisol and (iv) excessive exogenous cortisol in patients on prolonged treatment with corticosteroids.
- Cushing disease is the cause in 80% of women in ACTH-dependent cases. However, the commonest cause of all cases of Cushing is excessive exogenous treatment with corticosteroids.
- The differential diagnosis of Cushing disease/syndrome may include chronic alcoholism, obesity, primary hyperaldosteronism, diabetes mellitus and depression.
- The management goals: (i) Identify and manage the cause of excessive secretion of cortisol; (ii) manage the body changes caused by chronic secretion of corticosteroids such as osteoporosis; (iii) prescribe hormone replacement after surgical resection (e.g. pituitary adenoma, adrenalectomy); (iv) patients not suitable for surgical management are treated medically; and (v) provide patient education and symptomatic treatment as needed.

FURTHER READINGS

Biller BM, Grossman AB, Stewart PM, et al. Treatment of adrenocorticotropin-dependent Cushing's syndrome: a consensus statement. *J Clin Endocrinol Metab*. 2008;93(7):2454-2462. Review.

Loriaux DL. Diagnosis and differential diagnosis of Cushing's syndrome. *N Engl J Med*. 2017;376(15): 1451-1459. Review.

Newell-Price J, Bertagna X, Grossman AB, Nieman LK. Cushing's syndrome. *Lancet*. 2006;367(9522): 1605-1617.

Nieman LK, Biller BM, Findling JW, et al. The diagnosis of Cushing's syndrome: an Endocrine Society Clinical Practice Guideline. *J Clin Endocrinol Metab*. 2008;93(5):1526-1540.

Papanicolaou DA, Yanovski JA, Cutler Jr GB, Chrousos GP, Nieman LK. A single midnight serum cortisol measurement distinguishes Cushing's syndrome from pseudo-Cushing states. *J Clin Endocrinol Metab*. 1998;83(4):1163-1167.

Prague JK, May S, Whitelaw BC. Cushing's syndrome. *BMJ*. 2013;346:f945. Review.

Young Jr WF. Clinical practice. The incidentally discovered adrenal mass. *N Engl J Med*. 2007;356(6):601-610. Review.

CASE 5.4

'Too Tired ...'

Morrison Lawrence, a 59-year-old taxi driver, is brought to the emergency department because he is suffering from nausea, vomiting and diarrhoea for the past 16 hours. He gives a history of progressive fatigue, malaise and poor appetite for several months. He also has abdominal cramps, and has lost 6 kg in body weight over the past 5 months. On examination, his pulse rate is 100/min (standing 108/min) and blood pressure 100/68 mm Hg (standing 80/50 mm Hg). He is afebrile. His skin is tanned and he looks ill and dehydrated; his face, hands, extensor surfaces, chest and back are tanned. Cardiac examination shows normal first and second heart sounds, there are no murmurs or added sounds and the chest is bilaterally clear. On abdominal examination, there is diffuse tenderness on palpation. There is no rebound or localised guarding. Bowel sounds are hyperactive. Examination of the central nervous system is normal. Both chest X-ray and ECG are normal. Blood test results are shown in Table 5.4.1.

CASE DISCUSSION

Q1. On the basis of Morrison's presentation, what is your diagnosis?

Q2. What is your differential diagnosis?

Q3. What are the key clinical features of this disease? What are the scientific bases for these features?

Q4. What is the pathophysiology underlying these changes?

Q5. What are your management goals and management options?

ANSWERS

1. The findings of nausea, vomiting, diarrhoea, progressive fatigue, malaise, poor appetite, loss of body weight, tanned skin, orthostatic hypotension, low blood sodium, low blood glucose, high serum potassium, urea and creatinine are suggestive of the diagnosis of Addison disease (primary adrenocortical insufficiency).
2. The differential diagnosis includes the following:
   - Hyperpigmentation (tanned skin) – bronchogenic carcinoma and haemochromatosis
   - Weakness (progressive fatigue) – pseudopsychiatric disorders, myopathies, cardiac failure, renal insufficiency and hepatic and respiratory failure
   - Hypoglycaemia – fasting and overstimulation of insulin

Table 5.4.1 Morrison's blood test results

Blood test	Morrison's results	Normal range
Haemoglobin (Hb) (g/L)	106	123–157 (females) 140–174 (males)
White blood cell count (WBC) ($\times 10^9$/L)	6.60	4.0–10.0
Platelet count ($\times 10^9$/L)	250	130–400
Serum sodium (mmol/L)	128	135–145
Serum potassium (mmol/L)	5.9	3.5–5.0
Blood urea (mmol/L)	11.0	2.5–8.0
Serum creatinine (μmol/L)	140	70–120 (males) 50–90 (females)
Blood glucose (fasting) (mml/L)	3.0	3.3–5.8
Bicarbonate (HCO_3) (mmol/L)	20	24–30
Serum calcium (total) (mmol/L)	2.89	2.18–2.58

- Low serum sodium (hyponatraemia) – use of diuretics, inappropriate ADH secretion, salt-losing nephritis, oedema, heart failure, diarrhoea, hypothyroidism, cirrhosis and major surgery
- High serum potassium (hyperkalaemia) – chronic renal failure, gastrointestinal bleeding, rhabdomyolysis, angiotensin-converting enzyme inhibitor and spironolactone

The following are keys for the diagnosis of Addison disease:

- Weakness, anorexia, fatigability, nausea, vomiting, diarrhoea, abdominal pain and amenorrhoea
- Increased skin pigmentation, especially the skin of creases, pressure points, the nipples and scars of old surgery
- Hypotension and dehydration
- Low serum sodium and low blood glucose
- High serum potassium, urea and creatinine
- Low plasma cortisol level or failure to rise after administration of cosyntropin (synthetic adrenocorticotrophic hormone [ACTH])
- Elevated plasma ACTH levels

3. Clinical picture:

Symptoms:

- Asthenia
- Weakness
- Malaise
- Weight loss
- Anorexia
- Nausea

- Vomiting
- Diarrhoea
- Abdominal pain
- Depression
- Confusion
- Joint pains
- Amenorrhoea
- Syncope (postural drop of blood pressure)
- Hypotension
- Vitiligo
- Dehydration

Signs:

- Weight loss
- Generalised wasting
- Increased pigmentation of the skin, particularly palmar creases, scars and the areola, and buccal pigmentation
- Postural drop of blood pressure
- Dehydration

Adrenal crisis:

This is an emergency situation that needs hospital admission and immediate medical care. The patient presents with profound asthenia, severe pain in the abdomen, lower back and legs, peripheral vascular collapse, renal failure and azotaemia. The patient may be feverish or afebrile. Serum cortisol is low, and serum ACTH is raised.

4. Laboratory findings:
   - Moderate neutropenia, lymphocytosis and eosinophilic count >300/μL
   - Hyponatraemia
   - Fasting blood glucose level low
   - Hyperkalaemia
   - Hypercalcaemia
   - Raised blood urea and creatinine
   - Plasma cortisol level <100 nmol/L during the day, and ACTH >80 ng/L (are highly supportive of the diagnosis)
   - Antiadrenal antibodies detected in autoimmune Addison disease (detected in 50% of patients)
   - The short ACTH stimulation test: An absent or impaired cortisol response, which confirms the presence of hypoadrenalism (but this test has its limitations and cannot differentiate between Addison disease from ACTH deficiency and iatrogenic suppression from cortisol medication)
   - Radiological investigation:
     - Chest radiograph: Pulmonary tuberculosis, fungal infection or cancer
     - Abdominal CT scan: Noncalcified adrenal in autoimmune Addison disease; calcification of the adrenals noted in tuberculosis, haemorrhage, fungal infection and pheochromocytoma

Pathophysiology:

Both mineralocorticoids and glucocorticoids are deficient.

1. Mineralocorticoid deficiency:

   The physiological functions of mineralocorticoids are to stimulate sodium reabsorption and potassium excretion. The deficiency results in raised serum potassium and loss of sodium → postural drop of blood pressure, weakness, asthenia, decreased circulating volume and circulatory collapse.

   Note that when adrenal insufficiency is secondary to inadequate ACTH production (secondary adrenal insufficiency), the electrolyte levels are often normal or only mildly affected.

2. Glucocorticoid deficiency:

   The deficiency of glucocorticoids results in a number of dysfunctions including hypotension, severe insulin sensitivity and disturbance of fat and protein metabolism → decreased glycogen stored in the liver and hypoglycaemia.

   There is also decreased resistance to infection and decreased resistance to other stresses as well as decreased cardiac functions.

   The decreased glucocorticoids → stimulation of the pituitary gland → increased production of ACTH and increased blood beta-lipoprotein (has a melanocyte-stimulating action).

   These two substances, high ACTH and high blood beta-lipoprotein → increased pigmentation of the skin, darkness of the areola and darkness of the skin creases and scars.

5. Management goals:
   - Replacement of deficient hormones (glucocorticoids, mineralocorticoids and adrenal androgens)
   - Management of intercurrent illnesses
   - Patient education

BACK TO BASIC SCIENCES

Q1. What are the main differences between primary and secondary adrenal insufficiency?

Table 5.4.2 summarises the differences between primary adrenal failure and secondary adrenal failure.

Table 5.4.2 Differences between primary adrenal failure and secondary adrenal failure

Item	Primary adrenal failure (Addison disease)	Secondary adrenal failure
Causes	May be acute or chronic Destruction of the adrenal gland by autoimmune disease >90%, HIV/AIDS, tuberculosis, cytomegalovirus infection, lymphoma, amyloidosis, scleroderma, coccidioidomycosis	1. Hypothalamic–pituitary disease (inadequate ACTH production) 2. Long-term steroid therapy → suppression of hypothalamic–pituitary adrenal axis

Table 5.4.2 Differences between primary adrenal failure and secondary adrenal failure—cont'd

Item	Primary adrenal failure (Addison disease)	Secondary adrenal failure
ACTH	ACTH ↑↑↑	ACTH ↓↓↓
Hormonal deficiency	Mineralocorticoids, glucocorticoids and androgens are reduced	Mineralocorticoids are relatively preserved (serum sodium may be normal)
Skin/scars	Increased pigmentation of skin creases, scars and areola No loss of axillary and pubic hair	Usually is part of panhypopituitarism – white skin, loss of axillary hair and pubic hair

ACTH, adrenocorticotrophic hormone.

Q2. How would you explain increased pigmentation of skin creases in Addison disease?

The lack of production of glucocorticoids in Addison disease → increased production of ACTH and increased blood beta-lipoprotein → both result in increased pigmentation of the skin, scars and creases of the hands and areola.

In addition to elevated ACTH and elevated blood beta-lipoprotein, there is elevated melanocyte-stimulating hormone, which also contributes to increased pigmentation.

Q3. What are the main causes of Addison disease?

1. Autoimmune adrenal destruction (this is the most common cause in the United States, the United Kingdom and Australia; this disorder may be associated with other autoimmune disorders [hypoparathyroidism, type 1 diabetes mellitus, vitiligo, celiac disease, testicular failure, ovarian failure, pernicious anaemia])
2. Tuberculosis
3. Bilateral adrenal haemorrhage (sepsis, heparin-associated thrombocytopenia, antiphospholipid antibody syndrome, surgery, meningococcemia) (in case of haemorrhage due to meningitis caused by meningococcemia, the syndrome is known as Waterhouse–Friderichsen syndrome)
4. Combination of Addison disease and hypothyroidism (Schmidt syndrome)
5. Cytomegalovirus infection (in patients with AIDS)
6. Metastatic cancer
7. Lymphoma
8. Amyloid disease
9. Coccidioidomycosis
10. Scleroderma

Q4. What are the causes of acute adrenocortical insufficiency?

- Patients with chronic adrenal insufficiency (acute on top of chronic)
- Bilateral adrenal haemorrhage (e.g. use of anticoagulants)
- Bilateral adrenalectomy or removal of adrenal tumour that has suppressed the other adrenal glands
- Bilateral injury of adrenal glands

REVIEW QUESTIONS

Q1. Which *one* of the following is *not* correct about primary adrenocortical failure (Addison disease)?
A. A low serum cortisol at 09:00 hours
B. Elevated ACTH
C. Poor cortisol response to exogenous ACTH
D. Loss of axillary and pubic hair
E. Is an autoimmune disease

Q2. Which *one* of the following pairs (adrenal gland zone/area–substance produced) is *not* correct?
A. Zona glomerulosa–aldosterone
B. Zona reticularis–dehydroepiandrosterone
C. Zona fasciculata–cortisol
D. Zona glomerulosa–glucocorticoid cortisol
E. Adrenal medulla–adrenaline

Q3. Which *one* of the following is correct in secondary adrenal failure?
A. ACTH levels are increased.
B. Mineralocorticoids are relatively preserved.
C. The skin is hyperpigmented.
D. There is no loss of axillary hair.

Q4. Which *one* of the following is *not* a cause of Addison disease?
A. Autoimmunity
B. Tuberculosis
C. *E. coli* infection
D. Adrenal haemorrhage
E. Cytomegalovirus infection

Q5. Which *one* of the following biochemical changes is *less likely* to be found in Addison disease?
A. Hyperkalaemia
B. Low plasma renin
C. Type IV renal tubular acidosis
D. Low plasma glucose
E. Hypercalcaemia

ANSWERS

A1. **D.** There is no loss of axillary or pubic hair in primary adrenocortical failure. Loss of axillary and pubic hair may occur in secondary adrenal failure.

A2. **D.** The zona fasciculata produces glucocorticoids. The zona glomerulosa is responsible for secreting the mineralocorticoid hormones; involved in regulating fluid balance.

A3. **B.** In secondary adrenal failure, the mineralocorticoids are relatively preserved.

A4. **C.** *E. coli* infection is not a cause of Addison disease.

A5. **B.** Loss of mineralocorticoids in Addison disease → increased sodium loss → decreased sodium level → decreased extracellular fluid volume → hypotension → increased plasma renin. This may occur years before the corticosteroid deficiency.

Remember that in Addison disease, there is ↑ serum potassium + ↑ ACTH levels and ↑ blood renin.

TAKE-HOME MESSAGE

- The diagnosis of Addison disease is based on the following: (i) Clinical picture: weakness, anorexia, fatigability, nausea, vomiting, diarrhoea, abdominal pain and amenorrhoea; (ii) increased skin pigmentation, especially the skin of creases, pressure points, the nipples and scars of old surgery; (iii) hypotension and dehydration; (iv) low serum sodium and low blood glucose; (v) high serum potassium, urea and creatinine; (vi) low plasma cortisol level or failure to rise after administration of cosyntropin (synthetic ACTH); and (vii) elevated plasma ACTH levels.
- The three common causes of Addison disease are (i) autoimmune adrenal destruction: this is the most common cause in the United States, the United Kingdom and Australia; (ii) tuberculosis; and (iii) bilateral adrenal haemorrhage.
- It is important to differentiate between primary and secondary causes of adrenal failure.
- Management includes the following goals: (i) Replacement of deficient hormones (glucocorticoids, mineralocorticoids and adrenal androgens), (ii) management of intercurrent illnesses and (iii) patient education.

FURTHER READINGS

Achermann JC, Silverman BL. Dehydroepiandrosterone replacement for patients with adrenal insufficiency. *Lancet.* 2001;357(9266):1381-1382. Review.

Baker Jr JR. Autoimmune endocrine disease. *JAMA.* 1997;278(22):1931-1937. Review.

Davenport J, Kellerman C, Reiss D, Harrison L. Addison's disease. *Am Fam Physician.* 1991;43(4):1338-1342. Review.

Melby JC. Assessment of adrenocortical function. *N Engl J Med.* 1971;285(13):735-739. Review.

Stulberg DL, Clark N, Tovey D. Common hyperpigmentation disorders in adults: Part I. Diagnostic approach, café au lait macules, diffuse hyperpigmentation, sun exposure, and phototoxic reactions. *Am Fam Physician.* 2003;68(10):1955-1960. Review.

Stulberg DL, Clark N, Tovey D. Common hyperpigmentation disorders in adults: Part II. Melanoma, seborrheic keratoses, acanthosis nigricans, melasma, diabetic dermopathy, tinea versicolor, and postinflammatory hyperpigmentation. *Am Fam Physician.* 2003;68(10):1963-1968. Review.

CASE 5.5

'They Rushed Me to the Emergency Room ...'

Laura Collin, a 12-year-old primary school student, is brought by her parents to the emergency department because Laura has vomited and has upper abdominal pain and shortness of breath for the past 2 hours. She has been passing urine more frequently for the past few days. The mother responds to the emergency doctor's questions and says, 'Laura had an upper respiratory infection and mild loose bowel motions about 3 weeks ago and was seen by the general practitioner, and she was prescribed antibiotics.' Although she has recovered from the upper respiratory infection, she always feels tired. On examination, Laura looks ill; she seems confused with a fluctuation in her conscious state. Her pulse rate is 110/min, blood pressure 100/60 mm Hg, temperature 37.6°C and respiratory rate 28 (Kussmaul acidotic breathing). She is dehydrated (dry tongue, decreased skin turgor). Abdominal examination shows tenderness in the epigastrium, no rigidity and sluggish bowel sounds. Neurological examination shows drowsy pupils that are equal in size bilaterally and reactive. There is no focal neurological deficit. Blood test results are shown in Table 5.5.1.

Liver function tests: Normal
Urinalysis: Ketones 4+

CASE DISCUSSION

Q1. On the basis of Laura's presentation, what is your diagnosis?

Q2. What is your differential diagnosis?

Q3. What are the key clinical features of this disease? What are the scientific bases for these features?

Q4. What is the pathophysiology underlying these changes?

Q5. What are your management goals and management options?

ANSWERS

1. The findings of vomiting, upper abdominal pain, shortness of breath, passing urine more frequently, fluctuation of her mental state, history of upper respiratory tract infection 3 weeks earlier and loose bowel motions, clinical picture showing Kussmaul acidotic breathing, dehydration (dry tongue, decreased skin turgor), tenderness in the epigastrium, sluggish bowel sounds, drowsiness and no focal neurological signs together with the results of her blood tests showing high blood glucose, leukocytosis and presence of ketone bodies in urine and the changes of blood gases are all suggestive of diabetic ketoacidosis (DKA).

Table 5.5.1 Laura's blood test results

Blood test	Laura's test	Normal range
Haemoglobin (Hb) (g/L)	138	123–157 (female) 140–174 (male)
White blood cell count ($\times 10^9$/L)	13.0	4.0–10.0
Platelet count ($\times 10^9$/L)	410	130–400
Random blood glucose (mmol/L)	17.6	3.3–5.8
HbA$_{1c}$ (%)	14.2	4–6
Serum sodium (mmol/L)	137	135–145
Serum potassium (mmol/L)	4.4	3.5–5.0
Serum chloride (mmol/L)	95	98–106
Blood urea (mmol/L)	6.0	2.5–8.0
Blood creatinine (μmol/L)	77	70–120 (male) 50–90 (female)
Arterial blood gases pH pCO$_2$ HCO$_3^-$	7.2 12 mm Hg 9 mmol/L	7.35–7.45 35–45 mm Hg 22–26 mmol/L
Anion gap (mmol/L)	33.0	8–16

HbA$_{1c}$, haemoglobin A$_{1c}$.

While this is not the typical presentation of type 1 diabetes mellitus, DKA may be precipitated by infection and may be the first manifestation of type 1 diabetes mellitus. Type 1 diabetes presents initially with ketoacidosis in 15%–67% of cases.

2. The differential diagnosis includes the following:
- Hyperglycaemia: Type 2 diabetes mellitus, medications such as corticosteroids, Cushing syndrome, acromegaly, pheochromocytoma and glucagonoma
- Metabolic acidosis from other causes such as alcoholic ketoacidosis
- Renal glycosuria: Genetic, Fanconi syndrome, chronic kidney disease and pregnancy
- Polyuria: Diabetes insipidus, hypercalcaemia and psychogenic polydipsia

3. Symptoms and signs:
- Increased thirst (polydipsia)
- Increased urination (polyuria)
- Increased appetite (polyphagia)
- Weight loss
- Ketoacidosis (nausea, vomiting, abdominal pain)
- Blurred vision
- Kussmaul breathing
- Drowsiness

- Nocturnal enuresis
- Postural hypotension

4. Laboratory findings:

The World Health Organization diagnostic criteria for diabetes are as follows:
- Fasting plasma glucose ≥7.0 mmol/L
- Random plasma glucose ≥11.1 mmol/L
- Haemoglobin A_{1c} (HbA$_{1c}$) ≥6.5% (48 mmol/mol)

Pathophysiological features:
- DKA is usually precipitated by infection (30%), error in the management of type 1 diabetes (15%) and newly diagnosed type 1 diabetes (10%).
- DKA is a life-threatening medical condition requiring hospital treatment. It is the result of the development of metabolic acidosis with plasma bicarbonate less than 15 mmol/L.
- In patients newly diagnosed with type 1 diabetes mellitus, the absence of insulin is a triggering stimulus together with intercurrent infection → ↑ triglyceride breakdown (to provide energy instead of glucose) → ↑ ketone body production (as a result of the breakdown of triglyceride) + ↑ hepatic glucose output and inhibition of peripheral glucose uptake → hyperglycaemia + increased ketone bodies in blood + acidosis.
- Hyperglycaemia → thirst, polyuria, dehydration and drowsiness.
- Increased ketone bodies in the blood → physiological response to get rid of ketone bodies by secreting ketone bodies in the stomach, urine and other body fluids → presence of ketone bodies in the stomach irritates the stomach → abdominal pain, nausea and vomiting.
- Increased ketone bodies in blood → acidosis, changes in blood pH, increased respiratory rate and Kussmaul breathing (the aim is to get rid of ketone bodies via the lungs).
- Increased ketone bodies in blood → increased excretion of ketone bodies in urine (again as a protective mechanism).

5. Management goals:
- Correct dehydration and electrolyte imbalance.
- Control blood glucose level and maintain it within the normal range (soluble insulin + 5% glucose in a drip).
- Correct acidosis and maintain blood pH within the normal range.
- Control any infections (broad-spectrum antibiotics).
- Monitor the cardiorespiratory system, haemodynamic changes, fluid balance, renal functions and clinical improvement.
- Watch for complications.
- Educate the patient and family.
- Prepare the patient for discharge and general practitioner follow-up.

Different types of insulin that may be used in the management of patients with type 1 diabetes are shown in Table 5.5.2.

Table 5.5.2 Types of insulin

Insulin type	Generic name	Preprandial injection timing[a] (h)	Onset[a] (h)	Peak[a] (h)	Duration[a] (h)	Blood glucose (BG) nadir[a] (h)
Rapid acting	Lispro[b]	0–0.2	0.1–0.5	0.5–2	<5	2–4
	Aspart[c]	0–0.2	0.1–0.3	0.6–3	3–5	1–3
	Glulisine[d]	0–0.25 (15 min before a meal or within 20 min of starting a meal)	0.15–0.3	0.5–1.5	1–5.3	2–4
Short acting	Regular	0.5–1	0.3–1	2–6	4–8	3–7
Intermediate acting	Lente	0.5–1	1–2	4–12	≤16	Before next meal
	NPH	0.5–1	1–3	6–15	16–26	6–13
Long acting	Ultralente	0.5–1	4–6	8–30	24–36	10–28
	Glargine[e]	Once daily[f]; evening meal or bedtime: twice daily; 12 hourly	1.1–4	No peak	10.8 to >24	Before next dose
	Detemir	Once daily[f]; evening meal or bedtime: twice daily; 12 hourly	1.1–4	No peak	12–24	Before next dose
Human premixed NPH/regular	70/30	0.5–1	0.5–1	2–12	14–24	3–12
NPH/regular	50/50	0.5–1	0.5–1	2–5	14–24	3–12
Insulin analogue premixed Lispro protamine/lispro	75/25	0.25	0.15–0.25	1	14–24	–
Aspart protamine/aspart	70/30	0.25	0.15–0.3	2–4	24	–

70/30, 70% NPH, 30% regular or 70% NPL/30% aspart; 50/50, 50% NPH, 50% regular; 75/25, 75% NPL, 25% lispro; 70/30, 70% NPA, 30% aspart; NPA, neutral protamine aspart; NPH, neutral protamine Hagedorn; NPL, neutral protamine lispro.

Note: Do not mix glargine, detemir or ultralente insulins with other insulins.

[a] Time profiles depend on several factors, including dose, anatomic site of injection, method (subcutaneous, intramuscular or intravenous; above-mentioned profiles are for subcutaneous injections), duration of diabetes, types of diabetes, degree of insulin resistance, level of physical activity, presence of obesity and body temperature. Sometimes ranges are wide to include data from several separate studies. Preprandial injection timing depends on premeal BG values and insulin type. If BG is low, it may be necessary to inject insulin and eat immediately (carbohydrate portion of meal first). If BG is high, it may be necessary to delay meal after insulin injection and eat carbohydrate portion last.
[b] Insulin analogue with reversal of lysine and proline at positions 28 and 29 on the B-chain of the insulin molecule.
[c] Insulin analogue with substitution of aspartic acid for proline at position 28 on the B-chain of the insulin molecule.
[d] Insulin analogue with substitution of lysine for asparagine at position 3 on the B-chain and glutamic acid for lysine at position 29 on the B-chain of the insulin molecule.
[e] Insulin analogue with substitution of glycine for asparagine at position 21 on the A-chain and addition of two arginines to the carboxyl terminus of the B-chain of the insulin molecule.
[f] Administer at same time each day, unrelated to meals. Morning administration may result in greater glucose lowering and less nocturnal hypoglycaemia.
Source: Andreoli TE, Benjamin IJ, Griggs RC, Wing EJ; Andreoli and Carpenter's Cecil Essentials of Medicine. 8th ed. Philadelphia, PA: Elsevier; 2010.

BACK TO BASIC SCIENCES

Q1. What is the pathology underlying type 1 diabetes mellitus?
- In type 1 diabetes mellitus, there is hyperglycaemia secondary to inadequate production of insulin by the beta-cells of Langerhans.
- The destruction of beta-cells is the result of T-cell-mediated autoimmune destruction and is associated with circulating autoantibodies to beta-cell antigens.

Q2. What is the role of cellular autoimmunity in the pathogenesis of type 1 diabetes mellitus?
- The destruction of beta-cells in the pancreas is mediated by T-cells (CD4$^+$, CD8$^+$) that infiltrated the islets and cause 'insulitis'.
- The progression of the disease can be delayed with immunosuppressive drugs (inhibit T-cell functions).

Q3. What is the role of autoantibodies in the pathogenesis of type 1 diabetes mellitus?
- The role of autoantibodies in the pathogenesis of type 1 diabetes mellitus is uncertain.
- There is no evidence that autoantibodies are involved in the destruction of the beta-cells.
- These autoantibodies may include the following:
  - Islet cell antibodies (ICA)
  - Islet cell autoantigens (IAA)
  - Glutamate decarboxylase 65 (GADA)
  - Tyrosine phosphatase 1A-2 (1A2A)
- Measurement of IAA, GADA and 1A2A can detect autoimmunity in 80% of patients and the risk of developing type 1 diabetes mellitus.

Q4. What is the role of the HLA system in the development of type 1 diabetes mellitus?
HLA region on chromosome 6p21 (HLA-DR3, HLA-DR4), specifically HLA-DRB1-DO81 haplotypes), increases the susceptibility for the development of type 1 diabetes.

Q5. What are the essential features for the diagnosis of type 1 diabetes mellitus?
- Polyuria, polydipsia and weight loss
- A random plasma glucose ≥11.1 mmol/L
- Plasma glucose ≥7.0 mmol/L after an overnight fasting
- Ketonaemia and ketonuria

Q6. What are the complications of type 1 diabetes mellitus?
- Diabetic ketoacidosis
- Hypoglycaemia
- Diabetic retinopathy
- Nephropathy

- Diabetic atherosclerosis
- Neuropathy
- Cataract
- Dupuytren contracture
- Carpal tunnel syndrome

Q7. How would you explain nausea, vomiting and abdominal pain in DKA?

- Absence of insulin → shift in the metabolism to use fat as a source of energy instead of carbohydrates → breakdown of fat → ketone body formation.
- Ketone bodies are increased in the blood → change in blood pH → the body tries to get rid of ketone bodies by secreting them in urine → ketone bodies detected in urine + secretion of ketone bodies into the stomach → ketone bodies irritate gastric mucosa → nausea, vomiting and abdominal pain.
- Also, vomiting → get rid of stomach content and ketone bodies in the stomach → correction of blood pH.

REVIEW QUESTIONS

Q1. Regarding haemoglobulin A_{1c} (HbA_{1c}), which *one* of the following is *not* correct?
A. HbA_{1c} of ≥6.5% denotes an increased risk of diabetes.
B. It can be used as a diagnostic test for diabetes.
C. The HbA_{1c} target in diabetic children (<5-year-olds) is <9.0%.
D. The HbA_{1c} target in diabetic children (5- to 12-year-olds) is <8.0%.

Q2. Regarding factors interfering with achieving glycaemic target in adolescents with type 1 diabetes, which *one* of the following is *not* correct?
A. Family dysfunction
B. Adolescent noncompliance
C. Psychiatric disorders/eating disorders
D. Meal planning
E. Celiac disease

Q3. Regarding diabetic ketoacidosis (DKA), which *one* of the following is *not* correct?
A. In adults, fluids and insulin are calculated on a per kilogram basis.
B. DKA is the presenting feature in 15%–60% of children with type 1 diabetes.
C. The most serious complication of DKA in children is cerebral oedema.
D. Insulin omission during intercurrent infection is a common cause of DKA.

ANSWERS

A1. **A.** HbA_{1c} ≥6.5% is diagnostic of diabetes. HbA_{1c} of 5.7%–6.4% denotes an increased risk of diabetes.

A2. **D.** The factors interfering with achieving glycaemic target in adolescents may include insulin resistance of puberty, hypothyroidism/hyperthyroidism, celiac disease or malabsorption, chronic infections, inadequate knowledge about diabetes, lack of appropriate parental supervision, family dysfunction, adolescent noncompliance, psychiatric disorders, eating disorders and depression.

Meal planning and regular monitoring of blood glucose level should help in achieving the glycaemic target.

A3. **A.** In children, not adults, the fluid and insulin requirements are calculated on a per kilogram basis.

TAKE-HOME MESSAGE

- DKA may be precipitated by infection and may be the first manifestation of type 1 diabetes mellitus. Type 1 diabetes presents initially with ketoacidosis in 15%–67% of cases.
- The essential features for the diagnosis of type 1 diabetes mellitus are (i) polyuria, polydipsia and weight loss; (ii) a random plasma glucose $\geq$11.1 mmol/L; (iii) plasma glucose $\geq$7.0 mmol/L after an overnight fasting; and (iv) ketonaemia and ketonuria.
- HLA region on chromosome 6p21 (HLA-DR3, HLA-DR4), specifically HLA-DRB1-DO81 haplotypes), increases the susceptibility for the development of type 1 diabetes.
- Environmental factors play a role in the development of type 1 diabetes mellitus.
- The role of autoantibodies in the pathogenesis of type 1 diabetes mellitus is uncertain.
- These autoantibodies may include ICA, IAA, GADA and 1A2A.
- HbA_{1c} >6.5% is diagnostic of diabetes. HbA_{1c} of 5.7%–6.4% denotes an increased risk of diabetes.
- The management goals of DKA are (i) correct dehydration and electrolyte imbalance; (ii) control blood glucose level and maintain it within the normal range (soluble insulin + 5% glucose in a drip); (iii) correct acidosis and maintain blood pH within the normal range; (iv) control any infections (broad-spectrum antibiotics); (v) monitor cardiorespiratory system, haemodynamic changes, fluid balance, renal functions and clinical improvement; (vi) watch for complications; (vii) educate the patient and family; and (viii) prepare the patient for discharge and general practitioner follow-up.

FURTHER READINGS

Atkinson MA, Eisenbarth GS, Michels AW. Type 1 diabetes. *Lancet.* 2014;383(9911):69-82.
Jacobson AM. The psychological care of patients with insulin-dependent diabetes mellitus. *N Engl J Med.* 1996;334(19):1249-1253. Review.
Pickup JC. Insulin-pump therapy for type 1 diabetes mellitus. *N Engl J Med.* 2012;366(17):1616-1624. Review.
Rewers M, Ludvigsson J. Environmental risk factors for type 1 diabetes. *Lancet.* 2016;387(10035):2340-2348.

CASE 5.6

'Trying Hard to Lose Weight ...'

Maria Walker, a 55-year-old school manager, presents to her general practitioner because she is suffering from generalised fatigue and increased frequency of passing urine. She has been on treatment for high blood pressure and increased blood lipid for more than 7 years. She does not exercise, although sometimes she has time to go walking for a few kilometres during the weekends. She has not seen her general practitioner for the past 3 months. On examination, her pulse rate is 100/min (regular), blood pressure 160/90 mm Hg, temperature 36.8°C and respiratory rate 20/min. Her body weight is 95 kg, her height 165 and body mass index (BMI) 34.9 kg/m^2. Her waist circumference is 97 cm, hip circumference 106 cm and waist:hip ratio 0.91. Apart from her high blood pressure, the rest of the systemic examination is normal. Urinalysis shows glucose +++ and no ketone bodies. Blood test results are shown in Table 5.6.1.

Electrocardiogram: Normal

CASE DISCUSSION

Q1. On the basis of Maria's presentation, what is your diagnosis?

Q2. What is your differential diagnosis?

Q3. What are the key clinical features of this disease? What are the scientific bases for these features?

Q4. What is the pathophysiology underlying these changes?

Q5. What are your management goals and management options?

ANSWERS

1. The findings of generalised fatigue, increased frequency of passing urine, on a background of hypertension, hyperlipidaemia for 7 years and obesity (BMI of 34.9), increased waist circumference and hip circumference and a lack of exercise together with glycosuria +++ and a fasting blood glucose of 7.8 mmol/L are all suggestive of the diagnosis of metabolic syndrome and type 2 diabetes mellitus.

2. The differential diagnosis:
   - Hyperglycaemia – type 1 diabetes mellitus, Cushing syndrome, acromegaly, somatostatinoma, pheochromocytoma and drugs such as corticosteroids, phenytoin and oral contraception
   - Other causes of hyperglycaemia – subtotal pancreatectomy, chronic pancreatitis, haemochromatosis, cirrhosis and gestational diabetes
   - Glycosuria (nondiabetic) – Fanconi syndrome, chronic renal failure and pregnancy

Table 5.6.1 Maria's blood test results

Blood test	Maria's results	Normal range
Haemoglobin (Hb) (g/L)	135	123–157 (female) 140–174 (male)
White blood cell count ($\times$ 10^9/L)	6.0	4.0–10.0
Platelet count ($\times$ 10^9/L)	250	130–400
Fasting blood glucose (mmol/L)	7.8	3.3–5.8
Total cholesterol (mmol/L)	7.1	<5.2
HDL cholesterol (mmol/L)	0.88	>1.00
LDL cholesterol (mmol/L)	4.62	<2.00
Blood triglycerides (mmol/L)	3.5	<2.20
Blood urea (mmol/L)	5.7	2.5–8.0
Blood creatinine (μmol/L)	70	70–120 (male) 50–90 (female)

3. Symptoms and signs:
   - Polyuria
   - Polydipsia (increased thirst)
   - Weakness
   - Blurred vision
   - Obesity
   - Peripheral neuropathy
   - Often asymptomatic
4. Laboratory findings:
   - Fasting and 2-hour postprandial blood glucose level
   - HbA_{1c}
   - Urinalysis for microproteinuria
   - Blood urea
   - Creatinine
   - Blood electrolytes
   - Liver function tests
   - Ultrasound of liver (if the liver is palpable to assess fatty infiltration of the liver)
   - Blood cholesterol
   - Blood triglycerides

Pathophysiology of type 2 diabetes: The main pathophysiological defects in type 2 diabetes mellitus are as follows:
   - Delayed insulin secretion by the beta-cells
   - Abnormal postprandial suppression of glucagon secretion by alpha-cells

These two abnormalities explain the postprandial hyperglycaemia.

The pathophysiological changes in type 2 diabetes mellitus may include the following:
   - Amyloid deposition and decreased function of beta-cells
   - Increased apoptosis of beta-cells in diabetes and decreased functional mass of the function of the islet of Langerhans

- Abnormal regulation of glucagon secretion from an inherited defect of alpha-cells
- Probable decrease in the intra-islet insulin (because of beta-cell defect) → impaired suppression of alpha-cells (the alpha-cells are normally suppressed by insulin) → exacerbation of hyperglycaemia due to paradoxical hyperglucagonaemia → failure to counter-regulate high blood glucose → high blood glucose.

The early abnormalities in the pathogenesis of type 2 diabetes are as follows:

- Normally insulin is secreted in a pulsatile manner; this pulsatility is dysregulated in patients with type 2 diabetes and their first-degree relatives (it is an early abnormality in type 2 diabetes).
- The ability of insulin to stimulate glucose uptake and suppress glucose release is reduced (known as insulin resistance). This is the second early abnormality that contributes to the pathogenesis of type 2 diabetes.
- The genetic susceptibility affects beta-cell function rather than insulin signalling. There are still gaps in our understanding of the role of genetics in the development of type 2 diabetes mellitus.

Differences between type 1 and type 2 diabetes are shown in Table 5.6.2.

5. Management goals:
   - Weight loss and exercise
   - Nonpharmacological approach, nutrition education and lifestyle changes
   - Patient education about the nature of the disease, management options, complications and prevention issues
   - Bariatric surgical procedures for obese (restriction and bypass)
   - Oral hypoglycaemic agents (Table 5.6.3)
   - A combination of oral hypoglycaemic agents and insulin
   - Self-monitoring of blood glucose

Table 5.6.2 Key differences between type 1 and type 2 diabetes mellitus

	Type 1	Type 2
Age at onset	Childhood or early adulthood, but can be manifested at any age	Middle age or older, but can be manifested in obese children and adolescents
Family history/genetic factors	Genetic risk defined, but most cases are sporadic	Strong genetic component, polygenic in most cases
Environmental triggers	Largely unknown	Obesity, sedentary lifestyle
Requirement for insulin therapy	Universal	Variable
Frequency among people with diabetes	5%–10%	~90%
Associated disorders	Autoimmunity, especially thyroid, other endocrine disorders	Hypertension, dyslipidaemia, metabolic syndrome, polycystic ovary syndrome

Source: Goldman L, Schafer AI. Goldman-Cecil Medicine. 25th ed. Elsevier; 2016.

Table 5.6.3 Oral hypoglycaemic agents used in managing type 2 diabetes

	Sulphonylureas	Biguanides	α-Glucosidase inhibitors	Thiazolidinediones	Meglitinides	D-Phenyl alanine derivatives
Generic name	Glimepiride Glyburide: micronised, nonmicronised Glipizide, glipizide XL Chlorpropamide Tolbutamide	Metformin Metformin XR	Acarbose Miglitol	Rosiglitazone Pioglitazone	Repaglinide	Nateglinide
Mode of action	↑↑ Pancreatic insulin secretion chronically ↑ Tissue insulin sensitivity	↓↓ HGP ↓ Peripheral IR ↓ Intestinal glucose absorption	Delays PP digestion of carbohydrates and absorption of glucose leading to ↓↓ PP hyperglycaemia	↓↓ Peripheral IR ↑↑ Glucose disposal ↓ HGP	↑↑ Pancreatic insulin secretion acutely	↑↑ Pancreatic insulin secretion acutely
Preferred patient type	Diagnosis age >30 years, lean, diabetes <5 years, insulinopenic	Overweight, IR, fasting hyperglycaemia, dyslipidaemia	PP hyperglycaemia	Overweight, IR, dyslipidaemia, renal dysfunction	PP hyperglycaemia, insulinopenic	PP hyperglycaemia, insulinopenic
Therapeutic effects ↓ HbA$_{1c}$[a] (%)	1–2	1–2	0.5–1	0.8–1.6 (2.6 with 45 mg pioglitazone monotherapy, in newly diagnosed)	1–2	1–2
↓ FPG[b] (mg/dL)	50–70	50–80	15–30	25–50	40–80	40–80
↓ PPG[b] (mg/dL)	~90	80	40–50	–	30	30
Insulin levels	↑	–	–	–	↑	↑
Weight	↑	↓	–	↑	↑	↑
Lipids		↓ LDL ↓↓ TG	↓ TG	LDL$_3$, TG (rosiglitazone) ↓↓ TG (pioglitazone) ↑ HDL (both)		

Class	Agent	Mechanism of action	Side effects	Route of administration	Dose(s)/day	Maximum daily	Dose (mg)
			Hypoglycaemia, weight gain, GI side effects	Oral	1–3	Depends on agent	
			Diarrhoea, abdominal discomfort, lactic acidosis. Contraindicated: Cr >1.5 mg/dL (men), >1.4 mg/dL (women); hepatic disease; CHF; alcoholism	Oral	2–3	2550	
			Abdominal pain, bloating, flatulence, diarrhoea. Contraindicated: inflammatory bowel disease, bowel obstruction, cirrhosis, Cr >2.0 mg/dL	Oral	1–3	150 (>60 kg BW)	300 (>60 kg BW)
			Oedema, anaemia, weight gain. Contraindicated: ALT >2.5 upper limit of normal, NYHA class 3 or 4, hepatic disease, alcoholism	Oral	1–2	45 (pioglitazone)	8 (rosiglitazone)
			Hypoglycaemia (low risk), caution if moderate/severe liver disease, slight weight gain	Oral	1–4+	16	
			Hypoglycaemia (low risk), caution if moderate/severe liver disease	Oral	1–4+	360	
DPP-4 inhibitors	Sitagliptin phosphate	Inhibits DPP-4 resulting in ↑ levels of incretins (GLP-1, GIP)					
Amylin mimetics	Pramlintide	↓Glycaemic surges ↓PP glucagon secretion ↓TG fluxes Delays gastric emptying Inhibits ghrelin					
Incretin mimetics	Exenatide (GLP-1 agonist)	↑Glucose-dependent pancreatic β-cell insulin synthesis and secretion ↓Glucagon secretion Restores first-phase insulin release ↓FPG ↓Gastric emptying ↓PPG β-cell preservation (induction of β-cell neogenesis →Anti apoptosis →β-cell mass)					
Combination preparations	Glyburide/metformin; Glipizide/metformin; Rosiglitazone/metformin; Rosiglitazone/glimepiride		As for individual agents	As for individual agents			

Table 5.6.3 Oral hypoglycaemic agents used in managing type 2 diabetes—cont'd

	Sulphonylureas	Biguanides	α-Glucosidase inhibitors	Thiazolidinediones	Meglitinides	D-Phenyl alanine derivatives
	In combination with diet and exercise, metformin or TZD (Thiazolidinediones, also known as glitazones)	Advanced T2DM Obese Inadequate response to metformin and/or sulphonylurea Adjunct to oral medications				
	0.6–1.4					
	0.6–0.9	0.8–1.3	1.5	2.1	1.2	1.6
	25 51 ↑	14–25 (at 1 year) 63–71 →→				
	→→→↓TG					
	Nausea, headache, anorexia, early satiety, weight loss (↓ calorie intake; ↓ fat, protein, CHO), vomiting, indigestion, abdominal pain, tiredness, dizziness, hypoglycaemia (in combination with insulin and/or sulphonylurea) More common in T1DM	Nausea, vomiting, diarrhoea, headache, dose-dependent anorexia, ↓ food intake, weight loss Hypoglycaemia when in combination with sulphonylurea (dose dependent) DO NOT use in T1DM or DKA	Nasopharyngitis Upper respiratory tract infections Headache	As for individual agents (may be reduced because of lower individual component doses)	As for individual agents (may be reduced because of lower individual component doses)	As for individual agents (may be reduced because of lower individual component doses)

Oral	Subcutaneous injection (abdomen, thigh)	Subcutaneous injection (abdomen, thigh, arm)				
1	1–3	1–2	1–2	1–2	2	1
100	Type 1 (180 µg) Type 2 (360 µg)	10 µg	20/2000	20/2000	8/2000	8/8
Range/dose (mg)	Depends on agent	500–1000	25–50 (>60 kg BW) 25–100 (>60 kg BW), slow titration of dose	15–45 (pioglitazone) 4–8 (rosiglitazone)	0.5–4	60–120
Optimal administration time	30 min premeal (some with food, others on empty stomach)	With meal	With first bite of meal	With/without meal (breakfast)	Preferably <15 min premeal (omit if no meal)	Preferably <15 min premeal (omit if no meal)
Main site of metabolism/excretion	Hepatic/renal, faecal	Not metabolised/renal excretion	2% of acarbose absorbed/faecal, 50%–100% of miglitol absorbed/not metabolised renal	Hepatic/faecal	Hepatic/faecal, renal	Renal 80%. hepatic/faecal 10%

Source: Andreoli TE, Benjamin IJ, Griggs RC, Wing EJ. Andreoli and Carpenter's Cecil Essentials of Medicine. 8th ed. Philadelphia, PA: Elsevier; 2010.

↑, increased; ↓, decreased; –, unchanged; ALT, alanine aminotransferase; BW, body weight; CHF, congestive heart failure; CHO, carbohydrate; Cr, creatinine; DKA, diabetic ketoacidosis; DM, diabetes mellitus; DPP, Diabetes Prevention Program; FPG, fasting plasma glucose; GIP, gastric inhibiting peptide; GLP-1, glucagon-like peptide–1; HbA$_{1c}$, glycosylated haemoglobin; HDL, high-density lipoprotein; HGP, hepatic glucose production; IR, insulin resistance; LDL, low-density lipoprotein; LDL$_3$, large buoyant LDL; NYHA, New York Heart Association; PP, postprandial; PPG, postprandial plasma glucose; T1DM, type 1 diabetes mellitus; T2DM, type 2 diabetes mellitus; TG, triglyceride; XR and XL, extended release.

[a]Values combined from numerous studies; values are also dose dependent.

[b]Not yet approved by FDA.

BACK TO BASIC SCIENCES

Q1. What are the roles of incretins in the pathogenesis of type 2 diabetes?

- The incretins (e.g. glucagon-like peptide-1 [GLP-1] and gastric inhibiting peptide [GIP] produced by the endocrine cells in the small intestine) may play a role in the pathogenesis of type 2 diabetes.
- These incretins are low in concentration in type 2 diabetes and their deficiency may be linked with the pathogenesis of the disease. Also, the islet of Langerhans may become less sensitive to the effects of incretins.
- The physiological roles of incretins are (i) increasing insulin secretion, (ii) supporting postprandial glucagon secretion and (iii) reducing gastric emptying.
- In type 2 diabetes, the low concentration of incretins could contribute to low insulin secretion, lack of glucagon secretion and disturbance of communication between gastric emptying and insulin effect.

Q2. What is the role of weight loss and caloric restriction on the reduction of the incidence of diabetes?

The Diabetes Prevention Program (DPP) demonstrated that 7% weight loss as a result of caloric restriction and exercise leads to 58% reduction in the incidence of diabetes after 3 years.

Q3. Can weight loss after diagnosis of type 2 diabetes produce a remission?

The study by Eriksson and Lindgarde (1991) showed that in the early stages of diagnosis of type 2 diabetes, a moderate 3.7% reduction of body weight demonstrated a 52% remission rate at 6 years of follow-up.

Q4. What is the role of bariatric surgery and weight loss on type 2 diabetes mellitus?

It has been reported that the remission rate is between 40% and 90% following bariatric surgery. Also, there is evidence that weight loss improves glycaemic control.

Q5. What are the early changes observed in the pathogenesis of type 2 diabetes?

1. Disturbance of the pulsatile secretion of insulin
2. Reduction in the ability of insulin to stimulate glucose uptake and suppress glucose release (known as insulin resistance)

Q6. Provide examples of medications that can worsen glucose metabolism and type 2 diabetes.

- Corticosteroids cause hyperglycaemia and the effect is dose dependent. It interferes with gluconeogenesis and the insulin sensitivity.
- Antipsychotic drugs such as olanzapine and clozapine possibly increase body weight and hence the development of diabetes mellitus.

- Some immunosuppressive drugs such as cyclosporine and tacrolimus induce destruction or malfunction of beta-cells of Langerhans.
- Protease inhibitors used to treat HIV infection impair insulin-stimulated glucose uptake in skeletal muscles and adipocytes.
- Other drugs such as beta-blockers, thiazides and niacin can also worsen glucose metabolism and type 2 diabetes.

Q7. How would you explain the development of diabetes mellitus in patients with acromegaly?
Growth hormone stimulates gluconeogenesis and lipolysis resulting in increased blood glucose and free fatty acid concentration.

Q8. How would you explain hyperglycaemia in patients with pheochromocytoma?
Pheochromocytoma → stimulation of the adrenergic receptors on the pancreatic islands → suppression of insulin secretion→ hyperglycaemia

REVIEW QUESTIONS

Q1. Which *one* of the following statements about type 2 diabetes mellitus is correct?
A. It accounts for more than 10% of patients with diabetes.
B. It accounts for 20%–30% of patients with diabetes.
C. It accounts for 30%–40% of patients with diabetes.
D. It accounts for 50%–80% of patients with diabetes.
E. It accounts for more than 90% of patients with diabetes.

Q2. Which *one* of the following tests could differentiate type 1 from type 2 diabetes?
A. HbA_{1c} level
B. Salivary cortisol level
C. C-peptide concentration
D. Continuous glucose monitoring

Q3. In obese patients with type 2 diabetes, which *one* of the following is not recommended?
A. Bariatric surgery
B. Pancreatic lipase inhibitor
C. Metformin therapy
D. GLP-1 antagonist
E. Low-calorie diets

Q4. Which *one* of the following is *not* correct about metformin?
A. Reduces hepatic glucose output
B. Enhances peripheral tissue sensitivity
C. Stimulates GLP-1 secretion

D. Causes folate deficiency

E. Has a moderate effect on lipid profile

Q5. Which *one* of the following statements is *not* correct about incretins?

A. Incretins increase insulin secretion.

B. Incretins are elevated in type 2 diabetes.

C. Incretins support postprandial glucagon secretion.

D. Incretins reduce gastric emptying.

ANSWERS

A1. **E.** Type 2 diabetes accounts for more than 90% of patients with diabetes mellitus.

A2. **C.** The concentration of C-peptide is a surrogate marker of insulin concentration in the plasma. It is a useful test to differentiate type 1 from type 2 diabetes (e.g. in people aged 25 years and developing diabetes). C-peptide is usually undetectable up to 3 years after the diagnosis of type 1 diabetes.

A3. **D.** GLP-1 analogues such as liraglutide rather than antagonists can be used in the management of obesity in patients with or without diabetes.

A4. **D.** Metformin causes vitamin B12 deficiency. It is contraindicated in patients with moderate to severe kidney disease.

A5. **B.** Incretins are low in concentration in type 2 diabetes. The deficiency plays a role in the pathogenesis of type 2 diabetes.

TAKE-HOME MESSAGE

- The symptoms of type 2 diabetes include polyuria, polydipsia, weakness, blurred vision, obesity and peripheral neuropathy. However, it can be asymptomatic.
- The main pathophysiological defects in type 2 diabetes mellitus are (i) delayed insulin secretion by the beta-cells and (ii) abnormal postprandial suppression of glucagon secretion by alpha-cells.
- The pathophysiological changes in type 2 diabetes mellitus may include (i) amyloid deposition and decreased function of beta-cells, (ii) increased apoptosis of beta-cells in diabetes and decreased functional mass of the function of the islet of Langerhans, (iii) abnormal regulation of glucagon secretion from an inherited defect of alpha-cells and (iv) there may be a decrease in the intra-islet insulin (because of beta-cell defect).
- The DPP demonstrated that 7% weight loss as a result of caloric restriction and exercise leads to 58% reduction in the incidence of diabetes after 3 years.
- The goals and options of type 2 diabetes management are (i) weight loss and exercise; (ii) nonpharmacological approach, nutrition education and lifestyle changes; (iii) patient

education about the nature of the disease, management options, complications and prevention issues; (iv) bariatric surgical procedures for obese (restriction and bypass); (v) oral hypoglycaemic agents; (vi) a combination of oral hypoglycaemic agents and insulin; and (vii) self-monitoring of blood glucose.

FURTHER READINGS

Chatterjee S, Khunti K, Davies MJ. Type 2 diabetes. *Lancet*. 2017;389(10085):2239-2225. Review.

Eriksson KF, Lindgärde F. Prevention of type 2 (non-insulin-dependent) diabetes mellitus by diet and physical exercise. The 6-year Malmö feasibility study. *Diabetologia*. 1991;34(12):891-898.

Ismail-Beigi F. Clinical practice. Glycemic management of type 2 diabetes mellitus. *N Engl J Med*. 2012; 366(14):1319-1327. Review.

Lascar N, Brown J, Pattison H, Barnett AH, Bailey CJ, Bellary S. Type 2 diabetes in adolescents and young adults. *Lancet Diabetes Endocrinol*. 2017 Aug 25. pii: S2213-8587(17)30186-9. Review.

McCarthy MI. Genomics, type 2 diabetes, and obesity. *N Engl J Med*. 2010;363(24):2339-2350. Review.

Viner R, White B, Christie D. Type 2 diabetes in adolescents: a severe phenotype posing major clinical challenges and public health burden. *Lancet*. 2017;389(10085):2252-2260. Review.

Haematology System

CASE 6.1

'Looking Pale ...'

Ronald Pitt, a 40-year-old accountant, comes in to see his general practitioner because he is suffering from progressive tiredness and fatigue for the past 6–8 months. Mr Pitt has always been healthy and has regular exercise. He occasionally has knee pains for which he takes over-the-counter ibuprofen tablets. He noted that he becomes a little short of breath on mild exercise. He has no paroxysmal nocturnal dyspnoea, palpitations, ankle oedema, fever, nausea, vomiting, dysuria or bleeding per rectum. On examination, his pulse rate is 100/min, blood pressure 130/80 mm Hg, temperature 37°C and respiratory rate 18/min. He has no cyanosis or clubbing of fingers. He has pallor of conjunctivae and the palms of his hands. There is no lymphadenopathy. Cardiovascular and respiratory examinations are normal. The upper abdomen is soft and tender but not rigid. There is no hepatosplenomegaly or palpable masses. Bowel sounds are present. Mr Pitt's blood tests are summarised in Table 6.1.1.

CASE DISCUSSION

Q1. On the basis of Mr Pitt's presentation, what is your diagnosis?

Q2. What is your differential diagnosis?

Q3. What are the key clinical features of this disease? What are the scientific bases for these features?

Q4. What is the pathophysiology underlying these changes?

Q5. What are your management goals and management options?

ANSWERS

1. The findings of progressive tiredness, fatigue for the past 6 months, shortness of breath on mild exercise, pallor of both conjunctivae and the palms of his hands and tenderness of the upper abdomen, and the finding from the history of intake of over-the-counter ibuprofen together with the findings from investigations of low haemoglobin, low mean corpuscular volume, low serum iron, low serum ferritin and raised transferrin are all suggestive of iron-deficiency anaemia most likely related to gastritis and gastric bleeding caused by ibuprofen.
2. The differential diagnosis includes the following:
   - Anaemia of chronic disorders
   - Microcytic anaemia due to other causes

Table 6.1.1 Mr Pitt's blood test results

Blood test	Mr Pitt's results	Normal range
Haemoglobin (Hb) (g/L)	95	115–160
White blood cell count (WCC) ($\times 10^9$/L)	5.5	4.0–11.0
Platelet cell count ($\times 10^{12}$/L)	4.6	4.40–5.80
Mean corpuscular volume (MCV) (fL)	68	80.0–100.0
Serum iron (μmol/L)	5	9–30
Serum ferritin (μg/L)	4	10–120
Transferrin (g/L)	4.5	2.0–4.0
Iron saturation (%)	6	15–50

- Autoimmune haemolytic anaemia
- Lead poisoning
- Occult GI bleeding
- Thalassaemia traits
- Hereditary spherocytosis
- Sideroblastic anaemia
- Malabsorption
- Menstrual disorders

3. Symptoms and signs:

Symptoms:
- Progressive fatigue and diminished capacity to exercise
- Breathlessness
- Intermittent claudication
- Palpitations

Signs:
- Pallor
- Tachycardia and systolic flow murmur
- Heart failure in severe anaemia
- Brittle nails and spoon-shaped nails (koilonychias)
- Atrophy of the tongue papillae
- Angular stomatitis
- Brittle hair
- Dysphagia

Note that a rare syndrome known as 'Plummer–Vinson or Paterson–Brown–Kelly syndrome' is characterised by dysphagia in patients (usually women) with iron-deficiency anaemia due to the formation of an oesophageal web.

4. Laboratory investigations:
- Blood film: Characteristically the red cells are microcytic and hypochromic together with the presence of anisocytosis (variation in size) and poikilocytosis

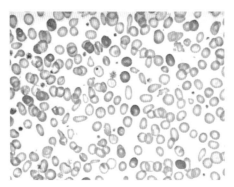

Figure 6.1.1 A blood film of microcytic, hypochromic anaemia. *(Source: Kumar V, Abbas AK, Fausto N, Mitchell R. Robbins Basic Pathology, 8th Edition. London, UK: Elsevier; 2007.)*

(variation in shape). Blood film usually shows no target cells (target cells are commonly present in thalassaemia). It also shows no intraerythrocytic crystals (seen in patients with haemoglobin c disorders). Fig. 6.1.1 shows a blood film of microcytic, hypochromic anaemia.

- Full blood count: Haemoglobin level is low; mean corpuscular volume and mean corpuscular haemoglobin concentration (MCHC) are below the normal range. Often the platelet count is elevated ($>450,000/\mu L$). The white blood cell count is within the normal range.
- Serum iron: The serum iron concentrations are low compared to normal.
- Total iron-binding capacity (TIBC): In iron-deficiency anaemia, TIBC is elevated.
- Serum ferritin: Serum ferritin reflects the amount of cellular stored iron. A low serum ferritin indicates low iron stores and this finding confirms iron-deficiency anaemia. However, serum ferritin is an acute-phase reactant and is raised in the presence of infection, inflammation, cancer and liver damage. In these patients, serum ferritin may be normal even in the presence of iron-deficiency anaemia (Namaste et al., 2017).
- Serum soluble transferrin receptors: In iron-deficiency anaemia, serum soluble transferrin receptors are elevated.
- Bone marrow examination: Perl's Prussian blue stain of bone marrow aspirate or trephine shows absent iron stores. It is rarely needed.
- Endoscopic evaluation (upper and lower gastrointestinal endoscopic examination): A recent report has shown that even in premenopausal women with iron-deficiency anaemia, for 28 out of 43 women (65.1%), a gastrointestinal source was the cause of their chronic blood loss suggesting that this population will benefit from bidirectional endoscopic evaluation of the gastrointestinal tract (Fireman et al., 2006).

5. Management goals:
- Educate the patient.
- Treat the underlying cause of iron-deficiency anaemia such as gastrointestinal bleeding.
- Oral medications: Ferrous sulphate 325 mg three times daily. It is recommended to start with one tablet daily and gradually increase to three tablets daily for

3–6 months. Gastrointestinal side effects and poor compliance, and poor iron absorption are the major challenges.

- Parenteral iron is recommended in patients who did not tolerate oral iron, were refractory to oral iron therapy or have a gastrointestinal condition interfering with oral iron absorption (e.g. inflammatory bowel disease).
- Recheck full blood count and compare response at 3 and 8 weeks after the commencement of treatment.

BACK TO BASIC SCIENCES

Q1. What is the definition of anaemia?
The term 'anaemia' means a drop of blood haemoglobin level below 130 g/L in men or below 120 g/L in females. This definition is meant for adults and does not include children or pregnant women.

Q2. What are the common causes of anaemia?
- Increased loss from the gastrointestinal tract (upper or lower gastrointestinal tract) and increased menstrual blood loss
- Bone marrow failure (e.g. fibrosis)
- Increased demand such as during pregnancy and in young children
- Impaired iron absorption (e.g. in malabsorption)
- Decreased intake of foods rich in iron

Q3. In a simple way, how would you clinically classify anaemia?
Anaemia can be classified into microcytic, normocytic or macrocytic types on the basis of mean corpuscular volume. Another way is to classify anaemia into acute anaemia (as in severe acute bleeding) or chronic anaemia (bleeding over a long duration).

Q4. What are the causes of iron-deficiency anaemia?
1. Occult gastrointestinal blood loss:
   - Peptic ulcer
   - Gastritis
   - Angiodysplasia
   - Gastrointestinal tumours (e.g. colorectal cancer)
2. Malabsorption:
   - Coeliac disease
   - Tropical sprue
   - Infection (e.g. giardiasis, TB)
   - Crohn disease

- Gastrectomy and bypass surgery (bariatric procedures)
- Radiation enteritis

3. Other causes (non-gastrointestinal loss):
   - Menorrhagia
   - Other gynaecological pathologies
4. Anorexia nervosa and vegetarians

Q5. Give examples of 'normocytic' anaemia.
- Anaemia of chronic diseases
- Renal failure
- Hypothyroidism
- Bone marrow failure
- Nutritional (mixed deficiency of iron, folate and B12)
- Acute blood loss

Q6. Give examples of 'macrocytic' anaemia.
- Nutritional (folate and B12 deficiency)
- Hypothyroidism
- Haemolysis/reticulosis
- Alcohol excess
- Drugs interfering with nuclear acid metabolism (5-fluorouracil, trimethoprim, methotrexate, zidovudine)
- Splenectomy
- Chronic liver disease
- Physiological (as during pregnancy)

Q7. How would you differentiate iron-deficiency anaemia from anaemia of chronic diseases?
- Iron-deficiency anaemia is characterised by a low concentration of serum iron, serum transferrin, serum ferritin and transferrin saturation but elevated transferrin. ESR and CRP are low in serum iron deficiency and hepcidin is also low.
- In anaemia of chronic disease, transferrin is low. ESR and CRP are raised because of associated inflammation in chronic diseases. Hepcidin is also elevated. Serum ferritin is elevated in anaemia of chronic diseases.

Q8. Explain how the laboratory blood test results can differentiate iron-deficiency anaemia from thalassaemia trait and sideroblastic anaemia.
Table 6.1.2 summarises the use of blood tests to differentiate iron-deficiency anaemia from other causes of microcytic, hypochromic anaemia.

Table 6.1.2 Use of blood tests to differentiate iron-deficiency anaemia from other causes of microcytic, hypochromic anaemia

Blood test	Iron-deficiency anaemia	Thalassaemia trait	Sideroblastic anaemia
MCV	Low	Low	Low
Serum iron	Reduced	Normal	Raised
Serum TIBC	Raised	Normal	Normal
Serum ferritin	Reduced	Normal	Raised
Iron in bone marrow	Absent	Present	Present
Serum soluble transfer receptor	Increased	Normal or raised	Normal or raised
Iron in erythroblasts	Absent	Present	Ring form

MCV, mean corpuscular volume; TIBC, total iron-binding capacity.

REVIEW QUESTIONS

Q1. Regarding iron metabolism, which *one* of the following statements is correct?
A. The average body iron is normally 100 mg/kg body weight.
B. Non-haeme iron is more readily absorbed than haeme iron.
C. Iron is mainly absorbed in the duodenum and proximal jejunum.
D. Approximately 90% of iron in an average diet is absorbed.

Q2. Regarding iron metabolism, which *one* of the following statements is *not* correct?
A. Iron circulates in the plasma bound to transferrin.
B. Approximately 30 mg/kg of iron is present within red blood cells as haemoglobin.
C. Approximately 90%–95% of iron in the body is recycled.
D. The majority of body iron is present in myoglobin in muscle tissues.

Q3. Which *one* of the following blood test results is expected to be elevated in iron-deficiency anaemia?
A. Mean corpuscular volume
B. Serum ferritin
C. Serum iron
D. Total iron-binding capacity

Q4. A healthy 58-year-old businessman is presenting to his general practitioner because he is suffering from progressive fatigue, pallor, shortness of breath on effort and palpitations. Clinical examination reveals tachycardia and pallor of the conjunctivae and the palms of hands. No other abnormalities are found. His haemoglobin is 75 g/L and blood film shows microcytic, hypochromic red blood cells with anisocytosis, poikilocytosis and no target cells. Other blood tests are consistent with iron-deficiency anaemia. At this stage what test would you order?

A. Stool for occult blood

B. Bone marrow examination

C. Lower and upper gastrointestinal endoscopy

D. Haemoglobin electrophoresis

Q5. Which *one* of the following is *not* a cause of microcytic, hypochromic anaemia?

A. Lead poisoning

B. Hypothyroidism

C. Sideroblastic anaemia

D. Thalassaemia

ANSWERS

A1. **C.** Iron is absorbed in the duodenum and the proximal jejunum through enterocytes. The average body iron content is approximately 40–50 mg/kg body weight.

Haeme iron and inorganic forms of iron are readily absorbed. Non-haeme iron is less absorbed compared to haeme iron (iron in meat).

Approximately 5%–10% of iron in an average diet is absorbed.

A2. **D.** The majority of body iron (about 75%; 30 mg/kg) is present within red blood cells as haemoglobin. Only 10% of body iron is present in myoglobin in muscle tissues (about 4 mg/kg).

A3. **D.** Total iron-binding capacity is elevated in patients with iron-deficiency anaemia.

A4. **C.** Faecal occult blood test is mainly used for screening, not for diagnosis. Upper and lower gastrointestinal endoscopy are recommended to find the cause of iron loss.

Bone marrow examination is of no help as the patient has iron–deficiency anaemia, and there are no changes in the platelet counts or white blood cells such as pancytopenia. Haemoglobin electrophoresis would be recommended if the changes are not consistent with iron-deficiency anaemia in the presence of microcytic, hypochromic anaemia.

A5. **B.** Hypothyroidism is associated with normocytic, normochromic anaemia. Iron-deficiency anaemia is the major cause of microcytic, hypochromic anaemia.

TAKE-HOME MESSAGE

- The term 'anaemia' means a drop of blood haemoglobin level below 130 g/L in men or below 120 g/L in females. This definition is meant for adults and does not include children or pregnant women.

- The symptoms of anaemia are progressive fatigue and diminished capacity to exercise, breathlessness, intermittent claudication and palpitations.
- The signs of iron-deficiency anaemia are pallor, tachycardia, systolic flow murmur, heart failure in severe anaemia, brittle nails, spoon-shaped nails (koilonychias), atrophy of the tongue papillae, angular stomatitis, brittle hair and dysphagia.
- Blood film: Characteristically the red cells are microcytic and hypochromic together with the presence of anisocytosis (variation in size) and poikilocytosis (variation in shape). Blood film usually shows no target cells (target cells are commonly present in thalassaemia). It also shows no intraerythrocytic crystals (seen in patients with haemoglobin c disorders).
- In serum iron deficiency, blood tests show low haemoglobin level, low serum ferritin, raised TIBC, low serum iron and reduced mean corpuscular volume.
- The goals and options in managing iron-deficiency anaemia are as follows: (i) Educate the patient; (ii) treat the underlying cause of iron-deficiency anaemia such as gastrointestinal bleeding; (iii) oral medications: ferrous sulphate 325 mg three times daily – it is recommended to start with one tablet daily and gradually increase the dose to three tablets daily for 3–6 months; (iv) parenteral iron is recommended in patients who did not tolerate oral iron or were refractory to oral iron therapy; and (v) recheck full blood count and compare response at 3 and 8 weeks after the commencement of treatment.

FURTHER READINGS

Camaschella C. Iron-deficiency anemia. *N Engl J Med.* 2015;372(19):1832-1843. Review.

Cantor AG, Bougatsos C, Dana T, Blazina I, McDonagh M. Routine iron supplementation and screening for iron deficiency anemia in pregnancy: a systematic review for the U.S. Preventive Services Task Force. *Ann Intern Med.* 2015;162(8):566-576. Review.

DeLoughery TG. Microcytic anemia. *N Engl J Med.* 2014;371(14):1324-1331. Review.

Fireman Z, Zachlka R, Abu Mouch S, Kopelman Y. The role of endoscopy in the evaluation of iron deficiency anemia in premenopausal women. *Isr Med Assoc J.* 2006;8(2):88-90.

Killip S, Bennett JM, Chambers MD. Iron deficiency anemia. *Am Fam Physician.* 2007;75(5):671-678. Review.

Lopez A, Cacoub P, Macdougall IC, Peyrin-Biroulet L. Iron deficiency anaemia. *Lancet.* 2016;387(10021): 907-916. Review.

Namaste SM, Rohner F, Huang J, et al. Adjusting ferritin concentrations for inflammation: Biomarkers Reflecting Inflammation and Nutritional Determinants of Anemia (BRINDA) project. *Am J Clin Nutr.* 2017;106(suppl 1):359S-371S. Review.

Piel FB, Steinberg MH, Rees DC. Sickle cell disease. *N Engl J Med.* 2017;376(16):1561-1573. Review.

'After Returning From a Holiday in Europe ...'

Mrs Patricia Bryson, a 48-year-old sales administrator, comes in to see her general practitioner after her return from a holiday in Europe. During the holiday, Mrs Bryson had back pain and pain in her right upper thigh. She also felt pains on and off in her arms and legs. She has become progressively fatigued and always feels thirsty. She has also noticed that she needs to wake up at night several times to pass urine. She was seen by a general practitioner during the holiday and a blood test showed that her haemoglobin was 80 g/L, and her fasting blood glucose was 5.3 mmol/L. On examination, her pulse rate is 90/min, blood pressure 130/85 mm Hg, temperature 36.6°C and her respiratory rate is 22/min. Her body mass index is 25 kg/m². Examination of her thyroid gland is normal. She has no palpable lymph nodes and the examination of the cardiovascular and respiratory systems is normal. X-ray of her back and the pelvis shows no fractures but several lytic lesions of the vertebrae and the pelvic bones. An X-ray of the skull is recommended together with blood tests.

CASE DISCUSSION

Q1. On the basis of Mrs Bryson's presentation, what is your diagnosis?

Q2. What is your differential diagnosis?

Q3. What are the key clinical features of this disease? What are the scientific bases for these features?

Q4. What is the pathophysiology underlying these changes?

Q5. What are your management goals and management options?

ANSWERS

1. The findings of progressive fatigue, back pain, bone pains of her arms and legs, anaemia, and increased frequency of urination even when blood glucose is normal, and severe lytic lesions of the vertebrae and the pelvis on radiological examinations suggest the diagnosis of multiple myeloma. The increased frequency of urination could be secondary to hypercalcaemia, and calciuria. Further investigations are needed to confirm the diagnosis and extent of her disease.

2. The differential diagnosis includes the following:
   - Metastatic bone disease
   - Monoclonal gammopathy of undetermined significance (MGUS)
   - Waldenström macroglobulinaemia
   - Malignant lymphoma
3. The clinical picture:
   Symptoms:
   - Bone pains, pathological fracture, fatigue, weakness, anaemia, infection, bleeding (thrombocytopenia), hypercalcaemia (confusion, constipation, nausea, thirst, increased frequency of urination), spinal cord compression and renal failure are present.
   - Most cases are detected during routine blood tests for other reasons.
   - Pathological fractures may be another reason for the diagnosis.
   - Two-thirds of patients may complain of bone pains and lower back pain.
   - Other sources of pain are long bones of the limbs, skull, pelvis or back.
   Clinical examination findings:
   - Eyes: Macular detachment, retinal haemorrhages, cotton-wool spots and pallor of conjunctivae
   - Skin: Ecchymosis or purpura (thrombocytopenia)
   - Bones: Tenderness and lytic pathological lesions
   - Neurological findings: Loss of sensations, neuropathy, myopathy, carpal tunnel syndrome (amyloid deposition) and confusion
   - Abdominal findings: Hepatosplenomegaly
   - Cardiovascular system: Cardiomegaly (immune deposition)
   - Other findings due to deposition of amyloid: Macroglossia and typical skin lesions (waxy papules or nodules on the ears and lips)
4. Laboratory investigations:
   - Blood tests: Full blood count – anaemia, thrombocytopenia and leukopenia. Reticulocyte count is low. Peripheral blood smears may show rouleaux formation.
   - ESR is significantly elevated.
   - Biochemical tests: These include total proteins, albumin, globulin, blood urea, creatinine, uric acid, electrolytes including calcium and magnesium, and liver function tests.
   - Urine tests: A 24-hour urine collection quantifies the Bence Jones proteins (lambda light chains) and creatinine clearance.
   - The finding of >1 g of proteins in 24-hour urine is a major criterion in the diagnosis.
   - Serum protein electrophoresis (SPEP): It helps to determine the type of each protein.
   - Urine protein electrophoresis (UPEP): It helps to identify the presence of Bence Jones proteins in urine.
   - Biochemical screening is done including calcium, creatinine, SPEP, immunofixation and immunoglobulin quantification (azotaemia, hypercalcaemia, elevated serum alkaline phosphatase and hypoalbuminaemia).

- Lactate dehydrogenase (LDH) is elevated.
- Quantitative immunoglobulin levels – IgG, IgM and IgA – are determined.
- Beta-2 microglobulin: Beta-2 microglobulin is increased in patients with renal failure without multiple myeloma and is useful in assessing prognosis.
- C-reactive protein: It is useful in assessing prognosis.
- IL-6 activity: It reflects plasma cell activity.
- Serum viscosity: The presence of central nervous system symptoms, nose bleeding or high M protein level may together indicate hyperviscosity syndrome.
- Radiological studies: (i) Plain X-rays, complete skeleton series at the diagnosis of multiple myeloma (skull, long bones, spine, pelvis and ribs). The skull is a common site affected in multiple myeloma showing lytic lesions and punched-out areas (Fig. 6.2.1A). These lesions may be demonstrated in the long bones of arms, pelvis and ribs. (ii) Computed tomography (CT) scans may show cortical involvement and risk of fractures. (iii) Magnetic resonance studies detect thoracic or lumbar spine and paraspinal involvement and early cord compression. (iv) Positron emission tomography: The use of whole-body MRI together with positron emission tomography has specificity and prediction validity of 100%.
- Aspiration and biopsy: Bone marrow aspiration and biopsy help in calculating the percentage of the plasma cells in the aspirate (bone marrow biopsy is better than aspiration). Usually plasma cells appear in sheets or clumps. Fig. 6.2.1B shows plasma cell myeloma.
- Histological studies: The presence of plasma cells (two to three times larger than normal lymphocytes) is characterised by the following features:
  - Eccentric nuclei
  - Smooth and rounded or oval nuclei
  - Clumped chromatin
  - Have a perinuclear halo or pale zone
  - Basophilic cytoplasm
  - Possibility of similar appearances of other cells such as Russell bodies and Mott cells (bone marrow examination is helpful)
- Cytogenic analysis of the bone marrow: Such examination is helpful in assessing prognosis. Most common is dilation of 17p13, which is associated with short survival and hypercalcaemia.

5. Management goals:
   - Eradicating symptoms
   - Prolonging and maintaining the quality of life
   - Supportive therapy
   - Psychotherapy
   - Management of complications

The treatment includes immunomodulating agents (lenalidomide, pomalidomide, thalidomide) and proteasome inhibitors.

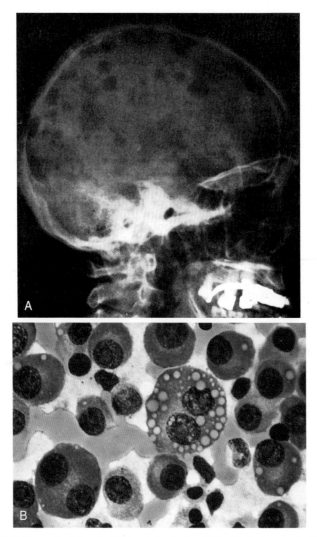

Figure 6.2.1 (A) Radiograph of the skull (lateral view) of a child with thalassaemia. Note the sharply punched-out bone defects. (B) Bone marrow aspirate. Normal bone marrow cells are replaced by atypical forms of plasma cells with multiple nuclei, prominent nucleoli and cytoplasmic droplets containing immunoglobulins. *(Source: Kumar V, Abbas AK, Fausto N, Mitchell R. Robbins Basic Pathology, 8th Edition. London, UK: Elsevier; 2007.)*

Supportive therapy: (i) bisphosphonates reduce the risk of bone events and monthly zoledronic acid; (ii) radiotherapy to target painful lytic lesions; (iii) analgesics for pains (use simple analgesics instead of opioids); and (iv) prophylaxis manage the side effects of chemotherapy.

Psychotherapy: It is important for patients and families. It includes peer support, education and social support.

BACK TO BASIC SCIENCES

Q1. What is multiple myeloma?

Multiple myelomas are plasma cell disorders (cloned plasma or lymphoplasmacytic cell disorders), which are characterised by the production of monoclonal antibodies (M protein) detected in serum and urine.

Q2. What is M protein?

The M protein is produced in multiple myeloma and consists of heavy chain (IgG, IgA, IgD or IgM) complexed with a κ or λ light chain or free light chains.

Q3. What is MGUS?

- The presence of a paraprotein (IgM, IgG and IgA) in the absence of myeloma, amyloid or lymphoma is known as MGUS.
- M protein in these patients is <3 g/dL.
- This may be an incidental laboratory finding but it is a premalignant condition with an annual risk of developing or progression to myeloma.
- MGUS has a prevalence of 5% in patients aged 70 years or older.

Q4. Briefly discuss the pathophysiology of multiple myeloma.

- Beta-cells residing in the bone marrow migrate to the germinal centre of lymph nodes → mature in response to antigens producing antigen-presenting cells
- Changes encoding the Ig heavy chain locus (on chromosome 14) occur.
- DNA changes, DNA breakage → repaired and possibly develop aberrant chromosomal translocations.
- These translocations may enhance oncogenes and enhance the Ig gene loci → increased expression.
- These deregulations → beta-cell immortalisation and malignant transformation.
- Interaction with inflammatory mediators (e.g. IL-6, insulin-like growth factor 1) → immortalisation of malignant plasma cells.
- Malignant plasma cells → genetic changes determining the evolution of MGUS to myeloma and the development of the clinical picture of multiple myeloma (anaemia, bone pains, renal insufficiency, hypercalcaemia, bone lytic lesion, pathological fracture and cloned bone marrow plasma cells $>60\%$).

Q5. What are the underlying mechanisms for anaemia in multiple myeloma?

- Bone marrow infiltration
- Renal impairment
- Anaemia of inflammation

It is usually normocytic, normochromic type of anaemia.

Q6. What are the underlying mechanisms for bone pains in multiple myeloma?
- Stimulation of osteoclasts and resorption
- Inhibition of osteoblasts and bone formation
- Osteolytic lesions and osteopenia as a result of above-mentioned two processes
- Development of osteolytic deposits and pathological fractures

Q7. What are the mechanisms underlying renal impairment in multiple myeloma?
- Light chains have direct toxic effects on the nephrons.
- Cast nephropathy leads to distal tubular blockage.
- Amyloid deposition occurs.
- Hypercalcaemia and dehydration exaggerate the deterioration of renal functions.
- Use of nonsteroidal anti-inflammatory drugs → inhibition of prostaglandin synthesis from arachidonic acid by nonspecific blocking of the enzyme cyclooxygenase → vasoconstriction → renal impairment (acute tubular necrosis and renal failure).
- Use of nonsteroidal anti-inflammatory drugs → interstitial nephritis and/or tubular necrosis → chronic renal failure.

Q8. What are the mechanisms underlying hypercalcaemia in multiple myeloma?
- Increased osteolytic activities
- Bone resorption
- Release of calcium from bones into extracellular tissues
- Impaired excretion of calcium by the kidneys because of renal damage

REVIEW QUESTIONS

Q1. Which *one* of the following is *not* among the clinical picture of multiple myeloma?
A. Renal failure
B. Hypocalcaemia
C. Recurrent infections
D. Hyperviscosity
E. Anaemia

Q2. Which *one* of the following explains why urinary participates in multiple myeloma are only light chains?
A. Majority of proteins produced in multiple myeloma are light chains.
B. Larger proteins release light chains in the renal collecting tubules.
C. Glomeruli allow the passage of only light chains.
D. Larger proteins are reabsorbed in the distal convoluted tubules.

Q3. Which *one* of the following is *less likely* to be the mechanism underlying anaemia in multiple myeloma?
A. Bone marrow infiltration
B. Inflammation

C. Renal impairment

D. Haemolysis

Q4. Which *one* of the following pathophysiological changes is *not* among those occurring in the transformation of MGUS to a malignant myeloma?

A. Mutation in RAS

B. Translocation involving chromosome 14

C. Apoptosis

D. Hyperdiploidy

E. Mutation of *TP*53

ANSWERS

A1. **B.** Hypercalcaemia and not hypocalcaemia is among the clinical picture of multiple myeloma.

A2. **C.** The glomeruli are unable to allow the passage of large chains. Only light chains are allowed.

A3. **D.** Haemolysis is not among the mechanisms commonly known to underlying anaemia.

A4. **C.** Apoptosis is a normal process. Inhibition of apoptosis is among the outcomes of transformation of MGUS to a myeloma.

TAKE-HOME MESSAGE

- Multiple myelomas are plasma cell disorders (cloned plasma or lymphoplasmacytic cell disorders), which are characterised by the production of monoclonal antibodies (M protein) detected in serum and urine.
- The M protein is produced in multiple myeloma and consists of heavy chain (IgG, IgA, IgD or IgM) complexed with a κ or λ light chain or free light chains.
- The differential diagnosis includes metastatic bone disease, MGUS, Waldenström macroglobulinaemia and malignant lymphoma.
- The management goals are (i) eradicating symptoms, (ii) prolonging and maintaining the quality of life, (iii) supportive therapy, (iv) psychotherapy and (v) management of complications.

FURTHER READINGS

Bladé J. Clinical practice. Monoclonal gammopathy of undetermined significance. *N Engl J Med.* 2006;355(26):2765-2770. Review.

Gerber DE. Targeted therapies: a new generation of cancer treatments. *Am Fam Physician.* 2008;77(3): 311-319. Review.

Kumar S, Paiva B, Anderson KC, et al. International Myeloma Working Group consensus criteria for response and minimal residual disease assessment in multiple myeloma. *Lancet Oncol.* 2016;17(8):e328-e346. Review.

Kyle RA, Rajkumar SV. Multiple myeloma. *N Engl J Med*. 2004;351(18):1860-1873. Review.

McCarthy M. Newer drugs for refractory and relapsed multiple myeloma are effective but costly, review finds. *BMJ*. 2016;353:i2725. Review.

Nau KC, Lewis WD. Multiple myeloma: diagnosis and treatment. *Am Fam Physician*. 2008;78(7):853-859. Review.

Palumbo A, Anderson K. Multiple myeloma. *N Engl J Med*. 2011;364(11):1046-1060. Review.

Raab MS, Podar K, Breitkreutz I, Richardson PG, Anderson KC. Multiple myeloma. *Lancet*. 2009; 374(9686):324-339. Review.

Rajkumar SV, Dimopoulos MA, Palumbo A, et al. International Myeloma Working Group updated criteria for the diagnosis of multiple myeloma. *Lancet Oncol*. 2014;15(12):e538-e548. Review.

Röllig C, Knop S, Bornhäuser M. Multiple myeloma. *Lancet*. 2015;385(9983):2197-2208. Review.

CASE 6.3

'Bleeding Gums ...'

Linda Allan, a 28-year-old nurse, presents to the emergency department with nasal and gum bleeding for a few hours. She gives no history of similar bleeding or bleeding per rectum, in urine or any other bleeding. She has no fever, chills, abdominal pain or bone pains. She noticed reddish spots or her left leg this morning while dressing to come to the hospital. She gives a history of upper respiratory tract infection 2 weeks earlier. On examination, she is conscious, but anxious. Her pulse rate is 105/min, blood pressure 120/80 mm Hg, respiratory rate 22/min and temperature 37°C. She has no jaundice and no palpable lymph nodes. She is bleeding from her nose and little oozing is noted from her gingiva. She has multiple flat reddish spots, each about 1 mm, on the skin of her upper left thigh. There is no hepatosplenomegaly or abdominal masses. Her blood haemoglobin level and white blood cell count are normal; her platelet count is low. Both her thrombin time and partial thromboplastin time are within normal limits.

CASE DISCUSSION

Q1. On the basis of Linda's presentation, what is your diagnosis?

Q2. What is your differential diagnosis?

Q3. What are the key clinical features of this disease? What are the scientific bases for these features?

Q4. What is the pathophysiology underlying these changes?

Q5. What are your management goals and management options?

ANSWERS

1. The findings of nasal and gum bleeding for a few hours, no lymph adenopathy, fever, bone pains or abdominal pains together with multiple flat reddish spots, each about 1 mm on the skin of upper thigh, and low platelet count, normal thrombin time and partial thromboplastin time are suggestive of the diagnosis of immune thrombocy-topenic purpura (ITP).

2. The differential diagnosis includes the following:
   - Myelodysplastic syndrome
   - Other causes of thrombocytopenia:
     a. Reduced platelet production:
        – Wiskott–Aldrich syndrome

- Chemicals, drugs, viral infections
- Haematological malignancies – leukaemia, myeloma, myelodysplasia, myelofibrosis
- Radiations
- Cytotoxic drugs and antibiotics (vancomycin)
- Alcohol excess
- Infections – HIV, cytomegalovirus, hepatitis B and C
- Bone marrow failure
- Congenital mutations of c-MPL, the thrombopoietin receptor

b. Increased platelet destruction:
- Secondary to systemic lupus erythematosus and lymphoma
- Infections: HIV, hepatitis B and C, malaria
- Drug-induced: Penicillins, sulphonamides, heparin, quinine
- Post-transfusion purpura
- Thrombotic thrombocytopenic purpura (TTP)
- Disseminated intravascular haemolysis

c. Abnormal distribution of platelets, e.g. splenomegaly:
- TTP

3. Clinical picture:

Symptoms and signs:
- Asymptomatic: Most patients are asymptomatic and present with low platelet count, bleeding, petechiae, bruises, mucosal bleeding (mouth, gums), bleeding from the nose and in urine or stool, and rarely intracranial haemorrhage

4. Laboratory findings:
- Full blood count (isolated thrombocytopenia; red blood cells and white blood cells are normal in shape and counts; if there is severe bleeding, haemoglobin may be low)
- Platelet size (uniformly large platelets may be found in Bernard–Soulier syndrome): Very small platelets are present in male infants and in the presence of eczema (Wiskott–Aldrich syndrome).

  In ITP, both small and large platelets are present.
- Renal and liver function tests
- Immunoglobulins
- Antiphospholipid antibody screening
- Anticardiolipin antibody
- ANA and double-stranded DNA
- Hepatitis B and hepatitis C screening tests
- HIV
- Thyroid function tests
- Ultrasound scan of the liver and spleen
- Bone marrow examination
- Antiplatelet antibodies

- Cytomegalovirus PCR (blood and urine)
- Epstein–Barr virus PCR
- Thrombopoietin (megakaryocyte growth and development factor [MGDF])
- *Helicobacter pylori* antibodies

Pathophysiological and laboratory features:

- ITP is mediated by the involvement of antibodies and T-cells. Antiplatelet antibodies are directed against both platelets and megakaryocytes. The antibodies coat the platelets and target their destruction (direct platelet lysis or via macrophages in the spleen).
- Antibodies also target the megakaryocytes and reduce platelet production.
- T-cells are reduced in ITP.
- Cytotoxic T-cells cause direct lysis of platelets and contribute to the thrombocytopenia.

5. Management goals:
   - Recently diagnosed patients (0–3 months) → steroids and IV immunoglobulin.
   - Persistent disease (3–12 months) → mycophenolate mofetil or thrombopoietin receptor agonists (TRAs) or rituximab.
   - Chronic disease (>12 months) → continue TRAs or repeated rituximab plus dexamethasone, continuous mycophenolate mofetil. Other treatment options include danazol, dapsone and splenectomy.
   - Patients with *H. pylori* antibodies should be given eradication treatment.

BACK TO BASIC SCIENCES

Q1. What is thrombopoietin?

Thrombopoietin is mainly produced by the liver and kidneys. It is a key regulator of platelet production by increasing the rate of megakaryocyte maturation and proliferation.

Q2. What is the normal platelet count?

It ranges between 150 and 400×10^9/L.

Q3. What are the possible mechanisms by which thrombocytopenia may occur?

- Reduction in platelet production (bone marrow failure)
- Increased destruction or consumption of platelets
- Abnormal distribution of platelets (as in splenomegaly)

Q4. Briefly discuss the clinical picture of drug-induced thrombocytopenia.

- Patients usually have symptoms such as light-headedness, chills, fever, nausea and vomiting often before the bleeding. They may have purpura and bleeding from the nose, gums, gastrointestinal tract or urinary tract (severe thrombocytopenia).
- Patients may present with disseminated intravascular coagulation or renal failure, haemolytic uraemic syndrome or TTP.

Q5. Give examples of drugs that pose a higher risk of developing thrombocytopenia.
- Trimethoprim–sulfamethoxazole
- Quinine–quinidine
- Abciximab
- Heparin
- Gold salts
- Rifampin
- Vancomycin
- Cimetidine

Q6. What are the mechanisms by which thrombopoietin regulates platelet production?
- Thrombopoietin, mainly produced by the liver, binds and activates the thrombopoietin receptors on the membrane of megakaryocyte and induces cytoplasmic signalling → platelet production.
- In patients with bone marrow failure and thrombocytopenia, the levels of thrombopoietin are raised.
- However, in most patients with immune thrombocytopenia, the levels of thrombopoietin are lower than expected.

Q7. What is the role of thrombopoietin in the management of ITP?
- The synthetic thrombopoietin has been developed and clinical trials have been carried out to assess its value in managing ITP.
- Examples of these agonists are (i) romiplostim and (ii) eltrombopag.
- Both drugs have been found to reduce bleeding complications in immune thrombocytopenia.

REVIEW QUESTIONS

Q1. Which *one* of the following is *not* among the clinical picture of immune thrombocytopenia?
A. Petechiae on the skin
B. Bruises
C. Mucosal bleeding
D. Lymphadenopathy

Q2. Which *one* of the following tests in a patient with immune thrombocytopenia is *not* routinely ordered as a first-line investigation?
A. *H. pylori* serology
B. Hepatitis C and B screening
C. Bone marrow examination

D. HIV
E. Thyroid function tests

Q3. Which *one* of the following is the treatment of choice in newly diagnosed immune thrombocytopenic purpura (0–3 months)?
A. Mycophenolate mofetil
B. Thrombopoietin receptor agonists
C. Steroids
D. Rituximab
E. Splenectomy

Q4. Which *one* of the following is *not* part of the pathophysiology of immune thrombocytopenia purpura?
A. Antiplatelet antibodies
B. Abnormalities in T-helper cells
C. Abnormalities in cytotoxic T-cells
D. Virus inhibition of megakaryocytes

ANSWERS

A1. **D.** Lymphadenopathy is not part of the clinical diagnosis of immune thrombocytopenia. It may suggest other haematological conditions such as leukaemia.

A2. **C.** Bone marrow examination is not carried out as a first-line investigation. It is recommended in adults if there is failure to respond to first-line treatment or when another underlying pathology is suspected.

A3. **C.** The treatment of choice in newly diagnosed patients is steroids or IV immunoglobulins.

A4. **D.** There is no evidence that a virus infection directly inhibits megakaryocytes in immune thrombocytopenic purpura.

TAKE-HOME MESSAGE

- The normal number of platelets ranges between 150 and 400 $\times$ 10^9/L.
- Thrombopoietin is mainly produced by the liver and kidneys. It is a key regulator of platelet production by increasing the rate of megakaryocyte maturation and proliferation.
- The mechanisms by which thrombocytopenia occur are (i) reduction in platelet production (bone marrow failure), (ii) increased destruction or consumption of platelets and (iii) abnormal distribution of platelets (as in splenomegaly).
- The management of ITP: (i) recently diagnosed patients (0–3 months) → steroids and IV immunoglobulin; (ii) persistent disease (3–12 months) → mycophenolate

mofetil or TRAs or rituximab; (iii) chronic disease (>12 months) → continue TRAs or repeated rituximab plus dexamethasone, continuous mycophenolate mofetil and other treatment options including danazol, dapsone or splenectomy; and (iv) patients with *H. pylori* antibodies should be given eradication treatment.

FURTHER READINGS

Aster RH, Bougie DW. Drug-induced immune thrombocytopenia. *N Engl J Med*. 2007;357(6):580-587. Review.

Cines DB, Blanchette VS. Immune thrombocytopenic purpura. *N Engl J Med*. 2002;346(13):995-1008. Review.

Diagnosis and treatment of idiopathic thrombocytopenia purpura. American Society of Hematology ITP Practice Guideline Panel. *Am Fam Physician*. 1996;54(8):2437-2447, 2451-2452. Review.

Hill LJ, Tung EE. From prednisone to pylori: a case of Helicobacter pylori-induced chronic immune thrombocytopenia. *BMJ Case Rep*. 2014;2014:bcr2014205786.

Imbach P, Crowther M. Thrombopoietin-receptor agonists for primary immune thrombocytopenia. *N Engl J Med*. 2011;365(8):734-741. Review.

Jansen AJ, Swart RM, te Boekhorst PA. Thrombopoietin-receptor agonists for immune thrombocytopenia. *N Engl J Med*. 2011;365(23):2240-2241.

Provan D, Newland AC. Guidelines for immune thrombocytopenia. *N Engl J Med*. 2011;364(6):580-581.

Rodeghiero F, Stasi R, Gernsheimer T, et al. Standardization of terminology, definitions and outcome criteria in immune thrombocytopenic purpura of adults and children: report from an international working group. *Blood*. 2009;113(11):2386-2393.

Von Drygalski A, Curtis BR, Bougie DW, et al. Vancomycin-induced immune thrombocytopenia. *N Engl J Med*. 2007;356(9):904-910.

CASE 6.4

'Unexpected Outcomes ...'

Tom Torres-Fleming, a 42-year-old cleaner, comes in to see his general practitioner because he is suffering from night sweats, fever and left upper quadrant abdominal pain. On examination, his pulse rate is 95/min, blood pressure 120/80 mm Hg, temperature 37.1°C and respiratory rate 20/min. There is no lymphadenopathy. Abdominal examination shows that the spleen is palpable 17 cm below the left costal margin, and there is no hepatomegaly. No other clinical findings were found. His blood test results are summarised in Table 6.4.1.

Liver function tests are normal; blood urea, creatinine and electrolytes are all within the normal range.

Bone marrow biopsy shows hypercellularity, loss of fat spaces and no bone marrow fibrosis. Chromosomal analysis: It shows Philadelphia (Ph) chromosome positive (typical translocation between chromosomes 9 and 22).

CASE DISCUSSION

Q1. On the basis of Tom's presentation, what is your diagnosis?

Q2. What is your differential diagnosis?

Q3. What are the key clinical features of this disease? What are the scientific bases for these features?

Q4. What is the pathophysiology underlying these changes?

Q5. What are your management goals and management options?

ANSWERS

1. The findings of night sweats, fever, left upper quadrant abdominal pain and splenomegaly of 17 cm below the left costal margin together with the results of investigations showing low haemoglobin, white blood cells reaching $160 \times 10^9/L$ (immature myeloid forms 12%, band neutrophils 59%, neutrophils 9%, lymphocytes 9%, monocytes 6%, basophils 5%, metamyelocytes 6%, myelocytes 5%, promyelocytes 3% and blast cells 2%), thrombocytosis ($588 \times 10^9/L$), lactate dehydrogenase (LDH) 1800 units/L, raised uric acid and bone marrow biopsy showing hypercellularity, loss of fat spaces, no bone marrow fibrosis and the presence of Ph chromosome (typical translocation between chromosomes 9 and 22) are suggestive of the diagnosis of chronic myeloid leukaemia (CML), Ph chromosome positive.

Table 6.4.1 Tom's blood test results

Blood test	Tom's results	Normal range
Haemoglobin (Hb) (g/L)	100	115–160
Packed cell volume (PCV)	0.35	0.37–0.47
White cell count (WBC) (×10⁹/L)	160	4.0–11.0
Differential counts	Immature myeloid forms 12% Band neutrophils 59% Neutrophils 9% Lymphocytes 9% Monocytes 6% Basophils 5% Metamyelocytes 6% Myelocytes 5% Promyelocytes 3% Blast cells 2%	0 <0.7 2–7 1.0–4.0 0.1–1.0 <0.10 0 0 0 0
Platelet count (×10⁹/L)	588	150–400
Lactate dehydrogenase (LDH) (units/L)	1800	100–190
Uric acid (μmol/L)	650	180–420

2. The differential diagnosis may include the following:
   - Acute myeloid leukaemia
   - Acute lymphoblastic leukaemia
   - Myelofibrosis
   - Chronic eosinophilic leukaemia
   - Essential thrombocytosis
   - Chronic neutrophilic leukaemia
   - Sepsis
3. Clinical picture
   - There are three phases in CML: the chronic, accelerated and blast phases.
   - Most patients present in the chronic phase and only 15% present in the more aggressive accelerated or blast phase.
   - The disease may be asymptomatic and is detected from a full blood count requested for routine examination or other reasons.

   Symptoms:
   - Anorexia
   - Shortness of breath
   - Abdominal discomfort and pain due to splenomegaly
   - Fever
   - Weight loss
   - Headache

- Priapism (due to leukocytosis $>100 \times 10^9/L$)
- Bruising
- Bleeding
- Infections

Signs:
- Pallor
- Splenomegaly
- Lymphadenopathy (uncommon)
- Retinal haemorrhage
- Recurrent severe infections

4. Investigations:
   - Full blood count: Haemoglobin is low. The anaemia is normocytic, normochromic anaemia; the white blood cell count is raised.
   - Blood film: It shows neutrophilia with whole mature myeloid precursors (immature forms, bands, neutrophils, lymphocytes, monocytes, basophils, metamyelocytes, myelocytes, promyelocytes and blast cells).
   - Increased number of blast cells is suggestive of accelerated phase or blast crisis.
   - Bone marrow aspiration/trephine: Cellularity is increased, and myeloid precursors are increased (Fig. 6.4.1). There is no bone marrow fibrosis. Loss of fat spaces occurs.
   - Cytogenetics: A t(9:22) translocation (Ph chromosome positive) occurs.

5. Management:
   The goals and options of management:
   - Reduce clonal disease burden and control CML.
   - Relieve symptoms.
   - Monitor/manage the side effects of chemotherapy.
   - Monitor for complications.
   - Educate the patient.
   - Treatment with imatinib, a tyrosine kinase inhibitor, has revolutionised the management of CML.

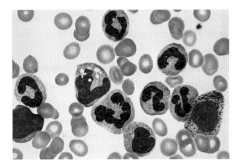

Figure 6.4.1 Bone marrow changes in chronic myelogenous leukaemia. *(Source: Kumar V, Abbas AK, Fausto N, Mitchell R. Robbins Basic Pathology, 8th Edition. London, UK: Elsevier; 2007.)*

- Mechanism of action of imatinib: Imatinib is a tyrosine kinase inhibitor → blocks the enzymatic and controlling function of the *BCR-ABL transcript* protein → completes haematological response in more than 95% of patients and 70% of patients with no cytogenetically deleted Philadelphia translocation (Ph) cells in the bone marrow.
- Imatinib enables patients to achieve 'a molecular remission'.
- Side effects of imatinib are headaches, nausea, abdominal pain, rashes, cytopenia and cardiac adverse effects.
- In the blast phase, most patients have a short life. Treatment here may include other chemotherapy as in acute leukaemia and stem cell transplantation.

BACK TO BASIC SCIENCES

Q1. What is chronic myeloid leukaemia (CML)?
- CML is a myeloproliferative disease characterised by the presence of Ph chromosome and driven by its products (the *BCR-ABL1* tyrosine kinase).

Q2. What is Philadelphia (Ph) chromosome?
- The Ph chromosome results from the fusion oncogene *BCR-ABL* owing to the juxtaposition of the 3′ portion of the Abelson (*ABL*) gene from the long arm of chromosome 9 with the 5′ portion of the breakpoint region (*BCR*) on the long arm of chromosome 22.
- The resulting fusion oncogene is an active tyrosine kinase; *BCR-ABL* is a 210-kDa protein.
- The Ph chromosome unregulated the proliferation of myeloid cells seen in CML.

Q3. What is imatinib?
- The *BCR-ABL* protein contains an active tyrosine kinase region of *ABL* producing a cytokine-independent, proliferative signal. These signals are responsible for the continuous cell growth and replication.
- Pharmacological inhibition of active tyrosine kinase located in the *BCR-ABL* protein has shown significant control of CML.
- Imatinib is an inhibitor of multiple tyrosine kinases, including *ABL*, *BCR-ABL*, platelet-derived growth factor receptor (PDGFR) and c-Kit.

Q4. How would you explain patients with CML not responding to imatinib?
- Imatinib selectively inhibits the signalling and the growth of *BCR-ABL*-positive cells, inducing apoptosis of these cells and control of CML.
- A single mutation in the *BCR-ABL* gene will result in changes in the *BCR-ABL* protein affecting the binding of imatinib with *BCR-ABL*. This may explain cases in which there is a resistance to imatinib.
- New medications, tyrosine kinase inhibitors, have been developed to overcome this resistance to imatinib. These new medications are dasatinib and nilotinib.

Q5. What are the side effects of imatinib?

The side effects of imatinib include headache, nausea, abdominal pain, skin rashes and serious cardiac effects.

REVIEW QUESTIONS

Q1. Which *one* of the following is the most likely genetic mutation in chronic myeloid leukaemia (CML)?

A. *EML4-ALK*
B. *BCR-ABL*
C. *PML-RAR*
D. *JAK2-V617F*

Q2. A 55-year-old male presents to his general practitioner because he is suffering from progressive fatigue, loss of appetite, weight loss, sweating and left upper quadrant abdominal pain. Clinical examination reveals that he is pale and has splenomegaly. There is no lymphadenopathy. The results of his blood investigations show low haemoglobin, and a peripheral blood smear demonstrates myelocytes, metamyelocytes and basophils. Bone marrow aspirates mimic his peripheral blood smear. Which *one* of the following is the most likely diagnosis?

A. Mantle cell lymphoma
B. Primary myelofibrosis
C. Acute promyelocytic leukaemia
D. Chronic myeloid leukaemia

Q3. Which *one* of the following statements about imatinib is correct?

A. It causes priapism.
B. It stimulates platelet-derived growth factor receptor (PDGFR).
C. It is a tyrosine kinase inhibitor.
D. It stimulates the *BCR-ABL* region.

Q4. In patients with chronic myeloid leukaemia who have failed to respond to two tyrosine kinase inhibitors, which treatment should be considered?

A. Blood transfusion
B. Cytarabine
C. Glucocorticoid
D. Allogeneic stem cell transplantation

ANSWERS

A1. **B.** CML is associated with *BCR-ABL* mutation.

A2. **D.** The clinical picture, the peripheral blood film and the bone marrow aspiration are consistent with CML.

A3. **C.** Imatinib acts by inhibiting tyrosine kinase located in the region of *ABL* of Ph chromosome.

A4. **D.** Patients with CML who fail to respond to treatment with two or more tyrosine kinase inhibitors should be considered for allogeneic stem cell transplantation as early as possible.

TAKE-HOME MESSAGE

- CML is a myeloproliferative disease characterised by the presence of Ph chromosome and driven by its products (the *BCR-ABL*1 tyrosine kinase).
- There are three phases in CML: The chronic, accelerated and blast phases.
- Most patients present in the chronic phase and only 15% present in the more aggressive accelerated or blast phase.
- The disease may be asymptomatic and is detected from a full blood count requested for routine examination or other reasons.
- The symptoms of CML include anorexia, shortness of breath, abdominal discomfort, pain due to splenomegaly, fever, weight loss, headache, priapism (due to leukocytosis >100 × 10^9/L), bruising, bleeding and infections.
- The signs of CML include pallor, splenomegaly, lymphadenopathy (uncommon), retinal haemorrhage and recurrent severe infections.
- The goals of management of CML are (i) reduce clonal disease burden and control CML; (ii) relieve symptoms; (iii) monitor/manage the side effects of chemotherapy; (iv) monitor for complications; and (v) educate the patient.

FURTHER READINGS

Apperley JF. Chronic myeloid leukaemia. *Lancet.* 2015;385(9976):1447-1459. Review.

Apperley JF. Part I: mechanisms of resistance to imatinib in chronic myeloid leukaemia. *Lancet Oncol.* 2007;8(11):1018-1029. Review.

Apperley JF. Part II: management of resistance to imatinib in chronic myeloid leukaemia. *Lancet Oncol.* 2007;8(12):1116-1128. Review.

Baccarani M, Deininger MW, Rosti G, et al. European LeukemiaNet recommendations for the management of chronic myeloid leukemia: 2013. *Blood.* 2013;122(6):872-884. Review.

Faderl S, Talpaz M, Estrov Z, O'Brien S, Kurzrock R, Kantarjian HM. The biology of chronic myeloid leukemia. *N Engl J Med.* 1999;341(3):164-172. Review.

Gambacorti-Passerini CB, Gunby RH, Piazza R, Galietta A, Rostagno R, Scapozza L. Molecular mechanisms of resistance to imatinib in Philadelphia-chromosome-positive leukaemias. *Lancet Oncol.* 2003;4(2):75-85. Review.

Goldman J. ABC of clinical haematology. Chronic myeloid leukaemia. *BMJ.* 1997;314(7081):657-660. Review. No abstract available. Erratum in: BMJ 1997 Mar 15;314(7083):812.

Goldman JM, Melo JV. Chronic myeloid leukemia—advances in biology and new approaches to treatment. *N Engl J Med.* 2003;349(15):1451-1464. Review.

Hehlmann R, Hochhaus A, Baccarani M, European LeukemiaNet. Chronic myeloid leukaemia. *Lancet.* 2007;370(9584):342-350. Review.

Schiffer CA. BCR-ABL tyrosine kinase inhibitors for chronic myelogenous leukemia. *N Engl J Med.* 2007;357(3):258-265. Review.

CASE 6.5

'Before Travelling to Congo in Africa …'

Elias Nicoletta, a 21-year-old student from Cyprus, is planning to travel to Congo in Africa for volunteer work. Today he visits his general practitioner who prescribes him primaquine tablets and advises him to take the antimalarial tablets as a preventive measure for malaria, endemic in the area he plans to visit. Three days after commencing primaquine, Elias develops generalised fatigue and is seen in the emergency department. On examination, pulse rate is 90/min, blood pressure 120/75 mm Hg, temperature 36.8°C and respiratory rate 20/min. He looks pale and there is a yellow tinge of his sclerae. The remainder of the clinical examination is unremarkable. The results of his blood tests are shown in Table 6.5.1.

CASE DISCUSSION

Q1. On the basis of Elias' presentation, what is your diagnosis?

Q2. What is your differential diagnosis?

Q3. What are the key clinical features of this disease? What are the scientific bases for these features?

Q4. What is the pathophysiology underlying these changes?

Q5. What are your management goals and management options?

ANSWERS

1. The findings of generalised fatigue, pallor, a yellow tinge of the sclerae, low haemoglobin, increased bilirubin, normal transaminases and alkaline phosphatase, and blood film using supravital stain showing Heinz bodies together with the history of intake of antimalarial tablets earlier are suggestive of the diagnosis of haemolytic anaemia most likely due to glucose-6-phosphate dehydrogenase (G6PD) deficiency.

2. The differential diagnosis includes the following:
   - Inherited haemolytic anaemias:
     - Haemoglobinopathies: Sickle cell anaemia (HbSS, HbSC disease, HbS β-thalassaemia)
     - The thalassaemias (α- and β-thalassaemia, thalassaemia intermediate)
     - Red cell membrane disorders (hereditary spherocytosis, hereditary elliptocytosis)
     - Red cell enzyme defects (G6PD deficiency, pyruvate kinase deficiency)

Table 6.5.1 Elias' blood test results

Blood test	Elias' results	Normal range
Haemoglobin (Hb) (g/L)	5.1	115–160
Packed cell volume (PCV)	0.36	0.37–0.47
White cell count (WBC) ($\times 10^9$/L)	12.0	4.0–11.0
Platelet count ($\times 10^9$/L)	180	150–400
Total serum bilirubin[a] (μmol/L)	35	<26

Reticulocytes are increased.

[a]All other liver function tests (serum albumin, AST, ALT, ALP, INR) are within the normal range. Urinalysis is normal. Blood urea and creatinine are within the normal range. Peripheral blood smear shows bite cells. Blood film using supravital stain shows Heinz bodies.

- • Unstable haemoglobin disorders
- • Methaemoglobinaemia
3. Clinical picture:
   - • The symptoms usually appear in response to a trigger. Triggers may be ingestion of fava beans and infections or intake of drugs or chemical agents.
   - • These drugs include pamaquine, primaquine, quinolones, chloroquine, sulfonamides, nitrofurantoin, methylthioninium chloride (methylene blue) or dapsone.
   - • Haemolysis usually occurs within 1–3 days from the time of exposure to the trigger.

Symptoms:
   - • Pallor
   - • Shortness of breath on exercise
   - • Tiredness
   - • Fatigue
   - • Jaundice
   - • Dark urine

Signs:
   - • Pallor
   - • Jaundice

4. Investigations:
   - • Full blood count – low haemoglobin
   - • Peripheral blood film – bite cells
   - • Blood film using supravital stain – Heinz bodies (seen as small, rounded inclusions within red blood cells)
   - • Bilirubin – mainly indirect bilirubin raised
   - • Transaminases and alkaline phosphatase – normal (AST may be raised due to haemolysis)
   - • LDH – raised (due to haemolysis)
   - • Reticulocytes – raised (due to haemolysis)

- Blood urea and creatinine – normal (however, in severe cases with haemolysis, acute renal failure may occur with raised blood urea and creatinine levels)
- A fluorescent spot-screening test for G6PD activity, which detects the formation of NADPH

Pathophysiology:

- G6PD enzyme catalyses the oxidation of glucose-6-phosphate and the reduction of nicotinamide adenine dinucleotide phosphate ($NADP^+$) to NADPH. The latter is responsible for maintaining glutathione in its reduced form in the red blood cells.
- Reduced glutathione is important in the detoxification of free radicals.
- Reduced glutathione acts as a scavenger for dangerous oxidative metabolites and thus maintains the integrity of the red blood cells' membranes and inhibits denaturation of the haemoglobin.
- In normal cells, NADPH is regenerated by G6PD during oxidative stress.
- Deficiency of G6PD prevents reduced glutathione recycling.
- These biochemical mechanisms explain the vulnerability of red blood cells to oxidative stress (such as antimalarial drugs) and their haemolysis in patients with G6PD deficiency.

5. Management goals:
   - Stop the trigger – withdraw or stop the exposure (drugs, chemicals, fava beans).
   - If the trigger is infection, appropriate antibiotics should be started.
   - Blood transformation is rarely needed.
   - Educate the patients about food, drugs and chemicals that they should avoid. Explain the nature of the disease.

BACK TO BASIC SCIENCES

Q1. What are the key differences between G6PD deficiency and pyruvate kinase deficiency?

Table 6.5.2 summarises the differences between G6PD deficiency and pyruvate kinase deficiency.

Table 6.5.2 Differences between G6PD deficiency and pyruvate kinase deficiency

Item	G6PD deficiency	Pyruvate kinase deficiency
Prevalence	The most common inherited condition affecting humans.	Less common (second common defect in RBC enzymes).
Inheritance	X-linked disorder.	Autosomal recessive disorder.
Biochemical defect	There is a defect in the pentose monophosphate shunt, which catalyses the oxidation of glucose-6-phosphate and reduction of $NADP^+$ to NADPH. NADPH is essential for maintaining glutathione.	It is an enzymatic defect in the glycolytic pathway that produces ATP.

Continued

Table 6.5.2 Differences between G6PD deficiency and pyruvate kinase deficiency—cont'd

Item	G6PD deficiency	Pyruvate kinase deficiency
Effects of the defect	A lack of glutathione production in the presence of oxidative stress (drugs, chemicals, fava beans) → red cell haemolysis and denaturation of haemoglobin.	The accumulation of intermediates of the glycolytic pathway → loss of red cell function. The defect results in accumulation of 2,3-diphosphoglycerides → right shift of the oxygen dissociation curve (affected individuals have enhanced exercise tolerance and fewer symptoms despite their anaemia).
Presentation	Acute (after exposure to a trigger).	Chronic. In neonates, hydrops fetalis can occur. During childhood – anaemia, jaundiced, splenomegaly. Symptoms can be exacerbated after parvovirus B19 infection → severe anaemia. Gallstones and leg ulcers may be present.
Blood film	Bite cells, Heinz bodies (supravital stain).	Speculated, small, dense cells.
Diagnosis	History, clinical examination, low haemoglobin, raised bilirubin, raised LDH, raised reticulocytes. Blood film: Bite cells, Heinz bodies (supravital stain).	History, clinical examination. Quantitative enzyme assay.
Management	Stop exposure to triggering agent. Rarely blood transfusion is needed. Patient education.	Folic acid, blood transfusion in severe cases; some patients require regular blood transfusion, splenectomy. Antibiotic prophylaxis, vaccination. Iron chelating therapy. Stem cell transplantation.

Q2. Briefly discuss glucose-6-phosphate enzyme deficiency.

- G6PD deficiency is the most common condition affecting humans; approximately 400 million people worldwide are affected. Its highest prevalence is in Africa, the Middle East, the Mediterranean and Asia. The patient in this case is from Cyprus in the Mediterranean area.
- It is an X-linked disorder (the gene is located on the long arm of the X chromosome) and thus manifests predominantly in males.
- The Mediterranean variant is the most prevalent.
- G6PD enzyme is part of the pentose monophosphate shunt.

Q3. Can females be affected in G6PD deficiency?

The deficiency of G6PD is more common in males than in females (it is an X-linked disease). However, the female heterozygote can have the clinical disease. This is because the heterozygous females have two populations of red blood cells, one with a normal X and the other with G6PD-deficient X chromosomes.

Q4. Do you think that patients with G6PD deficiency have the same degree of severity of haemolysis?

No, the degree of severity of haemolysis varies significantly. There are more than 400 structural types of G6PD and they are mostly due to single amino acid substitutes. The WHO classification grouped these types into type B+ (present mainly in Caucasians and 70% of black Africans), type A+ (present in 20% of black Africans) and type A− in which haemolysis is self-limited (the degree of G6PD deficiency is more in older RBCs and less in newly formed young RBCs).

Q5. Briefly discuss pyramidine-5-nucleotidase deficiency.

Pyramidine-5-nucleotidase enzyme is involved in the catabolism of ribonucleic acid from young red blood cells. The deficiency of pyramidine-5-nucleotidase enzyme is an autosomal recessive disorder characterised by chronic haemolytic anaemia. One of the clues of the diagnosis of this disorder is the presence of prominent red blood cells with basophilic stippling.

REVIEW QUESTIONS

Q1. The gene of the G6PD is located on
A. The long arm of the X chromosome.
B. The short arm of the X chromosome.
C. The short arm of chromosome 17 (17p13).
D. Chromosome 11.

Q2. Which *one* of the following haematological disorders is *not* an inherited haemolytic anaemia?
A. Sickle cell anaemia
B. Pyruvate kinase deficiency
C. α-Thalassaemia
D. Paroxysmal nocturnal haemoglobinuria
E. Pyramidine-5-nucleotidase deficiency

Q3. Which *one* of the following is *not* an oxidant drug that can precipitate haemolysis in a patient with G6PD deficiency?
A. Methylene blue
B. Glibenclamide
C. Nitrofurantoin
D. Atorvastatin
E. Primaquine

Q4. A 30-year-old man presents to the emergency department with shortness of breath and generalised tiredness for the past 24 hours. A few days ago, he had a history of urinary tract infection and dysuria for which his GP commenced him on nitrofurantoin twice daily. His blood test shows low haemoglobin, increased bilirubin, increased reticulocyte count and a peripheral blood film showing bite cells. Which *one* of the following is the most likely diagnosis?

A. Pyruvate kinase deficiency

B. Sickle cell anaemia

C. G6PD deficiency

D. Hereditary spherocytosis

E. Hereditary elliptocytosis

ANSWERS

A1. **A.** The gene for G6PD is located on the long arm of X chromosome. The short arm of chromosome 17 (such as 17p13) is the location of p53 gene. Chromosome 11 is one of the most gene-rich and disease-rich chromosomes.

A2. **D.** Paroxysmal nocturnal haemoglobinuria is an acquired haemolytic disease.

A3. **D.** Atorvastatin does not trigger haemolysis in patients with G6PD deficiency.

A4. **C.** The clinical picture together with the laboratory results is suggestive of the diagnosis of G6PD deficiency.

TAKE-HOME MESSAGE

- G6PD enzyme catalyses the oxidation of glucose-6-phosphate and the reduction of $NADP^+$ to NADPH. The latter is responsible for maintaining glutathione in its reduced form in the red blood cells.
- Reduced glutathione is important in the detoxification of free radicals.
- Reduced glutathione acts as a scavenger for dangerous oxidative metabolites and thus maintains the integrity of the red blood cells' membranes and inhibits denaturation of the haemoglobin.
- In normal cells, NADPH is regenerated by G6PD during oxidative stress.
- Deficiency of G6PD prevents reduced glutathione recycling.
- These biochemical mechanisms explain the vulnerability of red blood cells to oxidative stress (such as antimalarial drugs) and their haemolysis in patients with G6PD deficiency.
- The symptoms usually appear in response to a trigger. Triggers may be ingestion of fava beans and infections or intake of drugs or chemical agents.
- These drugs include pamaquine, primaquine, quinolones, chloroquine, sulfonamides, nitrofurantoin, methylthioninium chloride (methylene blue) or dapsone.
- Haemolysis usually occurs within 1–3 days from the time of exposure to the trigger.

- The goals of the management of G6PD deficiency: (i) stop the trigger: withdraw or stop exposure (drugs, chemicals, fava beans); (ii) if the trigger is infection, appropriate antibiotics should be started; (iii) blood transformation is rarely needed; and (iv) educate the patients about food, drugs and chemicals that they should avoid. Explain the nature of the disease.

FURTHER READINGS

Beutler E. Glucose-6-phosphate dehydrogenase deficiency. *N Engl J Med.* 1991;324(3):169-174. Review.

Beutler E, Duparc S, G6PD Deficiency Working Group. Glucose-6-phosphate dehydrogenase deficiency and antimalarial drug development. *Am J Trop Med Hyg.* 2007;77(4):779-789. Review.

Cappellini MD, Fiorelli G. Glucose-6-phosphate dehydrogenase deficiency. *Lancet.* 2008;371(9606):64-74. Review.

Dhaliwal G, Cornett PA, Tierney Jr LM. Hemolytic anemia. *Am Fam Physician.* 2004;69(11):2599-2606. Review.

Frank JE. Diagnosis and management of G6PD deficiency. *Am Fam Physician.* 2005;72(7):1277-1282. Review.

Ong KIC, Kosugi H, Thoeun S, et al. Systematic review of the clinical manifestations of glucose-6-phosphate dehydrogenase deficiency in the Greater Mekong Subregion: implications for malaria elimination and beyond. *BMJ Glob Health.* 2017;2(3):e000415.

Weatherall DJ. ABC of clinical haematology. The hereditary anaemias. *BMJ.* 1997;314(7079):492-496. Review.

CASE 6.6

'Sweating and Chills ...'

Michael West, a 42-year-old news reporter, returns from Africa where he was on a work mission. He comes in to see his general practitioner because of periodic spiking fever for the past 3 days. He gives a history of an episode of malaria approximately 2 years ago. On examination, his pulse is 100/min, blood pressure 150/90 mm Hg, temperature 39°C and respiratory rate 22/min. Peripheral oxygen saturation is 98% at room temperature. The abdomen is soft and not tender. There is no hepatosplenomegaly. Cardiovascular, respiratory and nervous systems are all normal. Chest X-ray is normal. Blood test results are shown in Table 6.6.1. Thick blood smear and malaria antigen test confirm the diagnosis of *Plasmodium falciparum*.

CASE DISCUSSION

Q1. On the basis of Mr West's presentation, what is your diagnosis?

Q2. What is your differential diagnosis?

Q3. What are the key clinical features of this disease? What are the scientific bases for these features?

Q4. What is the pathophysiology underlying these changes?

Q5. What are your management goals and management options?

ANSWERS

1. The clinical findings of periodic spiking fever that lasted for 3 days, a history of malaria about 2 years earlier, fever with temperature 39°C and sweating, together with the blood test results showing low haemoglobin, low platelet counts and the findings from thick blood film and malaria antigen test, confirm the diagnosis of *Plasmodium falciparum* parasitaemia.

2. The differential diagnosis includes the following:
   - Viral infection
   - Bacteraemia
   - Brucellosis
   - Cholera
   - Trypanosomiasis
   - Typhus
   - Hodgkin disease
   - Q fever

Table 6.6.1 Michael's blood test results

Blood test	Michael's results	Normal range
Haemoglobin (Hb) (g/L)	75	115–160
Packed cell volume (PCV)	0.37	0.37–0.47
White cell count (WBC) ($\times 10^9$/L)	4.0	4.0–11.0
Platelet count ($\times 10^9$/L)	85	150–400

- Dengue fever
- Encephalitis
- Hepatitis
- Meningitis
- Typhoid fever

3. Clinical picture:

Symptoms:

- High fever (after residing in an endemic region).
- Prodromal period of tiredness, fatigue and aching.
- The symptoms are abrupt with an initial feeling of cold and rigors, and shaking 'cold stage'.
- The 'hot stage' then follows – the patient becomes feverish (temperature reaches 40°C), and suffers from restlessness, nausea, vomiting and convulsions.
- This stage is followed by a 'sweating stage' – the patient sweats profusely all over. Usually the patient falls asleep at this stage.
- Other symptoms include the following:
  - Headache
  - Cough
  - Body aches
  - Myalgia
  - Sore throat
  - Nausea
  - Vomiting
  - Loose bowel motions
  - Mild jaundice
- These general symptoms are similar to those experienced in viral infections, upper respiratory tract infections, food poisoning, typhoid fever, viral hepatitis, malaria and infectious mononucleosis.
- In severe *falciparum* malaria, the patient may have the following symptoms as well:
  - Severe anaemia (normocytic anaemia)
  - Coma (cerebral malaria)
  - Renal failure
  - Respiratory distress (pulmonary oedema, adult respiratory distress syndrome)
  - Hypoglycaemia

– Drop of blood pressure
– Cardiorespiratory failure
– Spontaneous bleeding
– Failure of coagulation mechanisms

Signs:

- Patient looks ill, and not well
- High fever (temperature in the range of 39–40°C)
- Profuse sweating
- Drowsiness
- Confusion
- Delirium
- Loss of consciousness
- Pallor
- Jaundice
- Increased respiratory rate
- Drop of blood pressure
- Circulatory collapse
- Signs of pulmonary oedema
- Abdominal tenderness and no rigidity
- Palpable spleen

4. Investigations:

- Full blood count and differential count: There may be low haemoglobin, low platelet counts and normal white cell counts with relative lymphocytosis.
- Thick and thin blood film: If negative, this test should be repeated for 2–5 days particularly when the clinical picture is suggestive of malaria.
- Blood cultures: They help in detecting secondary infections or bacteraemia.
- C-reactive protein: It is raised.
- Serum sodium, calcium and albumin may be low.
- Serum bilirubin: It is raised.
- Liver function tests: They are usually within normal range. The picture is similar to that of haemolytic anaemia. If abnormal, further tests including screening for hepatitis should be ordered to exclude hepatitis.
- Blood glucose: It is low, particularly in children.
- CSF examination: It is needed in patients suspected to have cerebral malaria, and also to exclude meningitis.

The life cycle of malaria in human and mosquito is summarised in Fig. 6.6.1.

5. Management goals:

- Emergency treatment needed in severe cases – IV artesunate 4 mg/kg/day for 3 days
- Admission in intensive care facility, mechanical ventilation and dialysis
- Blood transfusion for severe anaemia
- Continuous monitoring – fluid balance, pulmonary oedema and prerenal failure
- Watching for hypoglycaemia (in patients with secondary infection and those treated with quinine)

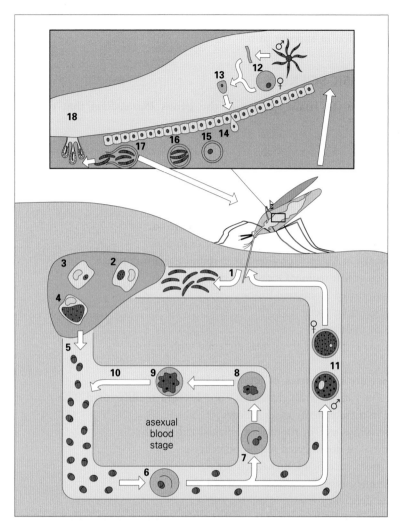

Figure 6.6.1 Life cycle of malaria in human and mosquito.

The Lower Part – The cycle in human body: 1. Sporozoites are injected into the human dermis through the bite of an infected *Anopheles* mosquito; 2. Sporozoites travel in the blood and infect liver cells; 3. Changes to hypnozoites; 4. Formation of hepatic schizont, then merozoites; 5. Release of merozoites from ruptured liver cells; 6. Merozoites penetrate red blood cells; 7, 8 and 9. Asexual reproduction; 10. Infect more red blood cells; 11. Development of male and female gametocytes.

The Upper part – The cycle in mosquito: 12. In a mosquito's stomach, a microgamete enters a macrogamete and forming a zygote; 13. The zygote becomes motile and elongated and developed into ookinete; 14. Ookinetes invade the midgut wall of the mosquito; 15. Ookinte changes to oocyst; 16. Oocyst grows; 17. Rupture and release of sporozoites; 18. Sporozoites travel to the mosquito's salivary glands.

(Source: Kumar V, Abbas AK, Fausto N, Mitchell R. Robbins Basic Pathology, 8th Edition. London, UK: Elsevier; 2007.)

- Spontaneous bacterial infection (blood culture and treat accordingly)
- Prevention in endemic area

BACK TO BASIC SCIENCES

Q1. What are the main species of the genus *Plasmodium* that cause malaria transmission?

- *P. falciparum*
- *P. vivax*
- *P. ovale*
- *P. malariae*

Q2. Briefly discuss how malaria is transmitted.

- By the bite of the female anopheline mosquitoes
- Sub-Saharan Africa: Consistent year-round transmission
- The Sahel belt region: Occasional transmission
- Contaminated blood transfusion
- Injecting drug users
- Airport malaria
- Returning travellers from areas endemic with malaria

Q3. What are the causes of anaemia in malaria?

Anaemia in patients with malaria is complex and multifactorial. The main causes of anaemia in these patients are as follows:

- Phagocytosis and/or rupture of infected red blood cells
- Removal of noninfected red blood cells
- Increased reticuloendothelial activity
- Splenomegaly and sequestration of red blood cells
- Folate deficiency
- Decreased red cell production (marrow hyperplasia in acute infection)
- Ineffective erythropoiesis
- Parvovirus B19 infection postulated as a cause of bone marrow aplasia in a few cases
- Genetic factors

Q4. What is black water fever?

Patients with black water fever have rapid intravascular haemolysis commonly associated with chronic *falciparum* malaria, most commonly in those who have taken antimalarial drugs, especially quinine, or are deficient in glucose-6-phospate dehydrogenase (G6PD).

Infection with *P. falciparum* may last for 6 months and in these patients haemolysis may occur suddenly involving parasitised and nonparasitised red blood cells. The mechanism of haemolysis is not clearly known. However, it may be related to autoimmunity. Patients with black water fever present with sudden, severe rigor, irregular fever, pain in the loins, epigastric pain, nausea, vomiting, profuse sweating, yellow skin and increased frequency of micturition. The urine is dark brown or cherry red and the spleen is usually palpable. Examination of peripheral blood reveals ring form of trophozoites of *P. falciparum*.

The patients with black water fever usually develop acute renal failure (usually because of renal vasoconstriction reflex). Also, they usually have cardiovascular collapse and decreased renal perfusion. They usually need haemodialysis for acute renal failure.

Q5. Briefly discuss the pathology of *P. falciparum*.
- In *P. falciparum*, there is widespread organ damage due to impaired microcirculation of body organs including the brain, kidney, gut and liver.
- At molecular level, *P. falciparum* erythrocyte membrane protein 1 (PFEMP1), its receptors, coagulation, host endothelial activation and inflammation of endothelium are all possible contributors to the development of cerebral malaria in patients infected with *P. falciparum*.
- Some people appear to have a genetic predisposition to develop **cerebral malaria** following infection with *P. falciparum*.
- The vast majority of malaria deaths are due to *P. falciparum*. Patients deteriorate rapidly and die within a few hours. The development of such complications is not related to a high parasitaemia (>1% of red blood cells are infected).
- Patients infected with *P. falciparum* may develop **black water fever** due to increased intravascular haemolysis of parasitised and nonparasitised red blood cells. These patients usually present with irregular fever, loin pains, epigastric pain, nausea and vomiting, yellow skin and dark brown urine.

REVIEW QUESTIONS

Q1. Which *one* of the following is responsible for the vast majority of malaria deaths?
A. *P. falciparum*
B. *P. ovale*
C. *P. malariae*
D. *P. vivax*

Q2. Which *one* of the following is at a high risk of overwhelming malaria?
A. Splenectomised patients
B. *P. ovale* infection
C. *P. malariae* infection
D. Iron-deficiency anaemia

Q3. Which *one* of the following is responsible for widespread organ damage?
A. *P. ovale* infection
B. *P. malariae* infection
C. *P. vivax* infection
D. *P. falciparum* infection

Q4. Which *one* of the following is associated with nephrotic syndrome?
A. *P. ovale* infection
B. *P. malariae* infection
C. *P. vivax* infection
D. *P. falciparum* infection

Q5. Which *one* of the following is associated with relapses for years after infection?
A. *P. vivax* or *P. ovale*
B. *P. malariae* or *P. falciparum*
C. Cerebral malaria
D. Black water fever

ANSWERS

A1. **A.** *P. falciparum* is responsible for the majority of deaths in malaria.

A2. **A.** Splenectomised patients and pregnant women are at a higher risk of overwhelming malaria.

A3. **D.** *P. falciparum* is usually associated with multiorgan damage.

A4. **B.** Patients infected with *P. malariae* are at risk of developing glomerulonephritis and nephrotic syndrome.

A5. **A.** Patients infected with *P. vivax* or *P. ovale* are at a higher risk of relapses for years after infection. This is because hypnozoites in the liver can cause relapses for many years after infection.

TAKE-HOME MESSAGE

- *P. falciparum* is responsible for the majority of deaths in malaria.
- *P. falciparum* is usually associated with multiorgan damage.
- Patients infected with *P. vivax* or *P. ovale* are at a higher risk of relapses for years after infection. This is because hypnozoites in the liver can cause relapses for many years after infection.
- The symptoms of *P. falciparum* may include high fever, sweating, feeling cold, nausea, vomiting, headache, cough, body aches, myalgia, loose bowel motions, convulsions and changes in the conscious state.
- The signs of *P. falciparum* may include the following: the patient looks ill and not well, high fever, drowsiness, confusion, delirium, loss of consciousness, pallor, jaundice, increased respiratory rate, drop of blood pressure, circulatory collapse, pulmonary oedema, abdominal tenderness and palpable spleen.
- Full blood count and differential count: There may be low haemoglobin, low platelet counts and normal white cell counts with relative lymphocytosis.

- Thick and thin blood film: If negative, this test should be repeated for 2–5 days particularly when the clinical picture is suggestive of malaria.
- Blood cultures: They help in detecting secondary infections or bacteraemia.
- The management of *P. falciparum* includes the following: (i) emergency treatment needed in severe cases – IV artesunate 4 mg/kg/day for 3 days; (ii) admission in intensive care facility, mechanical ventilation and dialysis; (iii) blood transfusion for severe anaemia; (iv) continuous monitoring – fluid balance, pulmonary oedema and prerenal failure; (v) watching for hypoglycaemia (in patients with secondary infection and those treated with quinine); (vi) spontaneous bacterial infection (blood culture and treat accordingly); and (vii) prevention in endemic area.

FURTHER READINGS

Baird JK. Effectiveness of antimalarial drugs. *N Engl J Med.* 2005;352(15):1565–1577. Review.

Croft AM. Malaria: prevention in travellers (non-drug interventions). *BMJ Clin Evid.* 2014;2014:0903.

Freedman DO. Clinical practice. Malaria prevention in short-term travelers. *N Engl J Med.* 2008;359(6): 603–612. Review.

Ong KIC, Kosugi H, Thoeun S, et al. Systematic review of the clinical manifestations of glucose-6-phosphate dehydrogenase deficiency in the Greater Mekong Subregion: implications for malaria elimination and beyond. *BMJ Glob Health.* 2017;2(3):e000415.

Phillips RE, Pasvol G. Anaemia of Plasmodium falciparum malaria. *Baillieres Clin Haematol.* 1992;5(2): 315–330.

Rosenthal PJ. Artesunate for the treatment of severe falciparum malaria. *N Engl J Med.* 2008;358(17): 1829–1836. Review.

Storm J, Craig AG. Pathogenesis of cerebral malaria—inflammation and cytoadherence. *Front Cell Infect Microbiol.* 2014;4:100.

Whitty CJ, Chiodini PL, Lalloo DG. Investigation and treatment of imported malaria in non-endemic countries. *BMJ.* 2013;346:f2900. Review.

SECTION 7

Renal System

CASE 7.1

'... After Severe Attack of Diarrhoea'

James Martin, a 75-year-old retired policeman, is brought by the ambulance to the emergency department of a local hospital because he is suffering from severe recurrent diarrhoea and vomiting. His stools are watery and he has abdominal pain all over. He has been on treatment for more than 2 years with furosemide (a loop diuretic) and enalapril (an angiotensin-converting enzyme inhibitor) for high blood pressure. His blood pressure is always in the range 130/80 to 140/90 mm Hg and his blood urea and creatinine are normal as per the results a month ago. He is also on naproxen (a NSAID) for chronic knee pain. On examination, his blood pressure is 90/60 mm Hg, pulse rate 130/min, respiratory rate 26/min and temperature 37.6°C. He is conscious, and there is no neurological deficit; cardiovascular and respiratory examinations show nothing significant; the abdomen is soft and is mildly tender but there is no rigidity. He received all emergency management including intravenous fluids. His blood urea and creatinine are raised and urine analysis shows granular and hyaline casts +++.

CASE DISCUSSION

Q1. On the basis of Mr Martin's presentation, what is your diagnosis?

Q2. What is your differential diagnosis?

Q3. What are the key clinical features of this disease? What are the scientific bases for these features?

Q4. What is the pathophysiology underlying these changes?

Q5. What are your management goals and management options?

ANSWERS

1. The findings of severe diarrhoea and vomiting (volume loss), possibly due to infectious gastroenteritis, may have contributed to reduced renal perfusion and glomerular filtration resulting in a rise in the blood urea and creatinine levels (acute renal failure). The finding that his blood urea and creatinine levels were normal a month earlier should exclude chronic renal failure. However, the presence of granular and hyaline casts in urinalysis raises the possibility of acute tubular necrosis. This change could be related to severe volume loss, together with the treatment with an angiotensin-converting

enzyme inhibitor, a diuretic and a NSAID. This triad (volume loss + NSAID + angiotensin-converting enzyme inhibitor) could have resulted in a decrease in renal blood supply to the kidney parenchyma and contributed to the development of acute tubular necrosis. Further assessment including urinary sodium, urine osmolality and urine specific gravity is needed.

2. The differential diagnosis includes the following (Fig. 7.1.1):
   - Prerenal causes (decreased kidney perfusion, decreased glomerular filtration rate)
     - Dehydration (e.g. repeated vomiting and diarrhoea)
     - Haemorrhage (e.g. gastrointestinal bleeding, trauma)
     - Heart failure/shock (decreased cardiac output)
     - Renal artery stenosis (e.g. fibromuscular dysplasia)
     - Burns (loss of plasma volume)
     - Third space loss (peritonitis, bowel obstruction, pancreatitis)
   - Renal disease (glomerulotubular or renal vessel disease)
     - Acute tubular necrosis (e.g. NSAIDs, contrast media, multiple myeloma, rhabdomyolysis, haemolysis, chemotherapy, cyclosporin A)
     - Ischaemia (prolonged prerenal insult, acute tubular necrosis)
     - Acute glomerulonephritis (immunoglobulin A nephropathy, systemic lupus erythematosus, cryoglobulinaemia, endocarditis)
     - Other causes of glomerulonephritis (microscopic polyarteritis, Goodpasture disease, anti-GBM glomerulonephritis)
     - Drugs (diuretics, NSAIDs, rifampin, phenytoin, β-lactams, allopurinol)
     - Infections (e.g. cytomegalovirus, *Streptococcus*)
     - Immunological disorders (systemic lupus erythematosus, Sjögren syndrome, sarcoidosis)
     - Vascular (malignant hypertension, thrombotic thrombocytopenic purpura)
   - Postrenal causes (urinary tract obstruction, back pressure affecting kidney functions)
     - Benign prostatic hyperplasia
     - Bladder tumour

   The following are the key features of acute renal failure:
   - A deterioration of the kidney functions resulting in a disturbance in the acid–base balance and the fluid and the electrolyte balance over hours or days
   - Inability to excrete nitrogenous waste resulting in sudden elevation of blood urea levels
   - Elevation of serum creatinine concentration
   - Oliguria (falling of urine output)
   - Development of symptoms reflecting the changes in the renal functions and the cause of failure (prerenal, renal or postrenal)
   - Deterioration may be on top of chronic renal failure

3. Clinical picture:
   Symptoms:
   - Nausea
   - Vomiting

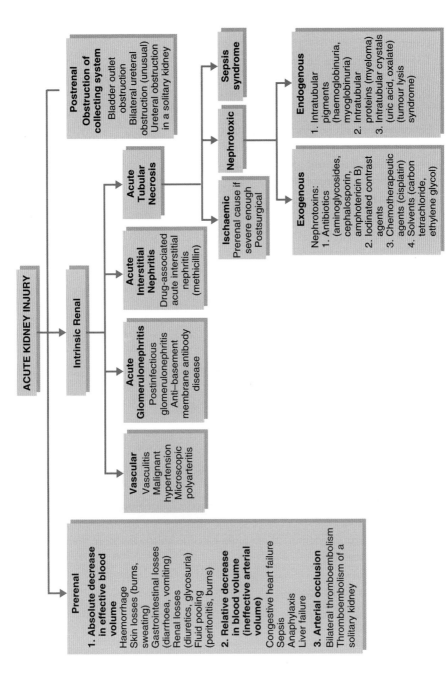

Figure 7.1.1 Causes of acute renal failure. *(Source: Andreoli TE, Benjamin IJ, Griggs RC, Wing EJ. Andreoli and Carpenter's Cecil Essentials of Medicine. 8th ed. Philadelphia, PA: Elsevier; 2010.)*

- Fatigue
- Tiredness
- Malaise
- Pruritus
- Loose bowel motions (in prerenal causes)
- Fever
- Decline in urine output
- Dark-coloured urine
- Shortness of breath (in heart failure, fluid overload)

Signs:
- Hypertension (malignant hypertension)
- Hypotension (in prerenal failure)
- Arrhythmias
- Signs of heart failure
- Pallor (in haemorrhage)
- Dehydration (in prerenal failure)
- Chest rales
- Pericardial friction rub
- Pericardial effusion, cardiac tamponade
- Bleeding
- Encephalopathy
- Oliguria <20 mL/h
- Distended jugular venous pressure (in heart failure, fluid overload)

4. Pathogenesis:

The pathogenesis of acute renal failure is shown in Fig. 7.1.2.

Laboratory findings:
- Full blood count – anaemia
- Elevated blood urea and serum creatinine
  - Stage 1: Serum creatinine 1.5–1.9 times baseline, urine output <0.5 mL/kg/h for 6–12 hours
  - Stage 2: Serum creatinine: 2–2.9 times baseline, urine output <0.5 mL/kg/h for 6–12 hours
  - Stage 3: Serum creatinine three times baseline, anuria for more than 12 hours
- Hyperphosphataemia
- Hypocalcaemia
- Anion gap (metabolic acidosis)
- Urine specific gravity:
  >1.020 (prerenal)
  <1.010 (intrinsic renal)
- Urine osmolality (mOsm/kg):
  >500 (prerenal)
  <500 (intrinsic renal)

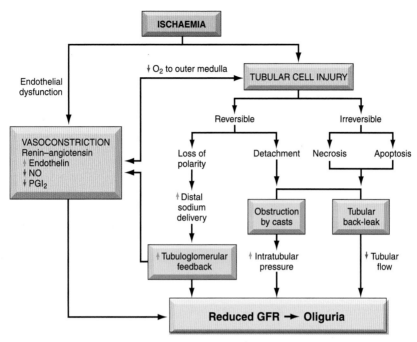

Figure 7.1.2 Pathogenesis of acute renal failure. *(Source: Kumar V, Abbas AK, Fausto N, Mitchell R. Robbins Basic Pathology, 8th Edition. London, UK: Elsevier; 2007.)*

- Urine sodium (mmol/L):
  <10 (prerenal)
  >20 (intrinsic renal)
- Fractional excretion of sodium $(FE_{Na}+)$ = Urine Na^+/plasma Na^+/urine creatinine/ plasma creatinine:
  $<1\%$ (prerenal)
  $>1\%$ (intrinsic renal)
- ECG: Changes suggestive of hypocalcaemia and hyperkalaemia
- Radiological studies: (i) Renal ultrasound – check the kidney size, exclude urinary back pressure in postrenal cases; (ii) CT or magnetic resonance imaging (MRI) to detect retroperitoneal fibrosis
5. Management goals:
   - Treat the cause – blood transfusion in case of haemorrhage, fluid replacement in case of dehydration, stopping drugs causing renal injury, relief of obstruction in postrenal failure.
   - Maintain haemodynamics, blood volume, cardiac monitor.
   - Monitor fluid in/out balance.
   - Correct the electrolyte imbalance and metabolic changes (haemodialysis, peritoneal dialysis), particularly in patients with the following:
     i. Severe metabolic acidosis
     ii. Uraemic symptoms

    iii. Fluid overload

    iv. Hyperkalaemia

    v. Severe acute renal failure (creatinine >500 μmol/L)

BACK TO BASIC SCIENCES

Q1. Give examples of drugs/chemicals that may cause renal tubular injury.

- Aminoglycosides
- Acyclovir
- Sulfonamides
- Cyclosporin A
- Amphotericin B
- Radiocontrast agents
- Toluene
- Cocaine
- HMG-CoA reductase inhibitors (e.g. statins)

Q2. Give examples of drugs that may cause acute interstitial nephritis.

- Diuretics (e.g. furosemide, hydrochlorothiazide)
- NSAIDs (e.g. ibuprofen, naproxen)
- Beta-lactam antibiotics (e.g. penicillin, cephalosporins, ampicillin, methicillin, nafcillin)
- Other antibiotics (e.g. vancomycin, rifampin)

Q3. Briefly discuss the mechanisms underlying ischaemic acute renal injury.

- Depletion of intravascular volume (e.g. haemorrhage, severe diarrhoea, vomiting, burns) → hypovolaemia → decreased glomerular perfusion → decreased glomerular filtration → decreased urine output
- Third space loss (e.g. bowel obstruction, peritonitis) → decreased effective intravascular volume → haemodynamic changes → decreased glomerular perfusion → decreased glomerular filtration
- Systemic vasodilation → maldistribution and haemodynamic changes → renal vasoconstriction → decreased glomerular filtration

Q4. How would you differentiate prerenal injury from ischaemic renal injury?

- Urine specific gravity:
  >1.020 (prerenal)
  <1.010 (intrinsic renal)
- Urine osmolality (mOsm/kg):
  >500 (prerenal)
  <500 (intrinsic renal)
- Urine sodium (mmol/L):
  <10 (prerenal)
  >20 (intrinsic renal)

- Fractional excretion of sodium $(FE_{Na}+)$ = Urine Na^+/plasma Na^+/urine creatinine/plasma creatinine:
  <1% (prerenal)
  >1% (intrinsic renal)

Q5. Can urinalysis (microscopic examination) help in differentiating prerenal injury from intrinsic renal injury?
Prerenal injury: Normal or hyaline casts may be seen.
Intrinsic renal injury: General casts, epithelial casts, eosinophil, red blood casts, RBCs and pus cells may be seen.

Q6. What are the possible causes for postrenal acute kidney injury?
- Bilateral urinary outflow obstruction
- A solitary kidney and a single urinary outflow obstruction
- Prostatic hypertrophy
- Prostatic or cervical cancer
- Retroperitoneal lymphadenopathy/fibrosis
- A neurogenic bladder
- Bilateral ureteric calculi or obstruction or blood clots
- Bladder cancer
- Retroperitoneal fibrosis
- Colorectal cancer, lymphadenopathy

REVIEW QUESTIONS

Q1. A delay in corrective medical management of prerenal azotaemia may result in
A. Sepsis.
B. Ischaemic acute kidney injury.
C. Microvascular congestion.
D. Increased glomerular filtration rate.

Q2. Which *one* of the following laboratory results is indicative of a prerenal injury rather than an intrinsic renal injury?
A. Presence of blood cell casts in urine microscopy
B. Urine sodium >20 mmol/L
C. Fractional excretion of sodium <1%
D. Urine specific gravity <0.010

Q3. Acute kidney injury is frequently first diagnosed from
A. Urine microscopy.
B. Patient symptoms.
C. Clinical examination.
D. Patient's biochemical profile.

Q4. Urine microscopy should be performed on a fresh urine sample because
A. Systemic alkalosis and high urinary bicarbonate are present.
B. Pus cells interfere with the examination.
C. Cellular elements degrade rapidly.
D. Inflammatory markers affect the examination.

ANSWERS

A1. **B.** Renal tubular epithelial cell injury, commonly termed acute tubular necrosis, occurs as a result of the delay in managing prerenal azotaemia. The underlying mechanism is related to the development of ischaemic changes (reduced renal blood flow) resulting in acute kidney injury.

A2. **C.** A fractional excretion of sodium of <1% is suggestive of prerenal injury.

A3. **D.** Acute kidney injury is frequently first diagnosed from the patient's biochemical profile. The patient's symptoms and signs are not specific or helpful in making the diagnosis. The urine microscopy cannot make such diagnosis.

A4. **C.** Cellular elements such as casts degrade rapidly with time and these elements are important in making the differentiation between prerenal injury and intrinsic renal injury.

TAKE-HOME MESSAGE

- Acute renal failure may be due to (i) prerenal causes, (ii) renal causes or (iii) postrenal causes.
- The symptoms of acute renal failure include nausea, vomiting, fatigue, tiredness, loose bowel motions and decrease in urine output.
- The signs in acute renal failure include dehydration (prerenal causes), pallor (haemorrhage), hypotension, hypertension, arrhythmias and signs of heart failure.
- Laboratory tests help in differentiating prerenal causes from renal causes.
- ECG: Changes are suggestive of hypocalcaemia and hyperkalaemia.
- Radiological studies: (i) renal ultrasound: check the kidney size, exclude urinary back pressure in postrenal cases; (ii) CT or magnetic resonance imaging (MRI) to detect retroperitoneal fibrosis.
- The goals and options: (i) treat the cause – blood transfusion in case of haemorrhage, fluid replacement in case of dehydration, stopping drugs causing renal injury, relief of obstruction in postrenal failure; (ii) maintain haemodynamics, blood volume, cardiac monitor; (iii) monitor fluid in/out balance; and (iv) correct electrolyte imbalance and metabolic changes (haemodialysis, peritoneal dialysis).

FURTHER READINGS

Bosch X, Poch E, Grau JM. Rhabdomyolysis and acute kidney injury. *N Engl J Med*. 2009;361(1): 62-72. doi:10.1056/NEJMra0801327. Review. No abstract available. Erratum in: *N Engl J Med*. 2011; 364(20):1982.

Hodgson LE, Sarnowski A, Roderick PJ, Dimitrov BD, Venn RM, Forni LG. Systematic review of prognostic prediction models for acute kidney injury (AKI) in general hospital populations. *BMJ Open.* 2017;7(9):e016591.

Kellum J, Leblanc M, Venkataraman R. Acute renal failure. *Am Fam Physician.* 2007;76(3):418-422. Review.

Klahr S, Miller SB. Acute oliguria. *N Engl J Med.* 1998;338(10):671-675. Review.

Naughton CA. Drug-induced nephrotoxicity. *Am Fam Physician.* 2008;78(6):743-750. Review.

Needham E. Management of acute renal failure. *Am Fam Physician.* 2005;72(9):1739-1746. Review.

CASE 7.2

'... Fluid Build-up in My Body'

Marium Mahmood, a 16-year-old student, presents, with her mother, to the emergency department because of swelling of Marium's face and shortness of breath. She gives a history of hospital admissions and recurrent swellings of her lower limbs. She was treated with steroids. Further assessment reveals that she neither is hypertensive nor has haematuria. Her full blood count, creatinine and electrolytes are within normal limits, and blood albumin is 24 g/L (n = 35–50 g/L). Her urine protein/creatinine ratio is >7 (normal <2). There is no hypocomplementaemia. A renal ultrasound shows symmetrically normal-sized kidneys. A renal biopsy is consistent with the diagnosis of minimal change disease. Because of poor response to prednisolone, she is placed on immunomodulator therapy.

CASE DISCUSSION

Q1. On the basis of Marium's presentation, what is your diagnosis?

Q2. What is your differential diagnosis?

Q3. What are the key clinical features of this disease? What are the scientific bases for these features?

Q4. What is the pathophysiology underlying these changes?

Q5. What are your management goals and management options?

ANSWERS

1. The findings of swellings of the face, recurrent swellings of the lower limbs and shortness of breath in her age group together with the absence of hypertension and haematuria, low serum albumin and raised urinary protein/creatinine ratio are consistent with the diagnosis of nephrotic syndrome. The renal biopsy indicates that she has minimal change disease, and such pathological diagnosis is consistent with the clinical findings.
2. The differential diagnosis of nephrotic syndrome includes the following:
   * Cirrhosis
   * Protein-losing enteropathy
   * Hypothyroidism
   * Malnutrition
   * Heart failure
   * Venous insufficiency

3. Key diagnostic features of nephrotic syndrome:
   - Proteinuria >3 g/day
   - Serum albumin <30 g/L
   - Oedema (peripheral, general, periorbital)
   - Renal insufficiency uncommon at presentation
   - Urine RBCs few and urine RBC casts unlikely
   - Hyperlipidaemia
   - Oval fat bodies in urine

   Clinical picture:
   Symptoms:
   - Weight gain
   - Peripheral oedema (may become generalised)
   - Shortness of breath (pulmonary oedema, pleural effusion, ascites)
   - Increased abdominal girth
   - Infections (increased susceptibility to infection because of urinary loss of immunoglobulins)
   - Increased risk of developing venous thrombosis (because of loss of anticoagulants in urine)

   Signs:
   - Hypertension
   - Proteinuria
   - Microscopic haematuria
   - Mild to moderate azotaemia
   - Hypoalbuminaemia
   - Intravascular volume depletion
   - Normal complement level

4. Laboratory investigations:
   - Serum albumin is <3 g/dL.
   - Serum protein is <6 g/dL.
   - Serum creatinine and blood urea are normal at the time of presentation.
   - Urinalysis: It shows proteinuria +++ (heavy proteinuria >3.5 g/day) and few casts and cells.
   - Oval fat bodies: They appear as 'grape clusters' under light microscopy.
   - Hyperlipidaemia is present.
   - Erythrocyte sedimentation rate (ESR) may be elevated.
   - Other investigations to identify the cause of nephrotic syndrome are (i) serum and urine protein electrophoresis, (ii) antinuclear antibodies and double-stranded DNA, (iii) serological tests for hepatitis, (iv) HIV tests and (v) blood glucose level, HbA_{1c}.
   - Renal biopsy is done in adults and if a primary renal disease is suspected. It is not recommended if the patient is diabetic or the blood urea is raised.

Pathophysiological features:

- Breaks in the glomerular capillary walls → haematuria → loss of selective barrier to particles and charge → proteinuria.
- In some glomerulopathies, there are structural changes in the walls of glomerular capillaries (e.g. in diabetes and amyloidosis) → adding to the pathophysiology.
- Other glomerulonephropathies show immune-mediated renal injury and deposition of immune complexes.
- Genetic-based changes and pathological changes in the glomerular podocytes may also contribute to proteinuria and changes in renal functions.
- The causes of glomerulonephritis are (i) diabetes mellitus, (ii) lupus nephritis, (iii) amyloidosis, (iv) HIV-associated nephropathy, (v) multiple myeloma and (vi) idiopathic.
- The glomerulonephritis could be the following:
    i. Minimal change disease (5%–10%) (Fig. 7.2.1)
    ii. Focal segmental glomerulosclerosis (20%–25%) (Fig. 7.2.2)
    iii. Membranous nephropathy (25%–30%) (Fig. 7.2.3)
    iv. Proliferative and sclerosing glomerulonephritides (15%–30%)
    v. Mesangiocapillary glomerulonephritis (5%)

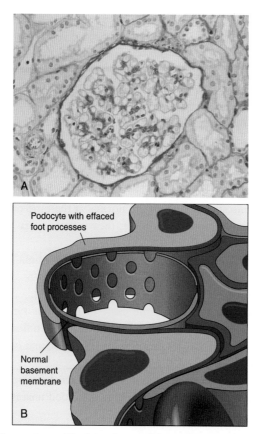

Figure 7.2.1 Minimal change disease. (A) a light micrograph image, (B) a two-dimensional diagram. *(Source: Kumar V, Abbas AK, Fausto N, Mitchell R. Robbins Basic Pathology, 8th Edition. London, UK: Elsevier; 2007.)*

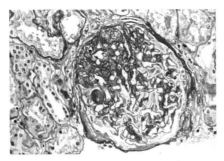

Figure 7.2.2 Focal segmental glomerulosclerosis; a light micrograph image. *(Source: Kumar V, Abbas AK, Fausto N, Mitchell R. Robbins Basic Pathology, 8th Edition. London, UK: Elsevier; 2007.)*

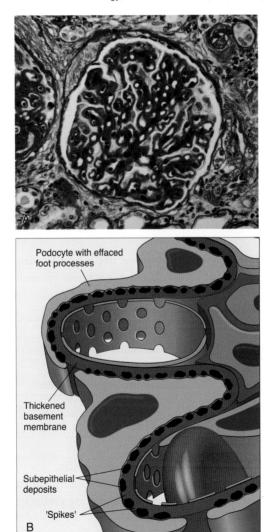

Figure 7.2.3 Membranous glomerulonephropathy. (A) a light micrograph image, (B) a two- dimensional diagram. *(Source: Kumar V, Abbas AK, Fausto N, Mitchell R. Robbins Basic Pathology, 8th Edition. London, UK: Elsevier; 2007.)*

5. Management goals:
   • Reduce oedema (salt restriction and diuretics).
   • Control high blood pressure (angiotensin-converting enzyme inhibitors or angiotensin II receptor blockers). These drugs delay the progression of the disease.
   • Manage hyperlipidaemia (statin).
   • Manage hypercoagulability by anticoagulation and warfarin for at least 3–6 months. Patients are at a high risk of developing deep venous thrombosis and pulmonary embolism. This is because of urinary loss of protein C and protein S.
   • Manage infections by the administration of systemic antibiotics and vaccination against encapsulated bacteria. Patients are at a higher risk of developing systemic infections because of hypogammaglobulinaemia.
   • Corticosteroids and cytotoxic drugs are indicated for primary renal disease.

BACK TO BASIC SCIENCES

Q1. List the systemic diseases in which glomerulonephritis may be a feature.
• Systemic lupus erythematosus and other connective tissue diseases
• Systemic vasculitis
• Infective endocarditis
• Diabetes mellitus
• Infectious diseases (hepatitis C, HIV, malaria, methicillin-resistant *Staphylococcus aureus*)
• Carcinoma/lymphoma
• Multiple myeloma
• Drugs such as nonsteroidal anti-inflammatory drugs and penicillamine

Q2. What are the key differences between nephrotic syndrome and nephritis?
Table 7.2.1 summarises the differences between nephrotic syndrome and nephritis.

Table 7.2.1 Differences between nephrotic syndrome and nephritis

Item	Nephrotic syndrome	Nephritis
Renal insufficiency at presentation	Uncommon	Common
Proteinuria	>3 g/day (In severe cases, >3.5 g/day)	Variable
Urine RBCs	Few	Predominant
Urine RBC casts	Unlikely	Present

Q3. Discuss the pathogenesis of glomerulonephritis.
• Main contributing factors are (i) genetic susceptibility, (ii) environmental factors (precipitants) and (iii) immune mechanisms triggering a number of changes resulting in the development of glomerulonephritis.
• The genetic factors include major histocompatibility complex HLA genes.

- The environmental factors (precipitants) include exposure to drugs, chemicals and infections.
- The immunological mechanisms are triggered as a result of inflammatory mediators, cellular immunity (T-cell macrophages), humoral immunity, antibodies, immuno-complexes and complement involvement.
- In the resulting pathophysiological processes, a number of changes occur depending on the subtype of glomerulonephritis including glomerular deposit of antibodies, circulating autoantibodies, immune complexes and complement deposition, particularly C3 (in mesangiocapillary glomerulonephritis (GN)).
- Abnormalities occur in serum complement (low C3 and C4) in poststreptococcal GN and in lupus nephritis.
- Deficiency of regulating protein 'factor H' occurs in haemolytic–uraemic syndrome and mesangiocapillary GN.
- Autoantibodies directed against complement (e.g. C3 nephritic factor C3NeF) occur in (i) mesangiocapillary GN (50% of patients), (ii) type II mesangiocapillary GN C3NeF and (iii) anti-C1q antibodies in lupus nephritis.

Q4. Discuss the differences between these subtypes of glomerulonephritis (minimal change GN, focal segmental glomerulosclerosis, membranous nephropathy and IgA nephropathy).

See Table 7.2.2.

Table 7.2.2 A comparison of subtypes of glomerulonephritis

Item	Minimal change nephropathy (minimal change disease)	Focal segmental glomerulosclerosis	Membranous nephropathy	IgA nephropathy
Presentation	• Most common in children • Causes 80% of nephrotic syndrome in children • No hypertension • No hypocomplementaemia • No haematuria • No cellular casts in urine • No persistent impairment in renal function	• Asymptomatic proteinuria or nephrotic syndrome • Associated with high blood pressure, microscopic haematuria, impaired renal excretory functions and cortisone resistance • Proteinuria is nonselective (albuminuria and high-molecular-weight protein)	• Asymptomatic proteinuria or nephrotic syndrome • Associated with hypertension, microscopic haematuria, impaired excretory renal function	• Most common type of GN • Presents with haematuria • Prognosis is good in patients with no heavy proteinuria, hypertension or impaired renal functions • End-stage renal disease (ESRD) in 25% of patients when there is proteinuria 1 g/24 h

Continued

Table 7.2.2 A comparison of subtypes of glomerulonephritis—cont'd

Item	Minimal change nephropathy (minimal change disease)	Focal segmental glomerulosclerosis	Membranous nephropathy	IgA nephropathy
Causes	• Occasionally secondary to use of NSAIDs • Secondary to malignancy/lymphoma	• Occurs after renal transplantation • Seen in extreme obesity • A variant seen in HIV infection	• Primary (idiopathic) form; approximately 70–80% of idiopathic form has autoantibodies to phospholipase A2 receptor (PLA2R); the PLA2R is absent in secondary forms • Secondary form (drugs, solid tumours, HepB, HepC, SLE, hypothyroidism) • Secondary form is associated with malignancy in 20% of patients (screening includes chest X-rays, mammography, colonoscopy, faecal occult blood, prostate-specific antigen) • Related to major histocompatibility complex (MHC), linked to HLA-DQA1 and chromosome 2 (PLA2R) gene	• Genetic, familial • Liver diseases such as cirrhosis, hepatitis B and C • Celiac disease • Dermatitis herpetiformis • Infections such as HIV infection and other infections

Table 7.2.2 A comparison of subtypes of glomerulonephritis—cont'd

Item	Minimal change nephropathy (minimal change disease)	Focal segmental glomerulosclerosis	Membranous nephropathy	IgA nephropathy
Biopsy	Light microscopy: Looks normal	• Scarring of glomeruli (focal) • Not all glomeruli are affected • Segmental – affects part of the individual glomeruli • Similar changes are seen after nephrectomy, ischemia and obesity	• There is 'thickening' of the vessel walls within the kidney • Scattered immune complex deposits	• IgA nephropathy is characterised by deposition of polymeric IgA in the glomerulus • The primary abnormality is in the IgA system, not in the kidney • 50% of patients have elevated serum IgA concentration; IgA is chemically abnormal
Treatment	• Approximately 90% of patients respond to high dose of corticosteroids (remission in 7–14 days to 16 weeks) • 50% of patients remain corticosteroid-dependent or cyclophosphamide or chlorambucil plus prednisolone for 8–12 weeks	• High corticosteroids up to 6 months • Cyclosporin A 3–4 mg/kg/day for 4–12 months • ACE inhibitors to reduce proteinuria • Obesity – reduce body weight	• Immunotherapy in idiopathic form	• In IgA nephropathy with ESRD, transplantation is recommended • Disease recurs in 50% of cases

REVIEW QUESTIONS

Q1. Autoantibodies to phospholipase A2 receptor (PLA2R) have been reported in the majority of patients with (*select one response*)
A. Minimal change nephropathy.
B. Focal segmental glomerulosclerosis.
C. IgA nephropathy.
D. Idiopathic membranous nephropathy.
E. Secondary forms of membranous nephropathy.

Q2. The glomerulonephropathy commonly seen after renal transplantation is (*select one response*)
A. IgA glomerulonephropathy.
B. Mesangiocapillary glomerulonephropathy.
C. Focal segmental glomerulosclerosis.
D. Membranous nephropathy.
E. Minimal change nephropathy.

Q3. The glomerular lesion that is similar to that of Henoch–Schönlein purpura in children is (*select one response*)
A. Focal segmental glomerulosclerosis.
B. Minimal change nephropathy.
C. IgA nephropathy.
D. Membranous nephropathy.

Q4. The most common type of glomerulonephritis is (*select one response*)
A. Membranous nephropathy.
B. Focal segmental glomerulosclerosis.
C. Minimal change nephropathy.
D. IgA nephropathy.

Q5. The autoantibodies directed against the complement C3 nephritic factor (C3NeF) is associated with (*select one response*)
A. Membranous nephropathy.
B. Mesangiocapillary glomerulonephritis.
C. IgA nephropathy.
D. Minimal change nephropathy.
E. Focal segmental glomerulosclerosis.

Q6. Deficiency in regulatory protein 'factor H' is associated with which *one* of the following conditions?
A. Minimal change nephropathy
B. Haemolytic–uraemic syndrome

C. IgA nephropathy

D. Focal segmental glomerulosclerosis

E. Membranous nephropathy

ANSWERS

A1. **D.** 70%–80% of idiopathic membranous nephropathy has autoantibodies to phospholipase A2 receptor. It is not reported in secondary forms.

A2. **C.** The focal segmental glomerulosclerosis may be seen after renal transplantation.

A3. **C.** IgA nephropathy is similar to that seen in Henoch–Schönlein purpura (vasculitis rash, arthritis, gastrointestinal inflammation).

A4. **D.** IgA nephropathy is the most common GN worldwide.

A5. **B.** C3NeF is associated with mesangiocapillary glomerulonephritis, particularly type II.

A6. **B.** Deficiency in regulating protein 'factor H' is associated with (i) haemolytic–uraemic syndrome and (ii) mesangiocapillary GN.

TAKE-HOME MESSAGE

- The symptoms of nephrotic syndrome are peripheral oedema (may be generalised), shortness of breath, increased abdominal girth, increased risk of infection and increased risk of deep venous thrombosis.
- The clinical signs of nephrotic syndrome are hypertension, proteinuria, microscopic haematuria, azotaemia, hypoalbuminaemia and intravenous volume depletion.
- Laboratory tests are important in the diagnosis.
- The glomerulonephritis could be (i) minimal change disease (5%–10%), (ii) focal segmental glomerulosclerosis (20%–25%), (iii) membranous nephropathy (25%–30%), (iv) proliferative and sclerosing glomerulonephritides (15%–30%) or (v) mesangiocapillary glomerulonephritis (5%).
- The goals and options of management: (i) Reduce oedema (salt restriction and diuretics); (ii) control high blood pressure (angiotensin-converting enzyme inhibitors or angiotensin II receptor blockers); these drugs delay the progression of the disease; (iii) manage hyperlipidaemia (statins); (iv) manage hypercoagulability by anticoagulation and warfarin for at least 3–6 months; patients are at a high risk of developing deep venous thrombosis and pulmonary embolism (this is because of urinary loss of protein C and protein S); (v) manage infections by administration of systemic antibiotics and vaccination against encapsulated bacteria; patients are at a higher risk of developing systemic infections because of hypogammaglobulinaemia; and (vi) corticosteroids and cytotoxic drugs are indicated for primary renal disease.

FURTHER READINGS

Buttgereit F, Burmester GR, Lipworth BJ. Optimised glucocorticoid therapy: the sharpening of an old spear. *Lancet*. 2005;365(9461):801-803. Review.

Hildebrandt F. Genetic kidney diseases. *Lancet*. 2010;375(9722):1287-1295. Review.

Hull RP, Goldsmith DJ. Nephrotic syndrome in adults. *BMJ*. 2008;336(7654):1185-1189. Review.

Kodner C. Nephrotic syndrome in adults: diagnosis and management. *Am Fam Physician*. 2009;80(10):1129-1134. Review.

Kodner C. Diagnosis and Management of Nephrotic Syndrome in Adults. *Am Fam Physician*. 2016;93(6):479-485. Review.

Maher JF. Diabetic nephropathy: early detection, prevention and management. *Am Fam Physician*. 1992;45(4):1661-1668. Review.

Orth SR, Ritz E. The nephrotic syndrome. *N Engl J Med*. 1998;338(17):1202-1211. Review.

Ronco P, Debiec H. Pathophysiological advances in membranous nephropathy: time for a shift in patient's care. *Lancet*. 2015;385(9981):1983-1992. Review.

CASE 7.3

'I Only Feel Tired …'

Fuller McCall, a 48-year-old high school teacher, comes in to see his general practitioner because he is suffering from generalised fatigue and muscle aches all over his body for about 6–8 months. He also gives a history of nausea, loss of appetite, changes in taste and numbness and tingling of his upper and lower limbs. Fuller is on treatment with an oral hypoglycaemic agent for type 2 diabetes mellitus and an angiotensin-converting enzyme (ACE) inhibitor for high blood pressure for over 18 years. On examination, there is pallor of conjunctivae, and the skin has a greyish, yellowish complexion. His blood pressure is 180/110 mm Hg, pulse rate 94/min, respiratory rate 19/min and temperature 36.7°C. His JVP is raised, and cardiac auscultation reveals normal first and second heart sounds. His abdomen is soft and not tender. Upper and lower limbs show glove-and-stocking hypoesthesia. Bilateral mild ankle oedema is also noted.

CASE DISCUSSION

Q1. On the basis of Mr McCall's presentation, what is your diagnosis?

Q2. What is your differential diagnosis?

Q3. What are the key clinical features of this disease? What are the scientific bases for these features?

Q4. What is the pathophysiology underlying these changes?

Q5. What are your management goals and management options?

ANSWERS

1. The findings of generalised fatigue and body aches are nonspecific for a particular disease. However, these symptoms taken together with other symptoms including nausea, loss of appetite, changes in taste and numbness and tingling in the upper and lower limbs, and the history of hypertension and diabetes mellitus for over 18 years are suggestive of chronic renal failure. The pallor of conjunctivae (possibly due to anaemia), the skin changes, the raised JVP, ankle oedema and high blood pressure are all suggestive of the diagnosis of chronic renal failure. Further assessment is needed including full blood count, blood film, platelet function, bleeding time, blood electrolytes, blood urea and creatinine levels, HbA_{1c}, urinalysis and ultrasound assessment of kidneys.

2. The differential diagnosis of chronic renal failure includes the following:
- Diabetic nephropathy
- Acute kidney injury
- Chronic glomerulonephritis
- Multiple myeloma
- Polycystic kidney disease
- Nephrolithiasis
- Renal artery stenosis
- Hypertensive nephrosclerosis
- Analgesic nephropathy
- Reflux/chronic pyelonephritis
- Sickle cell nephropathy

3. Clinical picture:

Symptoms:
- Patients are usually asymptomatic.
- Symptoms develop gradually and are nonspecific. These symptoms include the following:
  - Tiredness
  - Fatigue
  - Pruritus
  - Metallic taste
  - Anorexia
  - Nausea
  - Vomiting
  - Loss of concentration
  - Decreased libido
  - Erectile dysfunction
  - Dyspnoea
  - Retrosternal pain on inspiration (pericarditis)

Signs:
- Hypertension, which is a common sign
- Pallor of conjunctivae
- Friction rub
- Pleural effusion
- Peripheral neuropathy
- Myoclonus
- Looks ill
- Not well in general

4. Laboratory investigations:
- Elevated blood urea and creatinine concentration. Comparing the results with previous levels of creatinine and blood urea can help in differentiating chronic renal disease from acute kidney injury.

- Full blood count – low haemoglobin. Eosinophilia suggests vasculitis or allergic tubulointerstitial nephritis.
- Platelet dysfunction and prolonged bleeding time are present.
- Erythrocyte sedimentation rate (ESR) – markedly raised ESR suggests multiple myeloma.
- Blood film may show fragmented red blood cells (intravascular haemolysis).
- Arterial blood gases – metabolic disorder is present.
- Hyperphosphataemia occurs.
- Hypocalcaemia occurs.
- Hyperkalaemia occurs.
- Urinalysis – red cell casts, broad waxy casts are suggestive of glomerulonephritis.
- Proteinuria + + + occurs.
- Haematuria + + occurs.
- Glycosuria with normal blood glucose is common in chronic kidney disease.
- Immunological tests – these show low complement components C3 and C4 in systemic lupus erythematosus (SLE), mesangiocapillary glomerulonephritis, poststreptococcal glomerulonephritis and cryoglobulinaemia
- Autoantibodies – these are useful in SLE and scleroderma.
- Cryoglobulins – mesangiocapillary glomerulonephritis is present.
- Antibodies to hepatitis B and C (hepatitis B positive in polyarteritis or membranous nephropathy; hepatitis C protein in cryoglobulinaemia renal disease) are present.
- Antibodies to HIV are present.
- Antibodies to streptococcal antigens are present in poststreptococcal glomerulonephritis (Fig. 7.3.1 summarises the major manifestations of chronic renal failure).

Radiology:
- Ultrasound to assess the kidney size, hydronephrosis, anomalies
- CT scan to diagnose calculi and retroperitoneal fibrosis
- Magnetic resonance angiography to assess for renovascular disease

Pathophysiology of chronic renal failure: See Fig. 7.3.2.

5. Management goals:
- Manage acute hyperkalaemia – this is an emergency. Administer insulin with glucose intravenously, bicarbonate intravenously or calcium chloride or calcium gluconate intravenously.
- Manage acid–base disorders – maintain bicarbonate at >22 mmol/L.
- Manage high blood pressure – salt and water restriction, ACE inhibitors or angiotensin II receptor blockers, calcium channel-blocking agents or beta-blockers or diuretics.
- Manage heart failure – loop diuretics, ACE inhibitors and restriction of salt and water.
- Manage anaemia – mainly recombinant erythropoietin 50 units/kg, iron, B12 and folate.

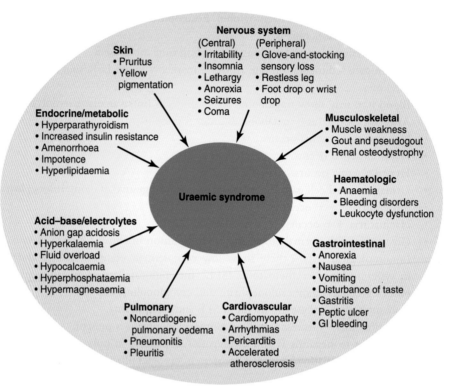

Figure 7.3.1 Major manifestations of chronic renal failure. *(Source: Andreoli TE, Benjamin IJ, Griggs RC, Wing EJ. Andreoli and Carpenter's Cecil Essentials of Medicine. 8th ed. Philadelphia, PA: Elsevier; 2010.)*

- Manage renal bone disease – oral phosphorous-binding agents, vitamin D or vitamin D analogues and calcitriol.
- Restriction of dietary phosphorous is of limited value.
- Restrict proteins in diet; restrict salt and water; restrict potassium and magnesium-containing laxatives.
- Manage coagulopathy.
- Dialysis – the aim is elimination of nitrogenous wastes, maintaining normal electrolyte balance, managing and correcting systemic acidosis, correcting the extracellular volume (types: (i) haemodialysis, (ii) haemofiltration and (iii) peritoneal dialysis).
- Renal transplantation is done.

BACK TO BASIC SCIENCES

Q1. What are the causes of chronic kidney disease?
- Primary glomerulonephritis
- Secondary glomerular disease:
    - Systemic lupus erythematosus
    - Amyloidosis

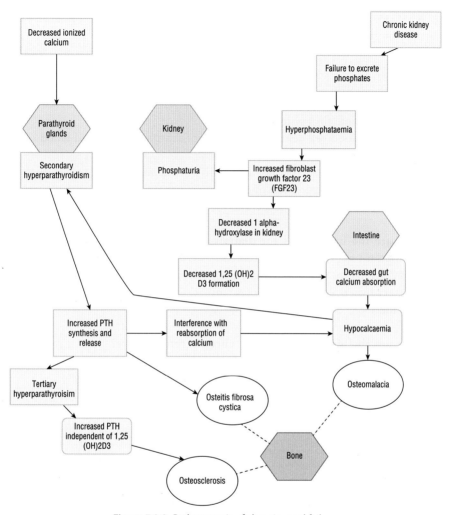

Figure 7.3.2 Pathogenesis of chronic renal failure.

- • Diabetic glomerulosclerosis
- • haemolytic-uraemic syndrome
- • Accelerated hypertension
- • Thrombotic thrombocytopenic purpura
- • Systemic sclerosis
- • Sickle cell disease
- • Tubulointerstitial disease (e.g. reflux nephropathy, tuberculosis, multiple myeloma, renal papillary necrosis, schistosomiasis)
- • Vascular diseases (e.g. renovascular disease)
- • Obstructive uropathy (e.g. prostatic disease, retroperitoneal fibrosis, calculus disease)

Q2. What are the mechanisms underlying anaemia in chronic renal disease?
Anaemia in chronic kidney disease is 'normocytic normochromic anaemia'. There are several mechanisms responsible for the development of anaemia in these patients:
1. Erythropoietin deficiency – main mechanism in chronic renal failure
2. Increased blood loss due to repeated blood loss in urine, with haemodialysis and from the gastrointestinal system
3. Increased red blood cell destruction because of short life span of red blood cells in chronic renal failure
4. Bone marrow suppression because of fibrosis of bone marrow due to hyperparathyroidism resulting in suppression of erythropoiesis
5. Deficiency of iron, B12 and folate, and protein loss

Q3. What are the indications for dialysis in chronic renal failure?
- Fluid overload not responding to diuretics
- Uraemic symptoms (e.g. pericarditis, encephalopathy and coagulopathy)
- Refractory hyperkalaemia (high potassium)
- Severe metabolic acidosis (pH < 7.20)

Q4. What are the aims of dialysis in chronic renal failure?
- Maintaining fluid volume and blood pressure control
- Maintaining electrolyte balance (sodium, potassium, calcium, phosphate)
- Maintaining normal pH and correcting metabolic acidosis

Q5. Discuss the mechanisms underlying bone disease in chronic renal failure.
Most patients with chronic renal disease have mixed bone disease; altered bone morphology may be summarised as follows:
- Osteomalacia – chronic kidney disease $\rightarrow$ hyperphosphataemia $\rightarrow$ increased fibroblast growth factor 23 (FGF23) by osteoblasts $\rightarrow$ decreased 1-alpha-hydroxylase in the kidney $\rightarrow$ decreased $1,25(OH)_2D_3$ $\rightarrow$ decreased calcium absorption from the intestine $\rightarrow$ hypocalcaemia $\rightarrow$ osteomalacia.
- Osteosclerosis – hypocalcaemia $\rightarrow$ stimulation of the parathyroid hormone (secondary hyperparathyroidism) $\rightarrow$ cystic formation and bone marrow fibrosis (osteitis fibrosa cystica) $\rightarrow$ development of tertiary hyperparathyroidism (increased production of parathyroid hormone (PTH) independent of $1,25(OH)_2D_3$) $\rightarrow$ osteosclerosis.
- Osteoporosis – steroids given after renal transplantation plus high to low bone turnover $\rightarrow$ osteoporosis.
- A dynamic bone disease – both bone formation and bone reabsorption are depressed together with hypercalcaemia (due to overtreatment with vitamin D), low PTH (after surgical parathyroidectomy) and normal levels of serum alkaline phosphatase. Dual-energy x-ray absorptiometry (DXA) in these patients shows osteopenia.

Q6. Discuss the risk factors for chronic kidney disease.

- Autoimmune disorders
- Diabetes mellitus – type 2
- Exposure to drugs (e.g. aminoglycosides, contrast media, sulfonamides, vancomycin, phenytoin, nonsteroidal anti-inflammatory drugs, amphotericin B and lithium)
- Familial history of chronic kidney disease
- Lower urinary tract obstruction
- Nephrolithiasis
- Reduction of kidney mass/malformation
- Systemic infection
- Urinary tract infection
- Exposure to chemicals (e.g. lead, cadmium, arsenic, mercury)
- Hypertension
- Neoplasia
- Complications of acute kidney disease
- Older age

REVIEW QUESTIONS

Q1. Which *one* of the following is *not* among the mechanisms responsible for anaemia in chronic kidney disease?
A. Erythropoietin deficiency
B. Increased blood loss
C. Intrinsic factor deficiency/defect
D. Bone marrow suppression
E. Increased red blood cell destruction

Q2. Which *one* of the following is *not* among the indications for dialysis in chronic kidney disease?
A. Pericarditis
B. Fluid overload despite diuretic treatment
C. Coagulopathy
D. Severe metabolic acidosis (pH < 7.20)
E. Refractory hypokalaemia

Q3. Which *one* of the following biochemical/hormonal changes is *not* found in chronic renal disease?
A. Hyperphosphataemia
B. Decreased fibroblast growth factor 23 (FGF23)
C. Decreased 1-alpha-hydroxylase in the kidney
D. Hypocalcaemia
E. Increased serum PTH

Q4. Which *one* of the following is *not* associated with decreased serum complement C3 and C4 proteins?
A. Systemic lupus erythematosus
B. Poststreptococcal glomerulonephritis
C. Cryoglobulinaemia
D. Mesangiocapillary glomerulonephritis
E. Minimal change nephropathy

Q5. Which *one* of the following is the definition of microalbuminuria?
A. Urinary albumin of 30–300 mg
B. Urinary albumin/creatinine ratio of 30–300 mg/g
C. Urinary albumin/serum albumin ratio of 30–300 mg/g
D. Albumin/blood urea ratio of 30–300 mg/g

ANSWERS

A1. **C.** Intrinsic factor defect or deficiency is not among the mechanisms responsible for anaemia in chronic kidney disease.

A2. **E.** Refractory hyperkalaemia not responding to medical treatment (not hypokalaemia) is an indication of dialysis in chronic kidney disease.

A3. **B.** The production of FGF23 is increased secondary to the presence of hyperphosphataemia resulting in phosphaturia.

A4. **E.** There are no changes in the complement components C3 and C4 in patients with minimal change glomerulonephropathy.

A5. **B.** Urinary albumin/creatinine ratio of 30–300 mg/g is an indication of microalbuminuria. Normally this ratio is <30 mg/g. If the ratio is >300 mg/g, we call this macroalbuminuria.

TAKE-HOME MESSAGE

- The symptoms in chronic renal failure develop gradually and are nonspecific. These symptoms include tiredness, fatigue, pruritus, metallic taste, nausea, vomiting, loss of concentration, decreased libido and erectile dysfunction.
- The clinical signs include hypertension, pallor, pleural rub and pleural effusion, and the patient does not look well.
- Blood urea and creatinine concentration are elevated. Comparing the results with previous levels of creatinine and blood urea can help in differentiating chronic renal disease from acute kidney injury.
- Laboratory investigations include renal function tests; full blood count; platelet count and function tests; ESR; blood film; blood gases; serum phosphate, calcium, sodium and potassium; and urinalysis.

- The aims of management in chronic renal failure include the following:

  (1) Manage acute hyperkalaemia, acid–base disorders, high blood pressure, heart failure, anaemia, bone disease and acid–base imbalance.

  (2) Manage heart failure-loop diuretics, ACE inhibitors and restriction of salt and water.

  (3) Manage coagulopathy.

  (4) Dialysis aims at elimination of nitrogenous wastes, maintaining normal electrolyte balance, managing and correcting systemic acidosis and correcting the extracellular volume (types: (i) haemodialysis, (ii) haemofiltration and (iii) peritoneal dialysis).

  (5) Renal transplantation is part of the management plan.

FURTHER READINGS

Bernal W, Jalan R, Quaglia A, Simpson K, Wendon J, Burroughs A. Acute-on-chronic liver failure. *Lancet*. 2015;386(10003):1576-1587. Review.

Grantham JJ. Clinical practice. Autosomal dominant polycystic kidney disease. *N Engl J Med*. 2008; 359(14):1477-1485. Review.

Himmelfarb J, Ikizler TA. Hemodialysis. *N Engl J Med*. 2010;363(19):1833-1845. Review.

Holick MF. Vitamin D deficiency. *N Engl J Med*. 2007;357(3):266-281. Review.

Meyer TW, Hostetter TH. Uremia. *N Engl J Med*. 2007;357(13):1316-1325. Review.

Ortiz A, Covic A, Fliser D, et al. Epidemiology, contributors to, and clinical trials of mortality risk in chronic kidney failure. *Lancet*. 2014;383(9931):1831-1843. Review.

Tonelli M, Pannu N, Manns B. Oral phosphate binders in patients with kidney failure. *N Engl J Med*. 2010;362(14):1312-1324. Review.

CASE 7.4

'Burning Pain on Passing Urine ...'

Hala Jordon, a 21-year-old university student, presents to her general practitioner because she is suffering from increased frequency of urination, pain on passing urine and a sense of incomplete voiding for about 2 days. She has no past history of similar symptoms and has always been healthy. She gives no history of fever, chills, urinary discharge or pain in her loins. On examination, her pulse rate is 80/min, blood pressure 120/80 mm Hg, respiratory rate 17/min and temperature 37.0°C. She has no abdominal rigidity or tenderness in her loins (costovertebral angle) but has some suprapubic tenderness. No pelvic examination was done. Urinary dipstick is positive for leukocyte esterase and nitrate. Urinalysis shows pus cells and an increased number of white and red blood cells. Urine Gram stain shows Gram-negative rods. Urine culture shows *Escherichia coli* growth.

CASE DISCUSSION

Q1. On the basis of Hala's presentation, what is your diagnosis?

Q2. What is your differential diagnosis?

Q3. What are the key clinical features of this disease? What are the scientific bases for these features?

Q4. What is the pathophysiology underlying these changes?

Q5. What are your management goals and management options?

ANSWERS

1. The findings of increased frequency of urination, pain on passing urine and a sense of incomplete voiding for about 2 days together with tenderness in the suprapubic area and positive urine dipstick for leukocyte esterase and nitrite are suggestive of lower urinary tract infection (UTI). UTIs are more common in females than in males mainly because of the short urethra. In this condition, the urinalysis and urine culture confirm the UTI with Gram-negative *E. coli*.
2. The differential diagnosis includes the following:
   * Urethritis
   * Vaginitis
   * Nonbacterial cystitis

- Interstitial cystitis
- Herpes simplex infection
- Urinary stones
- Chlamydia – genitourinary infection
- Bladder cancer
- Acute pyelonephritis
- Hypercalcaemic uropathy
- Increased urates in urine

3. Clinical picture: Symptoms and signs:
   A. Pyelonephritis:
   – Loin pain
   – Haematuria
   – Systemic symptoms (fever, rigor, vomiting, loss of appetite, tiredness, septic shock)
   – Blood culture positive in 20% of patients
   – Possibility of presence of symptoms of cystitis, in ascending infection (suprapubic pain/tenderness, increased frequency of urination, dysuria, urgency and offensive cloudy urine)
   B. Cystitis:
   – Dysuria
   – Increased frequency
   – Urgency
   – Suprapubic tenderness
   – Haematuria
   – Offensive cloudy urine
   C. Urethritis:
   – Dysuria
   – Urethral discharge
   – Fever, rigor usually absent
   – Usually sexually transmitted disease present (*Neisseria gonorrhoeae*, *Chlamydia trachomatis*, *Mycoplasma genitalium* or *Trichomonas vaginalis*)
   D. Prostatitis:
   – Perineal pain
   – Scrotal pain
   – Increased frequency
   – Urgency
   – Dysuria
   – May be acute or chronic (usually responsible for recurrent UTI in men)

UTI in children and elderly may not present with typical symptoms and the diagnosis can be easily missed.

4. Laboratory investigations:
   A. Urinary leukocyte esterase and nitrite (most Gram-negative bacteria can convert nitrate to nitrite)

    B. Microscopic analysis: Haematuria, pus cells, increased white blood cells in 75%–90% of patients

    C. Microbiological analysis:
- Bacterial count of >10^5 colony-forming unit/mL (CFU/mL) considered significant
- Gram stain
- Urinary white and red blood cells count per unit volume

    D. Urine culture: Indicated in complicated or recurrent infection and when risk of failure of treatment is higher, and in pregnant women presenting with UTI

    E. Other investigations:
- Ultrasonography with estimation of postmicturition bladder residual urine
- Abdominal X-ray
- Urodynamics
- Cystoscopy
- Micturition cystoscopy (in children)

Usually the investigations under item E are not routinely recommended. They are indicated in children, men with more than one infection and women with recurrent infections and in the presence of severe pyelonephritis.

Pathophysiology:

- The routes of infection could be (i) haematogenous infection and (ii) ascending infection – colonisation of the vaginal introitus, colonisation of the urethra or entry of the urinary bladder.

- Women are at an increased risk of developing UTI because of (i) short urethra, (ii) sexual intercourse and lack of postcoital voiding, (iii) oestrogen deficiency and (iv) the use of diaphragm and spermicide also possibly does not provide protection from infection.

- Factors that can increase the risk of UTI in both sexes may include (i) urethral strictures, (ii) renal calculi, (iii) incomplete bladder emptying, (iv) neurogenic bladder, (v) immunocompromised patients (use of cytotoxic drugs, transplant recipients and diabetic patients) and (vi) troubles with urine flow and changes in urine pH.

- Bacterial virulence factors: (i) Type 1 fimbriae (mediate binding to uroplakins, mannosylated glycoproteins on the surface of the bladder uroepithelial cells); (ii) P fimbriae (bind to galactose disaccharide on the surface of uroepithelial cells); (iii) P fimbriae bind to the P blood group antigen on red blood cells (responsible for most of recurrent UTIs in females); (iv) P fimbriae block phagocytosis; (v) P fimbriated *E. coli* is responsible for more than 95% of nonobstructive pyelonephritis in children: a higher density of receptors for P fimbriae on cells of the urinary tract and kidney plays an important role in infection in these patients; (vi) flagella enhance bacterial motility; and (vii) production of haemolysin induce pores in cell membrane and enhances spread of infection.

5. Management goals:
- Assess the severity, upper versus lower UTI.
- Treat the infection with antibiotics.

- Educate the patient.
- Prevent recurrence of infection.

A. Antibiotic treatment:

Men: They should be treated for at least 7 days to prevent complications such as prostatitis. A quinolone is preferable because of better tissue penetration in the prostate. Table 7.4.1 summarises antibiotic treatment for UTIs.

Women: Three-day treatment is preferred over one-dose treatment.

B. In mild pyelonephritis, treatment with oral antibiotics could be started empirically and reviewed in light of urine culture and sensitivity test. The patient is treated with ciprofloxacin for 7 days or with co-amoxiclav for 7-14 days.

C. For pregnant women, ciprofloxacin should be prescribed for 14 days.

D. In severe pyelonephritis, hospital admission for intravenous fluids and antibiotics should be commenced and then oral antibiotics continued when the clinical picture improves. Continue treatment for 14 days.

E. Educate the patient.

F. Prevent the recurrence of infection by increasing fluid intake and complete bladder emptying. In women, both long-term intake of low-dose antibiotics and postcoital antibiotics are effective.

Table 7.4.1 Oral antibacterial agents used in treating urinary tract infections

Antibacterial agent	Class of the agent	Comments
Co-amoxiclav	Beta-lactam + beta-lactamase inhibitor	Increased activity against organisms resistant by virtue of beta-lactamase production
Trimethoprim	Antimetabolite/nucleic acid synthesis inhibitor	Incidence of resistant strains increasing
Co-trimoxazole	Combination of trimethoprim with sulfamethoxazole (also antimetabolite nucleic acid synthesis inhibitor)	One of the most common 'first-line' therapeutic approaches; may be useful in 'blind' treatment but more toxic than trimethoprim alone; resistance also an issue
Nitrofurantoin	Urinary antiseptic	For uncomplicated UTI caused by *E. coli* and *Staphylococcus saprophyticus*; not active in alkaline pH (therefore not useful for *Proteus* infections)
Nalidixic acid	Quinolone	For uncomplicated UTI; Gram-negative infections only; not active against Gram-positive infections; increasing resistance an issue
Ciprofloxacin, gatifloxacin, levofloxacin, norfloxacin, ofloxacin, etc.	Quinolone	Very broad spectrum; not highly active against enterococci; increasing resistance an issue

Source: Goering R, Dockrell N, Zuckerman M, Wakelin D, Roitt I, Mims C, Chiodini P. Mims' Medical Microbiology. 4th ed. Lodon, UK: Elsevier; 2007.

Several different classes of antibacterial drugs [CE6] are available in oral formulations and suitable for treatment of UTI. Nitrofurantoin and nalidixic acid are useful only for lower UTIs as they do not achieve adequate serum and tissue concentrations to treat upper UTIs.

BACK TO BASIC SCIENCES

Q1. What are the common uropathogens responsible for UTIs?

- *E. coli* is the most common cause (in about 90% of cases) of community- and hospital-acquired urinary infections.
- Other pathogens are responsible for <10% of cases, which include the following:
  - *Proteus mirabilis*
  - *Staphylococcus saprophyticus*
  - *Klebsiella pneumoniae*
  - *Pseudomonas aeruginosa*

Q2. What are the possible risk factors for UTI?

- Anatomical anomalies in the urinary tract
- Incomplete bladder emptying
- Recent UTI
- Ureteric strictures
- Females at a higher risk compared to males (e.g. short urethra, oestrogen deficiency)
- Sexual intercourse
- Family history of UTI
- Use of diaphragm and spermicidal contraception
- Disruption of normal bacterial flora
- Postmenopausal alteration in vaginal flora
- Pregnancy
- Urinary stones
- Immune-compromised state or post-transplantation
- P-blood group antigen (nonsecretor status)

Q3. What are the possible causes for a negative urine culture despite the presence of urinary tract symptoms?

- Urinary tract malignancy
- Patients on antibiotics, or were started on antibiotics when urine was collected for culture
- Mycobacterial infection
- Viral infection
- Infection with *C. trachomatis*, *Gardnerella vaginalis* or *Ureaplasma urealyticum*
- Bladder stone/urates in urine
- Idiopathic interstitial cystitis
- Cyclophosphamide

Q4. What are the possible causes for the increased UTIs in older men?

- Acquired structural and functional abnormalities of the urinary tract
- Impaired normal voiding – e.g. benign prostatic hyperplasia, obstruction, turbulent urinary flow

- Acute, chronic and recurrent bacterial prostatitis
- Diabetes mellitus
- Urological coexisting conditions such as incontinence or urinary retention
- Increased exposure to urinary catheterisation
- Immobility, dementia, bacteria and increased number of multidrug-resistant strains

Q5. What does uncomplicated UTI mean?

Healthy people who develop acute cystitis or pyelonephritis without the presence of anatomical abnormalities of the urinary tract and, in case of females, healthy premeno-pausal and nonpregnant women are generally classified as uncomplicated UTI.
On the other hand, all other patients are classified as complicated UTI.

REVIEW QUESTIONS

Q1. The most common uropathogen responsible for UTI is
A. *Staphylococcus saprophyticus.*
B. *Klebsiella pneumoniae.*
C. *Proteus mirabilis.*
D. *Escherichia coli.*

Q2. Which *one* of the following is *not* a risk factor for UTI?
A. Sexual intercourse
B. Use of spermicides
C. Previous UTI
D. A new sex partner
E. Daily beverage consumption

Q3. Which *one* of the following antibiotics is recommended in the treatment of UTI in a patient with acute prostatitis?
A. Co-amoxiclav
B. A quinolone (e.g. ciprofloxacin)
C. Maxipime
D. Amoxicillin
E. Cefalexin

Q4. Regarding UTI, which *one* of the following statements is *not* correct?
A. It affects 40% of women at some point of their life.
B. It is caused by bacteria, fungal or viral infections.
C. Pyelonephritis is the most common UTI.
D. Uncomplicated UTI occurs in the absence of anatomical abnormalities of the urinary tract.

ANSWERS

A1. **D.** *E. coli* is responsible for >90% of UTIs in the community and in hospitals.

A2. **E.** Daily beverage consumption is not shown in case–control studies to be a risk factor for UTIs. Other factors that were shown *not* to be a risk factor:
- Frequency of urination
- Delayed voiding habits
- Tampon use
- Douching
- Use of hot tubs
- Type of underwear
- Body mass index
  (for further reading, Hooton, 2012)

A3. **B.** A quinolone (e.g. ciprofloxacin) is preferable in men with UTI as it penetrates into the prostate if there is underlying acute prostatitis.

A4. **C.** Cystitis is the most common UTI.

TAKE-HOME MESSAGE

- The routes of infection could be (i) haematogenous infection or (ii) ascending infection – colonisation of the vaginal introitus, colonisation of the urethra or entry of the urinary bladder.
- Women are at an increased risk of developing UTI because of (i) short urethra, (ii) sexual intercourse and lack of postcoital voiding, (iii) oestrogen deficiency and (iv) the use of diaphragm and spermicide also possibly does not provide protection from infection.
- Factors that can increase the risk of UTI in both sexes may include (i) urethral strictures, (ii) renal calculi, (iii) incomplete bladder emptying, (iv) neurogenic bladder, (v) immunocompromised patients (use of cytotoxic drugs, transplant recipients and diabetic patients) and (vi) troubles with urine flow and changes in urine pH.
- Bacterial virulence factors through a number of mechanisms also contribute to UTI.
- *E. coli* is the most common cause (in about 90% of cases) of community- and hospital-acquired urinary infections.
- Other pathogens are responsible for UTI (<10% of cases). These organisms are (i) *P. mirabilis*, (ii) *S. saprophyticus*, (iii) *K. pneumoniae* and (iv) *P. aeruginosa*.
- The goals of management of UTI: (i) Assess the severity, upper versus lower UTI; (ii) treat the infection with antibiotics; (iii) educate the patient; and (iv) prevent recurrence of infection.

FURTHER READINGS

Car J. Urinary tract infections in women: diagnosis and management in primary care. *BMJ*. 2006; 332(7533):94-97. Review.

Car J, Sheikh A. Recurrent urinary tract infection in women. *BMJ.* 2003;327(7425):1204. Review.

Fihn SD. Clinical practice. Acute uncomplicated urinary tract infection in women. *N Engl J Med.* 2003;349(3):259-266. Review.

Finer G, Landau D. Pathogenesis of urinary tract infections with normal female anatomy. *Lancet Infect Dis.* 2004;4(10):631-635. Review.

Hooton TM. Clinical practice. Uncomplicated urinary tract infection. *N Engl J Med.* 2012;366(11):1028-1037.

Knox K. Women should be able to get antibiotics for urinary tract infection without a prescription. *BMJ.* 2015;351:h3441.

Peleg AY, Hooper DC. Hospital-acquired infections due to gram-negative bacteria. *N Engl J Med.* 2010; 362(19):1804-1813.

Schaeffer AJ, Nicolle LE. Urinary tract infections in older men. *N Engl J Med.* 2016;374(6):562-571.

Wise GJ, Schlegel PN. Sterile pyuria. *N Engl J Med.* 2015;372(11):1048-1054.

INDEX OF CASES

INDEX